Drug and Alcohol Abuse

A Clinical Guide to Diagnosis and Treatment
Third Edition

CRITICAL ISSUES IN PSYCHIATRY
An Educational Series for Residents and Clinicians

Series Editor: Sherwyn M. Woods, M.D., Ph.D.
University of Southern California School of Medicine
Los Angeles, California

Recent volumes in the series:

CLINICAL DISORDERS OF MEMORY
Aman U. Khan, M.D.

CLINICAL PERSPECTIVES ON THE SUPERVISION OF
PSYCHOANALYSIS AND PSYCHOTHERAPY
Edited by Leopold Caligor, Ph.D., Philip M. Bromberg, Ph.D.,
and James D. Meltzer, Ph.D.

CONTEMPORARY PERSPECTIVES ON PSYCHOTHERAPY WITH
LESBIANS AND GAY MEN
Edited by Terry S. Stein, M.D., and Carol J. Cohen, M.D.

DIAGNOSTIC AND LABORATORY TESTING IN PSYCHIATRY
Edited by Mark S. Gold, M.D., and A. L. C. Pottash, M.D.

DRUG AND ALCOHOL ABUSE: A Clinical Guide to Diagnosis
and Treatment, Third Edition
Marc A. Schuckit, M.D.

EMERGENCY PSYCHIATRY: Concepts, Methods, and Practices
Edited by Ellen L. Bassuk, M.D., and Ann W. Birk, Ph.D.

ETHNIC PSYCHIATRY
Edited by Charles B. Wilkinson, M.D.

MOOD DISORDERS: Toward a New Psychobiology
Peter C. Whybrow, M.D., Hagop S. Akiskal, M.D., and
William T. McKinney, Jr., M.D.

NEUROPSYCHIATRIC FEATURES OF MEDICAL DISORDERS
James W. Jefferson, M.D., and John R. Marshall, M.D.

THE RACE AGAINST TIME: Psychotherapy and Psychoanalysis
in the Second Half of Life
Edited by Robert A. Nemiroff, M.D., and Calvin A. Colarusso, M.D.

STATES OF MIND: Configurational Analysis of Individual
Psychology, Second Edition
Mardi J. Horowitz, M.D.

TREATMENT INTERVENTIONS IN HUMAN SEXUALITY
Edited by Carol C. Nadelson, M.D., and David B. Marcotte, M.D.

A Continuation Order Plan is available for this series. A continuation order will bring
delivery of each new volume immediately upon publication. Volumes are billed only
upon actual shipment. For further information please contact the publisher.

Drug and Alcohol Abuse

A Clinical Guide to Diagnosis and Treatment

Third Edition

Marc A. Schuckit, M.D.

Professor of Psychiatry
University of California, San Diego School of Medicine
Director of the Alcohol Research Center and Treatment Program
Veterans Administration Hospital
San Diego, California

Plenum Medical Book Company • New York and London

Library of Congress Cataloging in Publication Data

Schuckit, Marc Alan, 1944-
   Drug and alcohol abuse: a clinical guide to diagnosis and treatment / Marc A.
Schuckit.—3rd ed.
   p.   cm.—(Critical issues in psychiatry)
   Includes bibliographies and index.
   ISBN 0-306-43041-X
   1. Drug abuse. 2. Alcoholism. I. Title. II. Series. [DNLM: 1. Alcoholism. 2. Substance
Abuse—diagnosis. 3. Substance Abuse—therapy. WM 270 S384d]
RC564.S33   1989
616.86—dc19
DNLM/DLC   88-39817
for Library of Congress   CIP

First Printing—January 1989
Second Printing—January 1990

© 1989 Plenum Publishing Corporation
233 Spring Street, New York, N.Y. 10013

Plenum Medical Book Company is an imprint of Plenum Publishing Corporation

Printed in the United States of America

To Sam, who taught me how to laugh;
Lil, who showed me how to love those close to me;
and to Judy, Dena, and Jordan, who keep me doing both.

Preface to the Third Edition

It is hard to believe that 10 years have passed since the publication in 1979 of the first edition of this text. In the interim, some drugs have become less popular (e.g., hallucinogens) and others have peaked in street popularity (e.g., PCP and cocaine), while the overall prevalence of use of "recreational" drugs has generally leveled off and even decreased slightly. Recent years have also witnessed the introduction of new nonbenzodiazepine antianxiety drugs that are not true CNS depressants, and we have enhanced our knowledge of some of the basic pharmacology of many of the drugs of abuse. Our field has also recognized more about the ability of many drugs, especially depressants and stimulants, to mimic psychiatric disorders as well as to intensify preexisting psychiatric syndromes in the "dual–diagnosis" patient.

This edition of *Drug and Alcohol Abuse* has been modified to reflect these changes as well as others. Thus, the book includes a marked expansion of the discussion of dual diagnoses; contains a new section describing the non-benzodiazepine antianxiety drugs; presents new data regarding the brain mechanisms of a variety of drugs, including the opiates; and presents an extensive update on alcohol detoxification as well as drug and alcohol rehabilitation programs. Consistent with the overall goals of this work to help the student and clinician stay up to date, more than 60% of the references offered at the end of the chapters have been updated to reflect data published since the appearance of the second edition in 1984.

Additionally, anyone involved with the delivery of health care to patients with drug or alcohol problems must deal with the *Diagnostic and Statistical Manual of Mental Disorders* published by the American Psychiatric Association. Therefore, beginning in Chapter 3 and continuing throughout the text, I have referred you to relevant codes in the revised third edition of that important manual.

Each time I carry out a revision of this text, I am newly surprised at how much work this entails. As has been true in the past, I am indebted to my colleagues at the University of California and Veterans Hospital in San Diego for their support. Even more importantly, my personal state of dependence on the love and serenity created by Judy, Dena, and Jordan is the driving force that makes all things possible for me.

MARC A. SCHUCKIT, M.D.

vii

Preface to the Second Edition

In the intervening years between the publication of the first and second editions, this book has been used as a text for teaching in medical schools, psychology and social work courses, nursing curricula, and so on. As a result of my own efforts in this area and of correspondence from teachers in different disciplines, revisions have been made in every chapter. The goal has been primarily to clarify questions raised by students and to expand into areas of need. Regarding the latter, two new chapters have been added, one dealing with phencyclidine to meet the increasing use of this drug over the years and the other dealing with the two most prevalent substances of misuse, caffeine and nicotine. Additional changes include a thoroughly revised chapter on rehabilitation.

This revision could never have been carried out properly without the help of Cheyvonne Frontiero, the editorial assistance offered by Plenum Press, as well as the encouragement of Sherwyn Woods and my colleagues at the University of California, San Diego. Of course, this book could never have been written were it not for the love and happiness generated by my wife, Judy, and children, Dena and Jordan.

MARC A. SCHUCKIT, M.D.

Preface to the First Edition

This book grew out of a series of lectures developed to help the nonpharmacologist make sense out of a complex literature. The core of my approach is to learn the characteristics of drug classes, understand the usual types of difficulties associated with drugs, and then apply these general rules in clinical settings. It is hoped that the text will be a beginning place for gathering knowledge about drug types in the classroom and also a first step in handling emergency problems in clinical settings.

So that the book may properly serve as a resource for survey courses and as an emergency handbook, I have kept my comments relatively short, attempting to relate the most essential material. In order to help the reader understand drugs of abuse in greater depth, each chapter is highly referenced in the hopes that he will further expand his knowledge in this area.

I have never read a perfect manuscript or book, and (the views of my mother aside) this is not one. As with any complex endeavor, a series of compromises must be made as one decides whether to pursue Road A or Road B. My aim is to have this text strike a proper balance between the immediate needs of the clinician and those of the student looking for an introduction to substances of abuse.

I wish to extend my appreciation to Jane Ramsey, Edna Glenn, and my colleagues at the Alcoholism and Drug Abuse Institute of the University of Washington, as well as to my wife, Judy, and my colleagues at the University of California at San Diego Medical School, Department of Psychiatry, for their help in preparing this manuscript.

MARC A. SCHUCKIT, M.D.

Contents

List of Tables and Figures

Tables

Figures

An Overview

1.1. INTRODUCTION

This book is written for the medical student, the physician in practice, the psychologist, the social worker, and other health professionals, or paraprofessionals, who need a quick, handy, clinically oriented reference on alcohol abuse and other drug problems.

This first chapter addresses the need to learn the drug *classes* and the relevant problem areas from which generalizations can be made. Chapters 2 through 12 each deal with a specific class of drugs. The discussion in each of these chapters is subdivided into general information sections on the drugs in that class and sections covering the problems faced in emergency situations. Chapter 13 deals with multi-drug misuse, Chapter 14 briefly outlines an approach to treatment in emergency situations, and Chapter 15 presents most of the material on rehabilitation.

The text can be used in at least two basic ways:

1. *If you are treating an emergency problem* and know the probable class of the drug involved, you will turn to the emergency problem section of the relevant chapter. If you do not know the drug and need some general emergency guidelines, you will use the appropriate subsections of this chapter and Chapter 14. Emphasis is placed on the most relevant drug-related material, and it is assumed that the reader already has some working knowledge of the more general issues such as counseling techniques and/or physical diagnosis, laboratory procedures, and the treatment of life-threatening emergencies.

Once the emergency has been handled, you will want to review the general information available on that class of drugs. At your leisure, then, you might review the general information presented in this chapter and go on to read the first section and some of the references cited in the bibliography of the relevant chapter. For each chapter, I present a series of literature citations updated from the previous edition of this book.

2. *If you are interested in learning about drug classes* and their possible emergency problems, you should begin by skimming all the chapters. After gaining some level of comfort with the general thrust of the material, you can then reread in

1

detail those sections of most interest to you, going on to the more pertinent references. The first section of each chapter contains as little medical jargon as possible.

To address these goals and to make each chapter as complete in itself as possible (in the emergency room you do not want to have to jump too much from chapter to chapter), there is some redundancy in the sections of the various chapters that deal with the same subjects. The abuse of drugs of different classes, for example, may give rise to problems that require similar treatment. I have tried, however, to strike a balance between readability and clinical usefulness.

No handbook can answer all questions about every drug. The emergency-oriented nature of this text also tends to lead to oversimplification of rather complex problems. I give general rules that will need to be modified in specific clinical situations. Although you will not know everything about drugs after finishing the text, it is a place to start learning.

To present the material in the most efficient way, I have used a number of shortcuts:

1. In giving the generic names of medications, I have deleted the suffixes that indicate which salt forms are used (e.g., *chlordiazepoxide hydrochloride* is noted as *chlordiazepoxide*) because they provide little useful information.
2. The specific medications recommended for treatment in the emergency room setting represent the idiosyncrasies of my personal experience as well as those of other authors in the literature. The physician will usually be able to substitute another drug of the same class so that he can use a medication with which he has had experience [for example, when I note the use of haloperidol (Haldol), the physician might substitute *comparable* doses of trifluoperazine (Stelazine)].
3. The dose ranges of medications recommended for treatment of emergency situations are *approximations only* and will have to be modified for the individual patient based on the clinical setting and the patient's characteristics.
4. Although the treatment discussions are frequently offered as a series of steps (as seen in most discussions of toxic reactions), the order offered is a general guideline that is to be modified for the particular clinical setting.
5. It must be noted that the appropriate place for treating most emergency problems recorded here is in a hospital.

I have attempted to use the limited space I have in a manner that reflects the frequency with which the nonspecialist clinician encounters drug problems. Therefore, the greatest amount of material is presented for the most clinically important drug, alcohol. Also, alcohol and opiates, drugs for which the most data on rehabilitation are available, are used as prototypes for the other discussions of rehabilitation.

The causes of substance abuse are not known, nor is there evidence that knowledge of specific etiologies would help the clinician address the rehabilitation of patients with substance problems. It is assumed that the genesis of most alcohol and drug problems rests with a complex interaction between biological and environmental factors. Regarding the former, there is evidence that genetic factors may influence smoking and other drug-taking behaviors,[1,2] and there is excellent evidence, which is briefly mentioned in Chapter 3, that genetic factors contribute to the genesis of alcoholism.[1,2] With rare exceptions, etiology is not covered in depth in this clinically oriented text.

Another important issue is the prevalence and patterns of substance-related problems in populations, that is, epidemiology.[3,4] The use of substances is widespread in most societies, and almost everyone has had some contact with nicotine and caffeine, a substantial majority have used alcohol, and a majority of younger people have tried the cannabinols, especially marijuana.[3-7] With the exception of these brief general comments, I have chosen to give epidemiological information as it relates to each specific class of drugs and thus offer no separate section on this topic.

Two final notes that reflect the sensitivities of our times are needed. To save time and space, male pronouns are used in the text for the most part, but are meant to refer to both genders. For similar goals of efficiency, the terms *client, patient,* and *subject* are used interchangeably.

1.2. SOME DEFINITIONS

Before we can begin, it is important to set forth a series of clinical concepts central to the discussion of substance abuse. The definitions that follow are not the most pharmacologically sophisticated, but they do represent, I think, the greatest potential for use in clinical situations. To arrive at these terms, I have borrowed from a wide variety of standard texts and published studies, attempting to blend them into a readily usable framework.

1.2.1. Drug of Abuse

A *drug of abuse* is any substance, taken through any route of administration, that alters the mood, the level of perception, or brain functioning.[8,9] Such drugs include substances ranging from prescribed medications to alcohol to solvents.[10-12] All these substances are capable of producing changes in mood and altered states of learning.

There are a number of other practices that I have considered for inclusion. For instance, there are parallels between obesity (i.e., the use of food to the point of abuse) and the misuse of the most usual drugs.[13,14] Similarly, the compulsion surrounding some forms of gambling has much of the "feel" of the obsessive behavior observed during substance abuse.[15] However, it is not possible for one text to cover everything, and expansion into these topics, interesting and related though they are, might jeopardize my attempts to cover clinically related topics succinctly and thereby help the clinician in his or her day-to-day practice.

1.2.2. Drug Abuse

Drug abuse is the use of a mind-altering substance in a way that differs from generally approved medical or social practices.[6] Written in another way, when the continued use of a mind-altering substance means more to the user than the problems caused by such use, the person can be said to be abusing the drug.

1.2.3. Dependence

Dependence, also called *habituation* or *compulsive use,*[12] connotes a psychological and/or physical "need" for the drug.[8,12] Whenever possible in this text, I will distinguish between physical and psychological dependence:

1. *Psychological dependence* is an attribute of all drugs of abuse[8] and centers on the user needing the drug in order to reach a maximum level of functioning or feeling of well-being. This is a subjective item that is almost impossible to objectively quantify and thus is of limited usefulness in making a diagnosis.
2. *Physical dependence* indicates that the body has adapted physiologically to chronic use of the substance, with the development of symptoms when the drug is stopped or withdrawn. Although initially this concept appears to be quite simple, there is evidence that behavioral conditioning and psychological factors are important in what is usually felt to be a physical withdrawal syndrome.[16,17] There are two important aspects to physical dependence:
   a. *Tolerance* is the toleration of higher and higher doses of the drug or, said another way, the need for higher and higher doses to achieve the same effects. The phenomenon occurs both through alterations in drug metabolism by which the liver destroys the substance more quickly (*metabolic tolerance*), and through alterations in the functioning of the target cells (usually in the nervous system) in the presence of the drug, by which tissue reaction to the drug is diminished (*pharmacodynamic tolerance*). Tolerance is not an all-or-none phenomenon, and an individual may develop tolerance to one aspect of a drug's action and not another. The development of tolerance to one drug of a class usually indicates *cross-tolerance* to other drugs of the same class.[12]
   b. *Withdrawal* or an *abstinence syndrome* is the appearance of physiological symptoms when the drug is stopped too quickly. This phenomenon was described first and most completely for drugs like opiates or drugs that tend to depress the action of the central nervous system. However, there is evidence that there are also withdrawal signs when drugs with different actions, such as stimulants, are used. Like tolerance, withdrawal is not an all-or-none phenomenon and usually consists of a syndrome comprising a wide variety of possible symptoms.[12]

1.3. GENERAL COMMENTS ABOUT DRUG MECHANISMS

The drugs discussed here all affect the brain or the central nervous system (CNS). Unfortunately for our simplistic discussion, the actions of these drugs on the CNS tend to be highly complex. These factors are mediated through different neurotransmitters acting through a myriad of intercellular communications that strike a balance between excitatory and inhibitory functions.[18] This highly complex level of interaction, along with the drive of the nervous system to achieve equilibrium, or homeostasis, makes it very difficult to generalize about specific mechanisms of drug actions. The same drug can have behavioral-stimulation effects at one dose but sedation at another, and the actue effects of a drug in the CNS may be the opposite of the changes seen after chronic exposure.

The problems of understanding what to expect with a specific drug are even more complex for drugs bought "on the street." Most of these substances are not pure, and many [almost 100% for such drugs as tetrahydrocannabinol (see Section (THC) 1.4.4)] do not even contain the purported major substances. Thus, one must apply the general lessons discussed in this text carefully, staying alert for unexpected consequences when treating drug abusers.

Specific drug actions depend on the route of administration, the dose, the presence or absence of other drugs, and the patient's clinical condition. Disposition, metabolism, and sensitivity to substances are also affected by genetic mechanisms, probably both through levels of end-organ sensitivity (e.g., in the CNS) and through the amount and characteristics of the enzymes of metabolism and the amount of protein binding. One important factor to consider in predicting reactions to drugs is age, as growing older is accompanied not only by increased brain sensitivity but also by a reduction in total drug clearance for many substances, especially for the CNS depressants.[19]

In summary, a clinically oriented text such as this one can make few valid generalizations about the mechanisms of drug actions. The reader is referred to general pharmacology texts, including one edited by Goodman and Gillman.[12,18]

1.4. ONE APPROACH TO DRUG CLASSIFICATION

It is possible to learn the characteristics of a drug class and then to apply the general rules to the specific case. There are many possible classifications, some of which are best used for research and some of which are the most pharmacologically correct. However, I present a breakdown of drugs into classes that have particular usefulness in clinical settings and in which the drug class is determined by the most prominent CNS effects at the usual doses.[18]

This drug classification is presented in Table 1.1, along with some examples of the more frequently encountered drugs of each particular class. The classes are discussed in the following sections.

Table 1.1
Drug Classification Used in This Text

Class	Some examples
CNS depressants	Alcohol, hypnotics, antianxiety drugs
CNS sympathomimetics or stimulants	Amphetamine, methylphenidate, cocaine, weight-loss products
Opiates	Heroin, morphine, methadone, and almost all prescription analgesics
Cannabinols	Marijuana, hashish
Hallucinogens or psychedelics	Lysergic acid diethylamide (LSD), mescaline, psilocybin
Solvents	Aerosol sprays, glues, toluene, gasoline, paint thinner
Over-the-counter drugs	Contain: atropine, scopolamine, weak stimulants, antihistamines, weak analgesics
Others	Phencyclidine (PCP)

1.4.1. General CNS Depressants

The most prominent effect of these drugs is the depression of excitable tissues at all levels of the brain, along with relatively few analgesic properties at the usual doses.[18] The CNS depressants include most sleeping medications and antianxiety drugs (also called *minor tranquilizers*), and alcohol. The antipsychotic drugs (also called *major tranquilizers*), such as chlorpromazine (Thorazine) or haloperidol (Haldol), are *not* CNS depressants, do not resemble the antianxiety drugs in their structures or predominant effects, are not physically addictive, and are rarely used to induce a "high."

1.4.2. CNS Sympathomimetics or Stimulants

The predominant effect of these drugs at the usual doses is the stimulation of CNS tissues through blockage of the actions of inhibitory nerve cells or by the release of transmitter substances (chemicals released from one brain cell to stimulate the next cell) from the cells, or by direct action of the drugs themselves. The substances most relevant to clinical situations include all the amphetamines, methylphenidate (Ritalin), and cocaine. The related substances nicotine and caffeine are discussed in separately in Chapter 12, as their pattern of associated problems is limited to panic and medical difficulties.

1.4.3. Opiate Analgesics

These drugs, also called *narcotic analgesics,* are used clinically to decrease pain, and they include morphine and other alkaloids of opium as well as synthetic morphinelike substances and semisynthetic opium derivatives. Prominent examples of these drugs include *almost all* painkilling medications, ranging from propoxyphene (Darvon) to heroin and including oxycodone (Percodan) and pentazocine (Talwin).

1.4.4. Cannabinols (Principally Marijuana)

The active ingredient in all these substances is tetrahydrocannabinol (THC), which has the predominant effects of producing euphoria, an altered time sense, and, at doses higher than those usually found in clinical situations, hallucinations. This is a "street" drug sold in the United States primarily as marijuana or hashish, as pure THC is almost never available on the "black market."

1.4.5. Hallucinogens or Psychedelics

The predominant effect of these substances is the production of hallucinations, usually of a visual nature. The hallucinogens have no accepted medical usefulness and are a second example of "street" drugs. Phencyclidine (PCP) is abused as a hallucinogen, but because of its unique actions and problems is discussed separately in Chapter 9.

1.4.6. Glues, Solvents, and Aerosols

These substances are used in various fuels, aerosol sprays, glues, paints, and industrial solutions. They are used as drugs of abuse in attempts to alter the state of consciousness, producing primarily light-headedness and confusion.

1.4.7. Over-the-Counter Drugs and Other Prescription Drugs

A variety of substances are sold without prescription for the treatment of constipation, pain, nervousness, insomnia, and other common complaints. The sedative or hypnotic medications are the most frequently abused, contain antihistamines, and are taken by the abuser to produce feelings of light-headedness and euphoria. Finally, there are a number of other prescription drugs that are much less likely than the aforementioned ones to be abused, including diuretics, antiparkinsonian drugs, laxatives, and some antipsychotics.

1.5. ALTERNATE CLASSIFICATION SCHEMES

An additional breakdown of these substances, addressing a series of "schedules" developed by the Federal Drug Enforcement Administration (DEA), is presented in Table 1.2.[20,21] The classification is based on both the degree of medical usefulness and the abuse potential of the substance, ranging from Schedule I, which includes those drugs with few accepted medical uses and a high abuse potential (e.g., heroin), to Schedule V, drugs that have a high level of medical usefulness and relatively little abuse potential. Unfortunately, it is not always possible to generalize from the schedule level to the actual drug dangers, as exemplified by the classification of marijuana and heroin at the same level and of ethchlorvynol

Table 1.2
DEA Drug Schedules with Examples[20,21]

Schedule	Examples
I (high abuse, low usefulness)	Heroin
	Hallucinogens
	Marijuana
	Methaqualone (Quäälude)
II	Opium or morphine
	Codeine
	Synthetic opiates [e.g., meperidine (Demerol)]
	Barbiturates [e.g., secobarbital (Seconal)]
	Amphetamines, methylphenidate (Ritalin), and phenmetrazine (Preludin)
	PCP
III	Aspirin with codeine
	Paregoric
	Methyprylon (Noludar)
	Glutethimide (Doriden)
IV	Chloral hydrate (Noctec)
	Ethchlorvynol (Placidyl)
	Flurazepam (Dalmane)
	Pentazocine (Talwin)
	Chlordiazepoxide (Librium)
	Propoxyphene (Darvon)
	Diethylpropion (Tenuate)
V (low abuse, high usefulness)	Narcotic–atropine mixtures (Lomotil)
	Codeine mixtures (<200 mg)

(Placidyl) and glutethimide (Doriden) in different categories, despite their marked similarities in medicinal uses and potential for abuse.

Another way of looking at these drugs is to attempt to classify them by their "street" names (Table 1.3). These names differ from one locale to another and at the same place over time; therefore, this table can be seen as only a brief list of some of the more relevant street names that are *usually* used. It is important to gain some knowledge of the specific use of drug names in your vicinity. In the table, drugs are divided into the major classes outlined in this chapter, and the street names are given alphabetically within each class. For ease of reference, this is one of the few places in this text where trade names rather than generic names are used.

1.6. A CLASSIFICATION OF DRUG PROBLEMS

All drugs of abuse cause intoxication, *all induce psychological dependence* (feeling uncomfortable without the drug), and all are self-administered by an individual to change his level of consciousness or to increase his psychological comfort. Indeed, if people did not begin to feel at least a psychological need for the drug, the drug would likely not have caused a problem. Each class of drugs has its dangers, with patterns of problems differing among drug classes. In this section, I present some general concepts that will be discussed in greater depth in each chapter.

Table 1.3
A Brief List of 'Street' Drug Names

CNS depressants[a]

Blue birds	Green and whites (Librium)	Seccy
Blue devil	Greenies	Seggy
Blue heaven	Nembies	Sleepers
Blues	Peanuts	T-bird
Bullets	Peter (chloral hydrate)	Toolies
Dolls[b]	Rainbows	Tranqs (Librium–type)
Double trouble	Red birds	Yellow jackets
Downs	Red devils	Yellows
Goofballs	Roaches (Librium)[b]	

Stimulants[c]

Bennies	Dexies	Pinks
Blue angels	Double cross	Roses
Chris	Flake (cocaine)	Snow (cocaine)
Christine	Footballs	Speed
Christmas trees	Gold dust (cocaine)	Speedball (heroin plus
Coast to coast	Green and clears	cocaine)
Coke (cocaine)	Hearts	Truck drivers
Copilot	Lip poppers	Uppers
Crisscross	Meth	Ups
Crossroads	Oranges	Wake-ups
Crystal (IV	Peaches	Whites
methamphetamine)[b]	Pep pills	

Analgesics

Heroin		Other	
Brown	Scat	Black (opium)	PG or PO (paregoric)
H	Shit	Blue velvet (paregoric plus	Pinks and grays (Darvon)
H and stuff	Skag	antihistamine)	Poppy (opium)
Horse	Smack	Dollies (methadone)[b]	Tar (opium)
Junk		M (morphine)	Terp (terpin hydrate or
		Microdots (morphine)	cough syrup with
			codeine)

(continued)

Table 1.3
(Continued)

Cannabinols				
Marijuanalike			Hashishlike (more potent)	
Acapulco gold	Lid	Rope	Bhang	Hash
Brick	Locoweed	Sativa	Charas	Rope
Grass	Mary Jane	Stick	Gage	Sweet Lucy
Hay	MJ	Tea	Ganja	
Hemp	Muggles	Texas tea		
Jive	Pot	Weed		
Joint	Reefer	Yesca		
Key or kee	Roach[b]			

Phencyclidine (PCP)		
Angel dust	Hog	Shermans
Aurora	Jet	Sherms
Bust bee	K	Special L.A. coke
Cheap cocaine	Lovely	Superacid
Cosmos	Mauve	Supercoke
Criptal	Mist	Supergrass
Dummy mist	Mumm dust	Superjoint
Goon	Peace pill	Tranq
Green	Purple	Whack
Guerrilla	Rocket fuel	

Hallucinogens		
Acid (LSD)	Crystal[b]	Mescal (mescaline)
Blue dots (LSD)	Cube (LSD)	Owsleys (LSD)
Cactus (mescaline)	D (LSD)	Pearly gates (morning glory seeds)

[a]Moderate length of action *like* secobarbital unless otherwise noted.
[b]Many drugs have the same name.
[c]A form of amphetamine unless otherwise stated.

There is a limited range of adverse reactions to the drugs of abuse, and it was thus possible to summarize in tabular form the drug classes and the problems most prominent for each (Table 1.4). This section of the chapter expands on the information in the table. For most types of problems (e.g., a panic), I first discuss the most usual history, then note the usual physical signs and symptoms and the most prominent psychological difficulties, and, finally, give an overview of relevant laboratory tests. The generalizations presented for panic reactions, flashbacks, psychoses, and organic brain syndromes are so constant among drug categories that only a brief discussion of the clinical picture is presented in each relevant chapter. On the other hand, the toxic reactions and the withdrawal pictures seen with the different drug

Table 1.4
Clinically Most Significant Drug Problems by Class

	Panic	Flashbacks	Toxicity	Psychosis	OBS	Withdrawal
Depressants	−	−	+ +	+ +	+ +	+ +
Stimulants	+	−	+ +	+ +	+	+
Opiates	−	−	+ +	−	+	+ +
Cannabinols	+	+	+	−	+	−
Hallucinogens	+ +	+ +	+	−	+	−
Solvents	+	−	+ +	−	+ +	−
Phencyclidine (PCP)	+	?a	+ +	a	a	?a
Over-the-counter	+	−	+	−	+ +	−

aMost PCP problems appear to be related to a toxic reaction and the subsequent stages of recovery.

classes are so distinct that a detailed discussion of the clinical picture of each is presented in each chapter.

It is important at this juncture to note that with the exception of toxicological screens of the urine (to determine *if* the drug has been taken in the last day to week) and blood (to determine *how much* of the substance, if any, is in the blood), there are few laboratory tests that help to establish a drug diagnosis. The normal laboratory result for each of the toxicological screens is at or near zero.

In the material that follows, a hierarchy has been established to help you address the most clinically significant problem first:

1. Any patient who has taken enough of a drug to seriously compromise his vital signs is regarded as having a *toxic reaction*. Associated symptoms of confusion and/or hallucinations/delusions can be expected to clear as the overdose is properly treated.
2. Patients who demonstrate a drug-related clinical syndrome with relatively stable vital signs, but show strong evidence of drug withdrawal (even if the syndrome includes confusion or psychotic symptoms) are labeled *withdrawal*.
3. Patients with stable vital signs and no signs of withdrawal, but with levels of drug-induced confusion, are regarded as having an *organic brain syndrome* (OBS), even if the hallucinations or delusions are part of the clinical picture. In this instance, the psychotic symptoms can be expected to clear as the OBS disappears.
4. Thus, patients who show stable vital signs, no evidence of clinically significant confusion, and no signs of withdrawal, but who show hallucinations and/or delusions without insight, are regarded as having a *psychosis*.
5. Most remaining patients are expected to be demonstrating a *panic reaction* or *flashbacks*.

1.6.1. Panic Reactions

1.6.1.1. Typical History

The patient is usually a naive user who has typically taken marijuana, a hallucinogen, or a stimulant.[22] Shortly after ingestion of the drug and the onset of the "typical" drug effects, the individual acutely develops fears that he is losing control, that he has done physical harm to himself, or that he is going crazy, and he is brought in for help by friends, relatives, or the police.

1.6.1.2. Physical Signs and Symptoms

Physical findings reflect fear, anxiety, and sympathetic nervous system overactivity (e.g., increased pulse and respiratory rates) occurring in the midst of a panic. This overactivity includes an elevated pulse (usually about 120 beats per minute), an elevated respiratory rate (over 20 or 25 per minute), and an elevated blood pressure. The patient may also demonstrate slightly dilated pupils and excess perspiration.

1.6.1.3. Psychological State

Fear of going crazy, developing uncontrollable behavior, or the occurrence of permanent brain or heart damage (e.g., having a heart attack) dominates the clinical picture.

1.6.1.4. Relevant Laboratory Tests

Depending on the patient's clinical picture, steps must be taken to rule out any obvious physical pathology. Thus, in addition to the establishing the level of the vital signs, it is necessary to evaluate the need for an *electrocardiogram* (EKG) and to draw routine baseline laboratory studies [e.g., red blood (cell) count (RBC); glucose, liver function, and kidney function tests; white blood (cell) count (WBC); and tests of skeletal or heart muscle damage, such as creatinine phosphokinase (CPK)]. Some of the more relevant tests, along with their abbreviations and *most usual* normal values, are presented in Table 1.5. Of course, when a drug reaction is suspected but no adequate history can be obtained, urine (approximately 50 ml) and/or blood (approximately 10 cc) should be sent to the laboratory for a toxicological screen to determine which, if any, drugs are present.

1.6.2. Flashback

A flashback, also most frequently seen with the cannabinols and the hallucinogens, is the unwanted recurrence of drug effects. This is probably a heterogeneous group of problems, including the presence of residual drug in the body, psychological stress, a behavioral "panic," or the possibility of a temporary alteration in brain functioning.

Table 1.5
A Brief List of Relevant Laboratory Tests and Usual Norms

	Name	Usual value
Abbreviation	Serum chemistry	
—	Amylase	20–90 U/liter
—	Bilirubin	Total < 1.2 mg/dl
		Direct ≤ 0.2 mg/dl
BSP	Bromsulphalein	< 5% retention at 45 min
BUN	Blood urea nitrogen	8.0–23.0 mg/dl
Ca	Calcium	9.0–10.6 mg/dl
—	Creatinine	0.8–1.2 mg/dl
CPK	Creatinine phosphokinase	0–175 U/liter
—	Glucose	70–110 mg/dl
LDH	Lactic dehydrogenase	25–200 U/liter
Mg	Magnesium	1.8–2.5 mg/dl
K	Potassium	3.4–4.5 mmole/liter
SGOT	Serum glutamic oxalacetic transaminase	10–45 U/liter
SGPT	Serum glutamic pyruvic transaminase	10–45 U/liter
Na	Sodium	135–145 mmole/liter
	Blood counts	
Hgb	Hemoglobin	Men: 14–18 g/dl
		Women: 12–16 g/dl
Hct	Hematocrit	Men: 42–52%
		Women: 37–47%
MCV	Mean corpuscular (RBC) volume	Volume 82–92 μ^3
WBC	White blood count	4.3–10.8 × 10^3 cells

1.6.2.1. Typical History

This picture is most frequently seen after the repeated use of marijuana or hallucinogens. The typical patient gives a history of past drug use with no recent intake to explain the episode of feeling "high."

1.6.2.2. Physical Signs and Symptoms

These depend on how the patient responds to the flashback, that is, his degree of "panic." Physical pathology is usually minimal and ranges from no physical symptoms to a full-blown panic as described above.

1.6.2.3. Psychological State

The patient most typically complains of a mild altered time sense or visual hallucinations (e.g., bright lights, geometric objects, or a "trailing" image seen when objects move). Symptoms are most common when the subject enters darkness or before he goes to sleep. The emotional reaction may be one of perplexity or a paniclike fear of brain damage or of going crazy.

1.6.2.4. Relevant Laboratory Tests

Except for the unusually intense or atypical case in which actual brain damage might be considered [which would require a brain-wave tracing, or electroencephalogram (EEG); an adequate neurological examination; X rays of the skull; and so on], there are no specific laboratory tests. The patient will probably be drug-free, and it is likely that even toxicological screens will not be helpful.

1.6.3. Toxic Reaction

A toxic reaction is really an overdose that occurs when an individual has taken so much of the drug that the body support systems no longer work properly. Clinically, this reaction is most frequently seen with the CNS depressants and opiates. A detailed discussion of this phenomenon is given in each relevant chapter, as the picture differs markedly among drug types. This diagnosis takes precedence even if signs of confusion or psychosis are present.

1.6.4. Psychosis

A *psychosis,* as used here, occurs when an awake, alert, and well-oriented individual with stable vital signs and no evidence of withdrawal experiences hallucinations or delusions *without insight.*

1.6.4.1. Typical History

Drug-induced psychoses are usually seen in individuals who have repeatedly consumed CNS depressants or stimulants.[23] The onset of symptoms is usually abrupt (within hours to days) and represents a gross change from the person's normal level of functioning. The disturbance is dramatic and may result in the patient's being brought to a psychiatric facility or to the emergency room by police.

1.6.4.2. Physical Signs and Symptoms

There are few physical symptoms that are typical of any particular psychotic state. It is the loss of contact with reality occurring during intoxication that dominates the picture. However, during the psychosis, an individual may be quite upset and may present with a rapid pulse or an elevated blood pressure.

1.6.4.3. Psychological State

A psychosis occurs with the development of either hallucinations (an unreal sensory input, such as hearing things) or a delusion (an unreal and fixed thought into which the individual has no insight). In general, the drug-induced psychotic state lasts for several days to weeks and is usually totally reversible. As discussed in greater depth in the appropriate chapters, there is little evidence, if any, of chronic or permanent psychoses being induced in individuals who have shown no obvious psychopathology antedating their drug experience.

1.6.4.4. Relevant Laboratory Tests

No specific laboratory findings are associated with the psychosis, as the patient may be drug-free and still out of contact with reality. For patients who abuse drugs intravenously, the stigmata of infection (e.g., a high WBC) and hepatitis (e.g., elevated SGOT, SGPT, CPK, and LDH) may be seen. It is also *possible* that a urine or blood toxicological screen will reveal evidence of a drug.

1.6.5. Organic Brain Syndrome

An organic brain syndrome (OBS) consists of confusion, disorientation, and decreased intellectual functioning along with stable vital signs in the absence of signs of withdrawal.

1.6.5.1. Typical History

Any drug can induce a state of confusion and/or disorientation (an OBS) if given in high enough doses, but at very high levels, the physical signs and symptoms of a toxic overdose predominate. There are a number of drugs, including the atropinelike substances, the CNS depressants, and PCP, that produce confusion at relatively low doses. There are, in addition, some factors that predispose a person to confusion, including physical debilitation (e.g., hepatitis), advanced age, a history of prior head trauma, or a long history of drug or alcohol abuse. These factors combine to explain the varied types of onset for organicities ranging from a very rapidly developing picture after PCP in a healthy young person to a slow onset (e.g., over days to weeks) of increasing organicity for an elderly individual taking even therapeutic levels of CNS depressants.

1.6.5.2. Physical Signs and Symptoms

As defined in this text, the OBS patient most often presents with a stable physical condition and a predominance of mental pathology. However, because an organicity is more likely to be seen in an individual with some sort of physical problem, any mixture of physical signs and symptoms can be seen.

1.6.5.3. Psychological State

The patient demonstrates confusion about where he is, what he is doing there, the proper date and time, or who he is. He has trouble understanding concepts and assimilating new ideas, but usually maintains some insight into the fact that his mind is not working properly. This, in turn, may result in a level of fear or irritability. The signs of an OBS may be accompanied by visual or tactile (i.e., being touched) hallucinations.

1.6.5.4. Relevant Laboratory Tests

The first step in treating any OBS is to rule out major medical problems. Although the OBS may continue beyond the length of action of any drug (especially in the elderly), a blood or urine toxicological screen may be helpful. It is also important to aggressively rule out all potentially reversible nondrug causes of confusion. Thus, in addition to a good neurological examination, blood tests should be drawn to determine the status of the electrolytes [especially Na, Ca, and K (see Table 1.5)], blood counts (especially the Hct and Hgb levels, as shown in the table) and liver and kidney function (including the BUN and creatinine for the kidney and the SGOT, SGPT, and LDG for the liver). It is also necessary to evaluate the need for skull X rays (to look for fractures and signs of internal bleeding), a spinal tap (to rule out bleeding, infection, or tumors of the CNS), and an EEG (to look for focal problems as well as general brain functioning).

1.6.6. Withdrawal or Abstinence Syndrome

The withdrawal or abstinence syndrome consists of the development of physiological and psychological symptoms when a *physically* addicting drug is stopped too quickly. *The symptoms are usually the opposite of the acute effects of that same drug.* For instance, withdrawal from drugs that induce sleep, that can be used to help achieve relaxation, and that decrease body temperature (e.g., the CNS depressants) consists of insomnia, anxiety, and increases in body temperature and respiratory rate. The length of the withdrawal syndrome varies directly with the half-life (the time necessary to metabolize one-half of the drug), and the intensity increases with the usual dose taken and the length of time over which it was taken. Treatment consists of giving a good medical evaluation, offering general support (e.g., rest and nutrition), and addressing the immediate cause of the withdrawal symptoms by administering enough of the substance (or any other drug of the same class) to markedly decrease symptoms on Day 1 of treatment and then decreasing the dose over the next 5–10 days (or longer for drugs of very long half-life).

Clinically significant withdrawal syndromes are seen with the CNS depressants, the opiates, and the stimulants. Because these syndromes differ for each specific kind of drug, the reader is encouraged to review each relevant chapter.

1.7. A GENERAL INTRODUCTION TO EMERGENCY AND CRISIS TREATMENT[24,25]

The emergency care of the drug-abusing patient is covered within each chapter and in a general review in Chapter 14. The treatment approaches represent common sense applications of the lessons learned about the particular drug category, the probable natural course of that class of difficulty, and the dictum, "First, do no harm."

1.7.1. Acute Emergency Care

One must first address the life-threatening problems that may be associated with toxic reactions, psychoses, organic brain syndromes, withdrawal, and medical problems. The approach to emergency care begins by first establishing an adequate airway, supporting circulation and controlling hemorrhage, and dealing with any life-threatening behavior.

1.7.2. Evaluation

After the patient has been stabilized, it is important to evaluate other serious problems by gathering a good history from the patient and/or a resource person (usually a relative), doing careful physical and neurological examinations, and ordering the relevant laboratory tests.

1.7.3. Subacute Care

1. It is then possible to begin the more subacute care, attempting to keep medications to a minimum, especially for symptoms of *panic* and *flashbacks,* which tend to respond to reassurance.

2. For *toxic reactions,* the subacute goal is to support the vital signs until the body has had a chance to metabolize the ingested substance adequately.

3. The transient nature of the *psychoses* indicates that the best care is suppression of any destructive behavior during the several days necessary for the patient to recover.

4. Evaluation of an *OBS* requires careful diagnosis and treatment of all life-threatening causes.

5. *Withdrawal* is usually treated by conducting an adequate physical evaluation to rule out associated medical disorders, giving rest and good nutrition, and slowly decreasing the level of the addictive substance.

6. *Medical problems* must be handled individually.

1.8. ONWARD

You have now been introduced to my general philosophy regarding drugs, drug problems, and their treatment. The next chapter proceeds with a detailed discussion of the CNS depressants and is followed by two chapters on alcohol and the treatment of alcoholism, these three chapters serving as a prototype for the remaining chapters. Each of the clinically relevant drug types is then discussed, and the two final chapters emphasize emergency problems of substance misusers in general and an introduction to rehabilitation.

REFERENCES

1. Schuckit, M. A., & Gold, E. O. A simultaneous evaluation of multiple markers of ethanol/placebo challenges in sons of alcoholics and controls. *Archives of General Psychiatry 45:*211–216, 1988.

2. Schuckit, M. A. Biological vulnerability to alcoholism. *Journal of Consulting and Clinical Psychology 55:*301–309, 1987.
3. Kozel, N. Epidemiology of drug abuse: An overview. *Science 234:*970–973, 1987.
4. Hilton, M. Drinking patterns and drinking problems in 1984. *Alcohol: Clinical and Experimental Research 11:*167–174, 1987.
5. Smart, R. G., Mora, M. E., Terroba, G., & Varma, V. K. Drug use among non-students in three countries. *Drug and Alcohol Dependence 7:*125–132, 1981.
6. Editorial: Screening for drugs of abuse. *Lancet 1:*365, 1987.
7. Schuckit, M. A. (Ed.). *Alcohol Patterns and Problems.* New Brunswick, New Jersey: Rutgers University Press, 1985.
8. Schuckit, M. Drug classes and problems. *Drug Abuse and Alcoholism Newsletter 17*(1):1–4, 1988.
9. Mello, N. K., and Griffiths, R. R.: Alcoholism and drug abuse: An overview. In H. Y. Meltzer (Ed), *Psychopharmacology: The Third Generation of Progress.* New York: Raven Press, 1987, pp. 1511–1514.
10. Cohen, S. (Ed.). Pharmacology of drugs of abuse. *Drug Abuse and Alcoholism Newsletter 5*(6):1–4, 1976.
11. Alford, G. S., & Alford, N. F. Benzodiazepine-induced state-dependent learning: A correlative of abuse potential? *Addictive Behaviors 1:*261–267, 1976.
12. Jaffe, J. H. Drug addiction and drug abuse. In A. G. Gilman, L. S. Goodman, T. W. Rall, & F. Murad (Eds.), *The Pharmacological Basis of Therapeutics* (7th ed.). New York: Macmillan, 1985, pp. 532–581.
13. Stunkard, A. J., Foch, T. T., & Hrubec, Z. A twin study of human obesity. *Journal of the American Medical Association 256:*51–54, 1986.
14. Wilson, G. T. Chapter 14: Current status of behavioral treatment of obesity. In N. A. Krasnegor (Ed.), *Behavioral Analysis and Treatment of Substance Abuse.* NIDA Research Monograph 25. Rockville, Maryland: Department of Health, Education, and Welfare, 1979.
15. Dickerson, J., Hinchy, J., & Fabre, J. Chasing, arousal and sensation seeking in off-course gamblers, *British Journal of Addiction 82:*673–680, 1987.
16. Wenger, J. R., Tiffany, T. M., Bombardier, C., *et al.* Ethanol tolerance in the rat is learned. *Science 213:*575–576, 1981.
17. Siegel, S., Hinson, R. E., & Krank, M. D. Morphine-induced attenuation of morphine tolerance. *Science 212:*1533–1534, 1981.
18. Bloom, F. E. Neurohumoral transmission and the central nervous system. In A. G. Gilman, L. W. Goodman, T. W. Rall & F. Murad (Eds.), *The Pharmacological Basis of Therapeutics* (7th ed.). New York: Macmillan, 1985, pp. 236–259.
19. Pomara, N., Stanley, B., Block, R., *et al.* Increased sensitivity of the elderly to the central depressant effects of diazepam. *Journal of Clinical Psychiatry 46:*185–187, 1985.
20. Drug Enforcement Administration. *Controlled Substances Inventory List.* Washington, D.C.: Drug Enforcement Administration, January, 1979.
21. Cohen, S. (Ed.). The drug schedules: An updating for professionals. *Drug Abuse and Alcoholism Newsletter 5*(3):1–4, 1976.
22. Weil, A. T. Adverse reactions to marihuana: Classification and suggested treatment. *New England Journal of Medicine 5:*1–4, 1976.
23. Tsuang, M. T., Simpson, J. C., & Kronfol, Z. Subtypes of drug abuse with psychosis: Demographic characteristics, clinical features, and family history. *Archives of General Psychiatry 39:*141–147, 1982.
24. Stewart, R. B., Springer, P. K., & Adams, J. E. Drug-related admissions to an inpatient psychiatric unit. *American Journal of Psychiatry 137:*1093–1095, 1980.
25. Campbell, J. W., & Frisee, M. (Eds.). *Manual of Medical Therapeutics* (24th ed.). Boston: Little, Brown, 1983.

Central Nervous System (CNS) Depressants

2.1. INTRODUCTION

The central nervous system (CNS) depressant drugs include a variety of medications, such as hypnotics, most antianxiety drugs (also called *minor tranquilizers*), and alcohol.[1] As discussed in greater depth in Section 2.1.1.4.4, a new group of nonbenzodiazepine antianxiety drugs have appeared in recent years, but these are not CNS depressants. The general anesthetics are not presented here, as time and space constraints forced me to limit the discussion to the substances most clinically important in drug abuse. One anesthetic agent, phencyclidine (PCP), is abused as a hallucinogen and is discussed in Chapter 9.

The CNS depressants all have clinical usefulness, and most have an abuse potential. When used alone, they cause an intoxication or "high" similar to alcohol intoxication, but they can also be mixed with other drugs, such as stimulants, in attempts to modify some of the effects or side effects of those drugs.

As indicated by the high rate of prescriptions, a major avenue of supply is through the physician. In addition, many of the legally manufactured depressants find their way into the street marketplace.

The prototypical depressant drug is the barbiturate. These medications have been available since the 1860s[1] and have been prescribed for a wide variety of problems. The generic names of all barbiturates in the United States end in *-al* and in Britain, in *-one*.[1] The most widely prescribed class of CNS depressants, the benzodiazepines (Bz's), have some unique characteristics. Therefore, whenever appropriate, they are discussed separately.

2.1.1. Pharmacology

2.1.1.1. General Characteristics

The different CNS depressants possess markedly different lengths of action, as discussed below. Blood levels depend on the physical redistribution of the drug among various parts of the body; metabolic breakdown of the substance, usually in the liver; and excretion via the kidneys.

2.1.1.2. Predominant Effects

With the possible exception of the Bz's, the specific pharmacological mechanisms by which these drugs exert their effects are not completely known, but theories are discussed in other texts.[1] The depressants result in reversible depression of the activity of all excitable tissues—especially those of the CNS—with the greatest effects on the synapse (the space between two nerve cells).[1,2] The resulting depression in activity ranges from a slight lethargy or sleepiness, through various levels of anesthesia, to death from breathing and heart depression. It should be noted that through a phenomenon called a *paradoxical reaction* the hypnotics and the antianxiety drugs sometimes cause extreme excitement when given to children and elderly patients.

2.1.1.3. Tolerance and Dependence

2.1.1.3.1. Tolerance

Tolerance of these drugs is clinically important and occurs through both increased metabolism of the drug after its administration (*drug dispositional* or *metabolic tolerance*) and apparent adaptation of the CNS to the presence of the drug (*pharmacodynamic tolerance*).[1] However, metabolic tolerance also results in the enhanced metabolism of a variety of other substances, including the anticoagulant medications, with resulting altered blood levels. As is true of all medications, tolerance is not an all-or-none phenomenon, and most individuals do not demonstrate enhanced toleration of lethal doses of the depressants (with the possible exception of alcohol).[2]

An important aspect of tolerance occurs with the concomitant administration of additional depressant drugs. If a second drug is administered when the body is free of the first drug, cross-tolerance will probably be seen, at least in part, because of the expansion of the liver's capacity to metabolize depressant drugs. However, if the second depressant drug is administered *at the same time as* the first, the two drugs compete for metabolism within the liver, neither is metabolized properly, and the toxic effects of the first drug appear to multiply the toxic effects of the second. As an example, the patient regularly abusing alcohol who undergoes surgery while in an alcohol-free state is likely to show significant cross-tolerance to preanesthetic and anesthetic medications. If, however, the same patient tries to abuse a barbiturate or an antianxiety medication while intoxicated with alcohol, he is likely to show potentiation of the effects of both drugs, with the possibility of a resulting unintentional toxic reaction or overdose. Therefore, even an individual with tolerance to one drug can have a fatal overdose with a concomitantly administered second drug, a common clinical circumstance with barbiturates and alcohol.

2.1.1.3.2. Dependence

All CNS depressants, including the benzodiazepines like chlordiazepoxide (Librium), diazepam (Valium), and alprazolam (Xanax), produce a withdrawal state when stopped abruptly after the relatively continuous administration of high doses. The withdrawal picture *resembles* a rebound hyperexcitability characterized by body changes in a direction opposite to that seen with the administration of the drug (which may not be the actual pharmacological mechanism).[2]

It is possible to see signs of withdrawal after several weeks of intoxication,[2] but in general, the severity of the withdrawal syndrome parallels the strength of the drug, the doses taken, and the length of administration.[1,3] The actual dosage varies with the drug and the individual, but for a drug like pentobarbital, for example, the administration of 400 mg a day for 3 months results in definite withdrawal electroencephalographic (EEG) changes in at least one third of the individuals taking the drug; 600 mg for 1–2 months results in a mild to moderate level of withdrawal in half the individuals, with 10% going on to severe withdrawal, including seizures; and 900 mg for 2 months results in seizures in 75% of the individuals, with most demonstrating a confusion–disorientation syndrome [organic brain syndrome (OBS)].[2,3] With a drug like meprobamate (Miltown or Equanil), one can see severe withdrawal in an individual taking 3–6 g daily over 40 days. As a general rule, abuse of 500 mg of a barbiturate or an equivalent dose of other drugs will result in a risk of withdrawal seizures.[4,5]

With the benzodiazepines, moderate withdrawal symptoms can be seen in individuals taking two or three times the usual clinical dose for a matter of weeks.[2,5] Symptoms of withdrawal from benzodiazepines are likely to include headaches and anxiety (in about 80%), insomnia (about 70%), and tremor and fatigue (each seen in about 60%), as well as perceptual changes, tinnitus, sweating, and decreases in concentration.[6,7] Similar to the picture that can develop during alcoholic withdrawal, abrupt abstinence after higher doses of benzodiazepines can precipitate delirium, sometimes with associated psychotic features, and seizures.[1,2,6–8] There is also compelling evidence that some of the more mild symptoms listed above are likely to occur following months of daily benzodiazepines in therapeutic doses; one recent review reported two or more such symptoms in 82% of patients who had taken daily benzodiazepines for a year or more.[9]

2.1.1.4. Specific Drugs

Tables 2.1 and 2.2 give numerous examples of members of the different classes of hypnotic and antianxiety drugs. The actions of members of two major subclasses of drugs can overlap greatly. For example, antianxiety drugs in high enough doses induce sleep, whereas the hypnotics for many years were labeled *hypnosedatives* and were administered to treat anxiety. In addition, some of the hypnotics are used as general anesthetic agents.

Table 2.1
Nonbenzodiazepine CNS Depressants[a]

Drug type	Generic name	Trade name
Hypnotics		
Barbiturates		
Ultrashort-acting	Thiopental	Pentothal
	Methohexital	Brevital
Intermediate-acting	Pentobarbital	Nembutal
	Secobarbital	Seconal
	Amobarbital	Amytal
	Butabarbital	Butisol
Long-acting	Phenobarbital	Luminal
Barbituratelike	Methaqualone	Quäälude
	Ethchlorvynol	Placidyl
	Methprylon	Noludar
	Glutethimide	Doriden
Others	Chloral hydrate	Noctec
	Paraldehyde	—
Antianxiety drugs		
Carbamates	Meprobamate	Miltown, Equanil
	Tybamate	Salacen, Tybatran

[a]See Table 2.2 for the benzodiazepines.

2.1.1.4.1. Hypnotics

As shown in these two tables, some commonly used hypnotics are the barbiturates, the barbituratelike drugs, the aldehyde hypnotics (Table 2.1), and several benzodiazepines (Table 2.2).

1. The first subclass of *barbiturates* consists of the rarely abused *ultrashort-*acting drugs (used to induce anesthesia) with lengths of action of minutes (e.g., thiopental and methohexital). The *short* to *intermediate* -acting barbiturates exert their major effect for a period of approximately 4 hours, so that they are ideal for helping people get to sleep. These include the drugs most frequently prescribed and abused as hypnotics, such as pentobarbital (Nembutal) and secobarbital (Seconal). Finally, the *long-lasting* drugs, exemplified by phenobarbital, are most often used to treat chronic conditions such as epilepsy. Abuse of these drugs is relatively uncommon.

2. The *barbituratelike drugs* [e.g., mathaqualone (Quäälude) and glutethimide (Doriden)] were almost all introduced as ''nonaddictive and safe'' substitutes for the barbiturates. They were developed in an attempt to overcome some of the drawbacks of barbiturate hypnotics, such as the morning-after ''hangover,'' residual sleepiness, drug-induced disturbances in sleep patterns [especially in rapid-

eye-movement (REM) sleep], and the highly lethal overdose potential of barbiturates. However, most barbituratelike hypnotics share the dangers of the barbiturates. Two drugs are *especially* dangerous in overdoses, as they are highly fat-soluble and resistant to excretion, offer few clinical advantages, and should be prescribed rarely, if at all: ethchlorvynol (Placidyl) and glutethimide (Doriden).[10] Another drug, methaqualone (Quāālude), has been especially widely abused.[11]

3. The third group of hypnotics discussed here is exemplified by chloral hydrate (Noctec) and paraldehyde, drugs that share most of the dangers outlined for the barbiturate and barbituratelike hypnotics.

4. Four other drugs, representing the only departure from the general drawbacks outlined above, are the benzodiazepines flurazepam (Dalmane), nitrazepam (Mogodan), temazepam (Restoril), and triazolam (Halcion). Overall, these drugs disturb the sleep EEG least of all, benefiting the patient by decreasing the sleep latency and the number of awakenings along with increasing the total amount of sleep. At the same time, the amount of sleep in stage 2 increases while the sleep spent in stages 3 and 4 tends to decrease, and moderate changes in REM sleep are likely to occur. These changes are, however, relatively mild compared to those observed with other types of sleep-inducing drugs.[5]

5. In summary, most hypnotics share serious drawbacks. They disturb the natural sleep pattern, they are extremely dangerous if taken in an overdose (with the exception of the benzodiazepines), and all have an abuse potential. Two of the drugs, ethchlorvynol and glutethimide, have additional dangers of delayed metabolism, which make their prescription even more dangerous than that of the usual drug.

Table 2.2
Benzodiazepines (Bz)[1,6]

Generic name	Trade name	Half-life (hr)	Usual adult daily dose (mg)[a]
Alprazolam	Xanax	11–15	0.75–4
Chlordiazepoxide	Librium	5–30	5–25
Clonazepam[b]	Clonopin	20–50	0.5–10+
Clorazepate	Tranxene	30–60	15–60
Diazepam	Valium	20–50	2–15
Flurazepam[c]	Dalmane	50–100	15–30 HS
Lorazepam	Ativan	10–20	2–6
Nitrazepam[c]	Mogodan	24	5–10 HS
Oxazepam	Serax	5–20	10–60
Prazepam	Verstran (Centrax)	50–80	20–60
Temazepam[c]	Restoril	4–8	15–30 HS
Triazolam	Halcion	3–5	0.25–0.5

[a]HS indicates use at bedtime (hour of sleep).
[b]Used only as an anticonvulsant.
[c]Used only as a hypnotic.

It appears that *all* hypnotic medications lose their effectiveness if taken nightly for more than 2 weeks.[1,12,13] Therefore, considering their potential as suicide agents and their limited time of efficacy when used daily, there is a serious question about the wisdom of prescribing these medications for anything more than a short-term, acute crisis. If a hypnotic is required for an acute anxiety situation, I use a benzodiazepine, but rarely for more than 2 weeks at a time.

Numerous other approaches to handling insomnia are available and are discussed in detail in other texts.[14,15] For instance, after carefully ruling out problems to which insomnia might be secondary,[15] I prescribe a schedule of going to bed and getting up at the same time each day, no caffeinated beverages, and no naps. Milk at bedtime can be a useful adjunct, perhaps because of its tryptophan content.

2.1.1.4.2. Antianxiety Drugs

The class of drugs most frequently prescribed for anxiety is the benzodiazepines [e.g., diazepam (Valium)] (Table 2.2). These drugs have been demonstrated to be highly effective in handling *acute* anxiety, but no well-controlled study has yet proved that they work for more than 1 or 2 months when taken daily.[13,16]

The major dangers include a disturbance in sleep pattern and a change in affect (increased irritability, hostility, and lethargy). The carbamates (Table 2.1) are highly lethal when taken in overdose. Most members of this drug subclass have a length of action that exceeds the usual time between the administration of doses. I never prescribe the carbamates (meprobamate or tybamate) because they have a much higher addictive potential and greater possibility of fatal overdosage than the benzodiazepines.

2.1.1.4.3. Benzodiazepines (Bz's)

Although the drugs in this antianxiety subclass are definitely CNS depressants, they are discussed separately because of our level of understanding of their mode of action, because of their widespread use, and because of their asset of producing significantly less physiological impairment and less intense toxic reactions or overdose. These drugs are used as muscle relaxants (e.g., after strains or disc disease), as anticonvulsants (usually for non-grand-mal seuzures and/or for status epilepticus), and as antianxiety agents.[1] Their usefulness in treating anxiety states is best limited to short-term help (2 or 3 weeks) for severe situational problems. The more long-term and chronic major anxiety disorders (e.g., agoraphobia or obsessive–compulsive disease) are not usual targets for Bz treatment, as these drugs are not effective over a long enough period of time, and there is a possible rebound increase in symptoms when the drugs are stopped. The limited use of the Bz's in treating anxiety is discussed elsewhere.[13,17]

The specific drugs are listed in Table 2.2. Although there are variations among the drugs (especially related to their half-lives), the Bz's have great clinical similarities.[13,17] Compared with most other types of sedative/hypnotics, these drugs are relatively safe in overdose, are less likely to lead to metabolic tolerance, induce less significant changes in sleep stages, and appear to be less likely to produce physical addiction. All drugs of this class can be administered orally, and most are better absorbed by mouth than by injection (diazepam can be given intravenously and lorazepam is well absorbed intramuscularly).[17,18] They usually reach peak blood levels in 2–4 hours after oral administration, and most have active metabolites (except lorazepam and oxazepam). The frequency of administration varies with the half-life, so that lorazepam and oxazepam may need to be given four times a day to be effective, whereas clorazepate and diazepam may be used once per day (usually at bedtime). With the exception of the Bz's that have shorter half-lives (which are the same drugs that have no active metabolites), most of these drugs tend to accumulate in the body, reaching a steady state in 7–10 days, with the result that clinicians must be certain that sedative side effects do not progressively interfere with life functioning.

The pharmacological mechanisms of the Bz's are interesting. A unique attribute relates to the discovery in the brain of high-affinity selective receptors for Bz substances with actions that correlate closely with levels of anxiety or seizure activity.[1,19] This discovery indicates the probable existence of endogenous ligands (probably purines) for those specific receptors.[20,21] The Bz receptors are probably distinct from but interact closely with receptors for a brain neurotransmitter, gamma-aminobutyric acid (GABA), with a mutual enhancement of effects.[1,19,21] Although a direct link between Bz receptors and the actions of other CNS depressants has not been found, there is evidence that in physiological doses, at least one barbiturate, pentobarbital, increases binding at Bz receptors.[22] As might be predicted from these data, recent studies have also identified Bz's that act at the Bz/GABA sites to inhibit and *antagonize* the actions of other Bz's—drugs that may prove important in treating overdoses with medications that affect this receptor complex.[23]

2.1.1.4.4. Nonbenzodiazepine Anxiolytics

A number of non-Bz anxiety-reducing agents are currently undergoing evaluation.[24,25] This search is spurred on by the recognition that Bz's are not perfect, having associated problems of abuse, physical dependence, cognitive impairment, and interactions with other brain depressants as described elsewhere in this chapter. Even thought these non-Bz agents are technically not CNS depressants, they are briefly discussed in this section because they are used in clinical situations historically reserved for benzodiazepines.

These agents have a variety of structures and potential activities. They include nabilone, a tetrahydrocannabinol homologue distinguished by its relationship to the active ingredient in marijuana, and fenobam, a potentially effective anxiolytic with few muscle-relaxant or sedative/hypnotic properties and minimal potential for interaction with other CNS depressants.[26,27] Zopiclone is an effective non-Bz hypnotic with few cognitive effects and no documented interaction with alcohol.[25]

The best-known and most thoroughly studied of the non-Bz anxiolytics is buspirone (Buspar), an unusual fat-soluble molecule of multiple rings with a structure unlike that of any other anxiolytic agent.[28,29] This drug has either weak actions or no actions on Bz receptors, and it does not replace Bz's from their binding sites, nor does it directly affect GABA binding.[30,31] Buspirone is known to interact with the serotonin, norepinephrine, and acetylcholine systems, with the most clinically relevant effect probably being on serotonin.

In controlled studies, buspirone shows no hypnotic effects, but demonstrates anxiolytic properties comparable to those of a number of comparison Bz's, at least after 2 weeks of administration.[24] At the same time, this non-Bz drug appears to offer fewer safety concerns, as there is little evidence of cognitive impairment with clinically relevant doses of this drug and little evidence that it interacts with other brain depressants such as alcohol.[32,33] Nor do animal or clinical studies demonstrate a high potential for abuse of this agent.[24,34–36] If clinical observations continue to support this latter claim, buspirone may be the first effective anxiolytic without a clinically significant addiction risk, but only time will tell.

2.1.2. Epidemiology and Patterns of Abuse

The CNS depressants are prescribed in great quantities, as approximately 90% of hospitalized medical/surgical patients receive orders for hypnotic and/or antianxiety medication during their inpatient stay,[37] and more than 15% of American adults use these drugs during any one year.[38] Supporting the conclusion of high prevalence of use are the results of a study demonstrating that more than 1 in 3 American adults had had symptoms of insomnia during the preceding year, with the result that 2.6% had used a prescribed hypnotic, an additional 1.7% utilized other prescription drugs to help them sleep, and approximately 3% took over-the-counter sleeping pills.[39] These figures include a total of 0.3% of the population (11% of users) who had taken the medication regularly over the last year,[39] with evidence from additional studies that many of those consuming a hypnotic for more than a year should probably never have received the drug in the first place.[9] It has been estimated that up to 10% of general medical/surgical patients and 30% of individuals with serious psychiatric histories have, at some time, *felt* psychologically dependent on antianxiety or hypnotic drugs, with outright abuse seen for between 5 and 10%.[40]

Among the CNS depressants, the Bz's receive the widest use. In one year, over 2 billion tablets of diazepam alone were prescribed in the United States.[40] In a recent study, 9% of adults had taken a Bz in the last year for at least 1 month, as had 13% of college students.[41] Although use is certainly widespread, these figures do not necessarily indicate abuse, as these drugs are very effective on a short-term basis.[37,42,43]

In simple terms, depressant-drug abusers fall into two classes—those who receive the drugs on prescription and those who (belonging to a "street culture") primarily misuse illegally obtained medications. One survey has revealed that between one fourth and one third of abusers of illegally obtained medications report using hypnotics or antianxiety drugs over the prior month, usually periodic inges-tion of 30–80 mg of diazepam (Valium), frequently in combination with other drugs. For both types of abusers, at least 10% of all "drug mentions" in emergency rooms and crisis clinics are of diazepam.[44] The brain depressants continue to be drugs of abuse among young people, with data showing that as many as 16% of high school seniors in the United States had at one time or another taken a depressant "recreationally" in the late 1970s, but with evidence that this figure has probably decreased by the mid-1980s.[45–47]

Thus, misuse of these drugs should be considered in the evaluation of almost any patient seen in a usual medical setting, an emergency room, or a crisis clinic. In light of the limited time that these medications stay effective when taken daily, there is rarely a valid clinical need to prescribe them for more than 2–4 weeks.

2.1.3. Establishing the Diagnosis

Identification of the individual misusing or abusing CNS depressants requires a high index of suspicion, especially for patients with an OBS or paranoid delusions and for all patients who insist on receiving prescriptions for any of these medica-tions. It is imperative that these drugs not be given to patients who are not known to the physician and that, when they are prescribed, the prescriptions should be only for relatively small amounts (both to decrease the suicide overdose potential[48] and to discourage misuse); that no "repeats" be allowed; that bottles be labeled as to contents; and that past records be evaluated to determine how long the patient has been on the medication.

2.2. EMERGENCY PROBLEMS

The outline given below follows the general format presented in Table 1.4, reviewing the possible areas of difficulty seen in emergency rooms, the outpatient office, and crisis clinics. The most common problems seen with the CNS depres-sants are toxic overdose, temporary psychosis, and withdrawal.

2.2.1. Panic Reactions (Possibly 305.40 or 292.89 in DSM-III-R) (see Sections 1.6.1, 5.2.1, 7.2.1, and 8.2.1)

Panic reactions (high levels of anxiety due to the fear of either going crazy or coming to physical harm as a result of the normal effects of the drug) are most frequently seen with stimulants and hallucinogenic drugs. They are rarely noted as part of the acute reaction to sedating drugs, such as CNS depressants and opiates, except as symptoms of an abstinence syndrome.

2.2.1.1. Clinical Picture

The closest one comes to seeing an acute panic reaction is the hyperexcitability (paradoxical reaction) seen in some children and elderly individuals receiving depressant drugs, in which the patient is frightened and excited, cannot sleep, and has excessive energy.[1,49] It is also possible that anger and panic will be seen in some younger individuals taking Bz's, perhaps because their inhibitions are decreased.[1,50] Problems are likely to begin in the first hour or so after the drug is taken and to remain for its length of action.

Another type of problem noted with all CNS depressants (see Section 4.2.6 for alcohol) is the acute and protracted abstinence syndrome. The patient with this syndrome is likely to show anxiety and insomnia and, at least following alcohol abuse, can even demonstrate severe panic attacks.[6,7,50] A prior history of misuse of brain depressants must therefore always be considered part of the differential diagnosis of almost any clinical picture of anxiety.[51]

2.2.1.2. Treatment

The paradoxical reaction tends to clear within hours, with only general support and reassurance. It is best to avoid administering other drugs. The protracted abstinence syndrome should be addressed with the behavior-modification approaches mentioned in Section 4.2.6.2.3 and discussed at greater length in Section 15.2.4.1.4.

2.2.2. Flashbacks

These are not known to occur with CNS depressants. If a patient reports them, other diagnoses (especially emotional or neurological diseases) should be considered.

2.2.3. Toxic Reactions (see Sections 4.2.3, 6.2.3, and 14.4)

The most usual toxic reaction seen with the depressant drugs occurs with either a deliberate or an inadvertent overdose.

2.2.3.1. Clinical Picture

2.2.3.1.1. History

The toxic reaction usually develops over a matter of hours, and the patient often presents in an obtunded state with or without evidence of recent drug ingestion. This reaction can be seen when an individual mixes depressants (usually alcohol and hypnotics), develops a confused organic state that results in inadvertent repeated administration of the drug (an automatism[52]), unintentionally takes too high a dose of a street drug, or makes a deliberate suicide attempt.

2.2.3.1.2. Physical Signs and Symptoms

Toxic reactions are characterized by various levels of anesthesia and decreased CNS, cardiac, and respiratory functioning. An overdose of a depressant drug is very serious. The physical signs must be carefully evaluated in a manner similar to that reported in Section 6.2.3 for opiates and as suggested by other authors.[1,53] Examination includes:

1. A careful evaluation of the vital signs and the reflexes, with the findings depending on the drug dose, the time elapsed since ingestion, and any complicating brain conditions, such as hypoxia.[1,53]

2. The neurological exams will help establish the degree of coma. Important aspects include:

   a. *Pupillary reflexes:* Usually midpoint and slowly reactive, except with glutethimide (Doriden), with which pupils tend to be enlarged.

   b. *Corneal reflexes:* Present only in mild coma.

   c. *Tendon reflexes and pain reflexes:* Tend to be depressed.[53]

3. Cardiac arrhythmias may be present, especially with the short-acting barbiturates.[53]

4. The lungs may be congested from heart failure or from positional or infective pneumonia.

2.2.3.1.3. Psychological State

Because the patient often presents in a stupor or a coma, there are usually few other distinctive psychological attributes.

2.2.3.1.4. Relevant Laboratory Tests (see Section 6.2.3.1.4)

As with any shocklike state or comparable medical emergency, it is important to carefully monitor the vital signs and the blood gases (arterial oxygen and CO_2) to evaluate the need for a respirator. A toxicological screen on either urine (50 ml) or blood (10 cc) should also be carried out to determine the specific drug involved and the amount of the substance in the blood, and baseline blood chemistries and blood counts should be taken as outlined in Table 1.5. If the cause of the stupor or coma is not obvious, a thorough neurological evaluation for ancillary damage (including an EEG, skull X rays, a spinal tap, and so on) must be done.

2.2.3.2. Treatment (see Section 6.2.3.2)

Treatment begins with emergency procedures to guarantee an adequate airway, to make sure that the heart is functioning, and to deal with any concomitant bleeding.[1] The general goal is to support the vital signs until enough of the drug has been metabolized so that the patient is stable[54,55] following the general approach presented in Table 2.3. The specific emergency maneuvers will depend on the patient's clinical status. These maneuvers may range from simple observation for mild overdoses to starting an intravenous (IV) infusion, placing the patient on a respirator, and admitting him to an intensive care unit.

Although toxic reactions involving the Bz's should not be taken lightly, the clinical picture tends to be relatively mild, and fewer than 5% of patients require intensive-unit care for 48 hours or more.[56] Deaths are relatively rare (fewer than 1%), and especially rapid recovery is to be expected with the short-acting Bz's such as lorazepam and oxazepam, even if the blood levels are initially high.[56,57]

Table 2.3
Treatment of the Depressant
Toxic Reaction

Diagnose	History, clinical signs
First steps	Airway, assist respiration Cardiac Check electrolytes Treat shock Lavage (use cuff if obtunded; activated charcoal; castor oil?)
Consider	Forced diuresis (limited value) Hemodialysis
Avoid	CNS stimulants

The steps for approaching the patient with a toxic reaction to CNS depressants, not necessarily to be taken in the numbered order, include these:

1. Establish a *clear airway, intubate* if needed (using an inflatable cuff in case you want to do a gastric lavage), and place on a *respirator* if necessary. The respirator should use compressed air (oxygen can decrease the respiratory drive) at a rate of 10–12 breaths per minute.
2. Evaluate the *cardiovascular status* and control *bleeding;* treat shock with plasma expanders, saline, dextran, or the relevant drugs[55]; administer *external cardiac massage/defibrillation/intracardiac adrenaline,* if needed.
3. Begin an IV (large-gauge needle), replacing all fluid loss (e.g., urine), *plus* 20 ml for insensible loss (from respiration and perspiration), each hour.
4. Establish a means of measuring *urinary output* (bladder catheter, if needed). Send 50 ml of urine for a toxicological screen.[55]
5. Carry out *gastric lavage* with saline if oral medication was taken in the last 4–6 hours.[55] Continue lavage until you get a clear return. You may give 60 ml of *castor oil* via the stomach tube, especially if fat-soluble drugs like glutethimide (Doriden) were taken.[52,55]
6. There are recent data to indicate that repeated administration of activated charcoal or similar agent (e.g., 12–20 g or more of activated charcoal suspended in water and administered every 1–12 hours over the first 2 days) appears to help increase the rate of elimination of the brain depressants.[1,58,59]
7. Recognizing that analgesics can cause a similar picture and that the patient may have ingested more than one type of medication, consider the possibility of a narcotic overdose. This is easily tested for through the admin-

istration of a narcotic antagonist such as *naloxone* (Narcan) at a dose of 0.4 mg, given either intramuscularly (IM) or IV. If the patient has ingested narcotic analgesics to the point of obtundation, a rapid reversal of the picture should be demonstrated.

8. Carry out a more thorough *physical* and *neurological exam*—which must include *pupils, corneal reflexes, tendon reflexes,* presence of *pathological reflexes* (e.g., snout reflex), *pain perception* (use Achilles tendon), and *awake/alert status* (see Sections 6.2.3.2 and 14.4.3).

9. Draw *bloods* for arterial blood gases, general blood tests to evaluate liver and kidney functioning, blood counts, and toxicological screen.

10. Gather a thorough *history* of:
    a. Recent drugs (type, amount, time)
    b. Alcohol
    c. Chronic diseases
    d. Allergies
    e. Current treatments
       Obtain this information from the patient and/or any available resource person.

11. For the comatose patient, protect against *decubitus ulcers* (bedsores) by frequent turning, and *protect the eyes* by taping the lids closed if necessary.

12. Establish a *flow sheet* for:
    a. Vital signs
    b. Level of reflexes [Point (8) above]
    c. Urinary output
    d. IV fluids
       These should be recorded every 30 minutes. An example is given in a reference text.[4]

13. Consider *forced diuresis*. This is not needed for patients with stable vital signs or for those who present deep tendon reflexes (e.g., Grade I or II coma[53]) and rarely helps for chlordiazepoxide (Librium) or diazepam (Valium).[4] If either diuresis or dialysis is used, special care must be taken to maintain proper electrolyte levels and to avoid precipitating congestive failure. If diuresis is needed, you may use:
    a. Furosemide (Lasic), 40–120 mg, as often as needed to maintain 250 ml or more per hour.
    b. IV fluids, with the general approach being to give enough saline and water with glucose to maintain urinary output in excess of 250 ml per hour.

14. Hemodialysis or peritoneal dialysis can be considered for the patient in a deep coma, but is rarely needed. Hemoperfusion may be helpful for patients who have Grade IV coma with associated apnea and hypotension, for patients who show deterioration despite supportive treatment, for patients in prolonged coma with cardiorespiratory complications, or for patients with very high plasma drug levels.[56]

15. Evaluate the need for *antibiotics. Do not* use them prophylactically.
16. *Do not* use CNS stimulants.
17. For the unresponsive patient who requires admission to an intensive-care unit, it is possible to establish a prognosis by observing the levels and the degree of change in systolic pressure, the central venous pressure, and the acid–base balance (pH), as described in an excellent article.[55] A special word of warning is required regarding the ability of the depressant drugs to produce a temporary flat electroencephalogram (EEG), which reverses within a matter of days.[2]
18. There are some special CNS depressant pictures, but most of the generalizations outlined here would hold for any drug. However, one might expect a longer period of coma with the fat-soluble drugs like glutethimide (Doriden) and ethchlorvynol (Placidyl). Patients experiencing toxic reactions to those drugs may enter an emergency room looking alert or may be treated in a hospital and appear to come out of their coma only to relapse into a deep level of obtundation.

2.2.4. Psychosis (Possibly 292.11 in DSM-III-R) (see Sections 1.6.4, 4.2.4, and 5.2.4)

2.2.4.1. Clinical Picture

The depressant drugs can produce a temporary psychosis characterized by an acute onset, a clear sensorium (the patient is alert and oriented), auditory hallucinations, and/or paranoid delusions (e.g., thinking that someone is plotting against or trying to harm him). This picture has been more clearly described as it relates to alcohol and thus is discussed in greater depth in Section 4.2.4. However, similar pictures can be expected with the abuse of any CNS depressant.[60–62] It is probable that the generalizations presented for alcohol hold for the other depressants as well.

2.2.4.2. Treatment

The psychosis will probably clear within 2 days to 2 weeks with supportive care. Medications should not be given unless the paranoia and/or hallucinations create a serious danger to the patient or those around him. Then, antipsychotic drugs—e.g., haloperidol (Haldol), 1–5 mg four times a day [QID (Latin *quater in die*)], or thioridazine (Mellaril), 25–100 mg QID—can be used *until* the clinical picture clears.

2.2.5. Organic Brain Syndrome (Possibly 292.00, 292.83, or 292.90 in DSM-II-R) (see Section 1.6.5)

The OBS can result as part of an increased sensitivity to brain depressants, intoxication, an *overdose,* or during withdrawal. The confusion associated with intoxication tends to be mild and transient and thus is not discussed here in great depth.

2.2.5.1. General Comments

One special case of OBS needs further discussion. Individuals with decreased brain functioning (e.g., the elderly and those who have had previous brain damage as a result of trauma, infections, or other causes) are probably more sensitive to the effects of all CNS depressants, including the Bz's.[63] Thus, such individuals might be expected to show a clinically significant and relatively persistent, although rarely permanent, state of confusion whenever they take hypnotics, alcohol, or antianxiety drugs. Use or abuse of CNS depressants should be considered as part of the differential diagnosis for all confused states of recent onset or for anyone demonstrating a rapid deterioration in his usual state of cognition.

Another important topic involves the recognition of possible neuropsychological deficits in abusers of CNS depressant drugs. Clinical and anecdotal information reveals significant memory problems in many Bz- and hypnotic-drug abusers. These observations are corroborated by the demonstration of psychological test deficits (e.g., on the Halstead–Reitan Battery) in approximately a third or more of depressant abusers—deficits that remain after 3 weeks to 3 months of abstinence.[64] Interference with memory and learning can be demonstrated with these drugs even after a single dose.[65]

The treatment of an OBS induced by a CNS depressant involves a series of common sense steps. First, the patient should be evaluated for any life-threatening causes of the OBS: trauma (e.g., a subdural hematoma), serious infections in the CNS or elsewhere, blood loss, electrolyte imbalances, hypoglycemia, and so on. Next, all CNS depressants should be stopped, and the patient should be observed over the next several weeks to document possible improvement. As with alcohol, it is possible that some patients may demonstrate more permanent neuropsychological deficits, although this possibility has not been documented.

The discussion now highlights two specific categories of OBS in greater detail.

2.2.5.2. OBS Caused by Overdose

2.2.5.2.1. Clinical Picture

An overdose syndrome short of a coma is characterized by abnormal vital signs and confusion, disorientation, decreased mentation, and impaired memory processing. This picture closely resembles that seen during high-level alcohol intoxication. It may develop at even low doses in individuals at high risk for confusion, such as the elderly.[63,66]

2.2.5.2.2. Treatment

The confusional state is best treated with observation, usually in an inpatient setting where the patient is protected from wandering or harming himself. For younger individuals, the confusion usually clears within a matter of hours to days, but for older people, it might require an extended treatment period of 2 weeks or longer. In either instance, it is best to avoid the concomitant administration of any drug.

2.2.5.3. OBS during Withdrawal

2.2.5.3.1. Clinical Picture

A rapidly evolving OBS can be seen during withdrawal from these drugs.[8] It is usually temporary, rarely lasting more than a few days even without treatment. When it develops, signs of withdrawal are usually prominent, but one must take care to rule out other potentially lethal causes of OBS, including trauma, occult bleeding, and brain damage.

2.2.5.3.2. Treatment

Treatment of OBS during withdrawal is discussed in Section 2.2.6.2.

2.2.6. Drug Withdrawal Syndrome (e.g., 292.00 in DSM-III-R) (see Sections 4.2.6 and 6.2.6)

The depressant withdrawal syndrome consists of a constellation of symptoms that *might* develop in an individual taking any of these drugs daily in excessive doses. The final clinical picture is usually a mixture of any or all of the possible symptoms, running a time–course that tends to last 3–7 days for the short-acting drugs like alcohol (the most frequently abused CNS depressant[6,67]), but may be longer for longer-acting drugs like diazepam (Valium).

Although probably less likely to cause physical addiction than other depressants, all the Bz's can do so.[68] As new Bz's were introduced to the market, it was hoped that they might be less addicting or produce a more mild abstinence syndrome, but this has not proved to be the case for any of the new drugs of this class, including alprazolam (Xanax).[69–71] In fact, there is evidence that when administration of Bz's is continued for more than a month or so, even at doses in the therapeutic range, mild but disturbing withdrawal symptoms are likely to be seen.[32,35,71]

The Bz's are less often selected as the "street" drug of choice, tend to be avoided by drug-naive college students in experimental settings, and have a low but measurable level of self-administration when offered to animals IV.[41,68] As is true of all CNS depressants, the development of physical dependence relates to the drug dose and the period of time over which it was administered. Thus, physical withdrawal has been reported with diazepam in clinical dose ranges (e.g., 10–20 mg/day), as well as alprazolam or lorazepam (4 mg/day or less) when taken over a period of weeks to months.[41,71] When 2–3 times the normal maximal doses are ingested, physical dependence can probably be induced in a matter of days to weeks.[41]

2.2.6.1. Clinical Picture

2.2.6.1.1. History

A CNS-depressant withdrawal syndrome must be considered in any individual who presents with autonomic nervous system (ANS) dysfunction along with agitation and who asks the physician for a CNS depressant drug. This syndrome can be seen in the "street" addict, who may be abusing the drug either orally or IV, the middle-class abuser who obtains the drug on prescription but takes more than prescribed, and the medical user who has taken the drug daily for more than a month or so. The syndrome begins slowly over a period of hours and may not peak until Day 2 or 3 for alcohol and Day 7 for the short- to intermediate-half-life Bz's.

The time–course for the withdrawal of barbiturates, such as pentobarbital, or a drug like meprobamate (Miltown or Equanil) is outlined in Table 2.4. This table can be used as a general outline for what might be expected, showing the beginning of symptoms within a half day of stopping or decreasing the medications, a peak intensity at 24–72 hours, and disappearance of acute symptoms some time before Day 7. The time–course of withdrawal is probably a good deal longer for the longer-acting barbiturates and the antianxiety drugs, such as chlordiazepoxide (Librium), for which it has been reported that seizures and delirium can begin as late as Day 7 or 8.[3]

The wide range of half-lives for the Bz's demonstrates the correlation between the length of drug action and the timing of withdrawal symptoms. Thus, with the

Table 2.4
Time Course of Acute Withdrawal from Short/Intermediate Barbiturates and Meprobamate[2-4]

Time (after last dose)	Symptom	Severity
12–16 hours	Intoxicated state *Onset:* Anxiety, tremors, anorexia, weakness, nausea/vomiting, cramps, hypotension, increased reflexes	Mild
24 hours	Weakness, tremors, increased reflexes, increased pleading for drug High risk for grand mal seizures Delirium	Mild Severe
24–72 hours	Peak intensity	Greatest
3–7 days	Symptoms gradually disappear	Diminishing
1 week–6 months	Some anxiety, sleep disturbance, ANS irregularities	Mild

longer-acting Bz's, such as chlordiazepoxide, withdrawal can be expected to begin on Day 3 or 4, to peak on Days 5–8, and to disappear on Days 9–14,[72,73] but secondary abstinence symptoms of lesser severity may continue for months. The shorter-acting Bz's without known potent active metabolites (e.g., lorazepam and oxazepam) might demonstrate a time–course more similar to that of alcohol, with symptoms such as nausea beginning within hours, the withdrawal syndrome peaking on Day 2 or 3, and a great deal of improvement by Day 4 or 5.[41,72]

2.2.6.1.2. Physical Signs and Symptoms

The withdrawal symptomatology consists of a strong mixture of both psychological and physical problems. The patient usually develops a fine *tremor, gastrointestinal (GI) upset, muscle aches,* and problems of the *autonomic nervous system* (e.g., increased pulse and respiration rates, a fever, and a labile blood pressure).[40,41] More atypical withdrawal syndromes can also be seen, especially with the Bz's, and may include headache, malaise, and abrupt weight loss.[41] With any CNS depressant, but especially the barbiturates, somewhere between 5 and perhaps 20% of individuals will develop grand mal *convulsions*—usually one or at most two fits and rarely going on to demonstrate a state of repeated and continuous seizures known as *status epilepticus.*

2.2.6.1.3. Psychological State

The withdrawal symptomatology includes moderate to high levels of *anxiety* and a strong drive to obtain the drug. In addition, somewhere between 5 and 15% of individuals develop an OBS and/or a *hallucination–delirium* state. With the barbiturates, probably at least one half of people showing convulsions during withdrawal go on to a delirium if not treated.[3] Similar problems as well as hallucinations or delusions can be noted during withdrawal from Bz's.[41,74] The withdrawal psychotic states differentiated from the CNS-depressant-induced temporary psychosis described in Section 2.2.4.1 by the ANS dysfunction and the confusion seen during the withdrawal syndrome.

2.2.6.1.4. Relevant Laboratory Tests

Because the CNS withdrawal syndrome is potentially *more severe than any other type of drug withdrawal,* it is essential that an adequate physical examination be carried out and that all baseline laboratory tests (including most of the chemistries and blood counts listed in Table 1.5) be considered. A toxicological screen (10 cc blood or 50 ml urine) may or may not reveal evidence of the drug, depending on the length of time since the last drug dose and the specific substance involved. It is imperative that the physical condition be carefully monitored throughout the acute withdrawal syndrome.

2.2.6.2. Treatment (see Sections 4.2.6 and 6.2.6.2)

An important aspect of treatment is prevention. Thus, patients should never be placed on a daily CNS depressant for more than 2–3 weeks; even then, the drug should be tapered off slowly rather than stopped abruptly.[6,41]

The treatment of depressant withdrawal follows a relatively simple paradigm, consisting of a good *physical evaluation, general supportive care,* and *treatment of the withdrawal itself* (including recognition that symptoms may have occurred because a depressant drug was stopped too quickly).[2,4,75] The comments below apply to syndromes caused by withdrawal from depressants other than alcohol. Alcoholic withdrawal is discussed in Section 4.2.6.

1. Because of the possibility of the development of an OBS or convulsions, it is probably safest to carry out withdrawal in a *hospital setting*[3] (see Section 4.2.6.2.5 for an exception).
2. The poor physical condition of many drug abusers necessitates that each patient receive an adequate *physical examination* and general *screening laboratory procedures.*
3. Assuming that there has been a good physical evaluation and that the patient is being provided with good nutrition, rest, and *multivitamins,* treatment of the *withdrawal itself* can begin. The two most usual withdrawal regimens (neither of which is clearly superior) are outlined in Table 2.5. At this point, it is a good idea to develop a *flow sheet* of all symptoms as evaluated every 4 hours, along with the drug doses given.[4]
   a. The pentobarbital (short- to intermediate-acting barbiturate) method[4,75] comprises the following steps:

Table 2.5
Treatment of Depressant
Withdrawal[4,67,75]

I. Pentobarbital method
  Test dose: 200 mg
    If patient falls asleep, no treatment needed.
    If no reaction, repeat dose Q[a] 2 hr.
    Determine dose for 24 hr. Divide QID.
    Stabilize for 2 days.
    Decrease by 100 mg/day.
II. Phenobarbital method
  Calculate needed dose. Give 32 mg
    phenobarbital for each 100 mg pentobarbital
    or equivalent.
  Stabilize for 2 days.
  Give QID.
  Decrease by 30 mg each day.

---

[a]The Q alone stands for Latin *quaque* ("every").

    i. Administer an *oral test dose of 200 mg* of the drug (usually pentobarbital) and evaluate the patient 1–2 hours later. If he is sleeping at that time, he is probably not addicted to depressant drugs, and no active medication will be needed.[4]

    ii. If, after 2 hours, the patient is showing severe tremors, orthostatic hypotension, or other signs of withdrawal, it is assumed that severe withdrawal is imminent, and an alternate schedule of withdrawal is established, as discussed under (v) below.

    iii. If, at 2 hours, the patient looks normal, it is possible to wait 2–5 hours, retest with 200 mg of an oral intermediate-acting barbiturate, and continue with test doses during the day to establish the final level needed during the first 24 hours.

    iv. In this instance, the barbiturate is then withdrawn by approximately 100 mg each day. If serious withdrawal symptoms recur, withdrawal is proceeding too quickly, and the patient should be administered an extra 200-mg dose of the barbiturate IM; he should be restabilized at the needed dose, and withdrawal then reinitiated.

    v. For those patients who demonstrate severe signs of withdrawal after the administration of a 200-mg short- to intermediate-acting barbiturate test dose, Sapira and Cherubin[4] recommend that the patient be given 400 mg of an oral barbiturate, be reevaluated every 2 hours, and be carefully titrated to determine the dependent dose—which is probably high.

  b. The second withdrawal regimen utilizes a *longer-acting barbiturate, phenobarbital* (Luminal), which has a half-life of 12–24 hours.[76] This approach is based on the ease with which stable blood levels of this longer-acting drug can be reached—but suffers the drawback of some difficulty in titrating the original dose accurately.

    i. One begins by estimating the dose of the drug abused and giving approximately 32 mg of phenobarbital for each 100 mg of estimated abused barbiturate, for each 250 mg of a drug like glutethimide (Doriden), for each 400 mg of meprobamate (Equanil), for each 5 mg of diazepam (Valium), or for each 25 mg of chlordiazepoxide (Librium). The total dose of phenobarbital is divided into portions to be given four times per day (QID), with extra given if the patient begins to demonstrate signs of withdrawal.

    ii. One or two doses (or more) are withheld if the patient appears too sleepy or demonstrates some signs of intoxication, such as nystagmus[44] or ataxia.

    iii. The required dose is then utilized for 2 days, given in divided doses at 6 A.M., noon, 6 P.M., and midnight—the largest dose (approximately 1.5 times the other dose) being given at midnight.

    iv. After this, the dose is decreased by approximately 30 mg per day—a 200-mg IM dose is used if needed to control the emergence of serious withdrawal symptoms.[76] If the patient looks sleepy or confused, the next dose should be withheld until he clears.[44]

In utilizing either regimen, it has not been shown that it is necessary to include phenytoin (Dilantin).[77] It must also be emphasized that the information presented in Table 2.5 is a rough outline and that the individual dose must be titrated for the specific patient. The goal is to reach at 24 hours a drug level that decreases withdrawal symptomatology without intoxicating the patient or making him overly sleepy. As with any drug that has a half-life of more than a few hours, it is important to recognize that the drug could accumulate in the body over time. This danger is especially relevant in elderly patients.

c. Other authors suggest that one might use the drug of abuse itself as an appropriate withdrawal agent, gradually tapering the doses over an approximate 8-week period (although this regimen does not always result in a disappearance of major symptoms).[6,69] More data must be gathered to clarify the conflicting evidence as to whether an alpha agonist such as clonidine (Catapres) in doses of approximately 0.1–0.2 mg three times a day [TID (Latin *ter in die*)] is an appropriate treatment for the CNS-depressant withdrawal syndromes discussed in this chapter.[7,71] There are few data to support the use of beta blockers such as propranalol (Inderal) in the treatment of these syndromes.[7]

2.2.7. Medical Problems

There are few medical disorders known to be unique to depressant abusers. The conditions developed depend on the specific drug taken and the route of administration. A few "special" problems are discussed in this section.

1. There is much anecdotal information on the ability of these drugs to *impair memory* over an extended period of time—perhaps even permanently. However, this phenomenon has not been well worked out, although there is a possibility of permanent neurological damage.[78,79]

A related problem is the anterograde amnesia that can sometimes follow the acute administration of even modest doses of Bz's, without impairing long-term memory or causing any evidence of permanent damage.[80–82] Anecdotally, this is said to be especially likely with even clinically relevant doses of the very short half-life hypnotic Bz triazolam. In any event, these temporary problems with encoding of memory must be recognized as a possible danger in patients, and there is evidence that use of some Bz's might create minor problems in memory and recall that could even interfere with performance among students.[81]

2. IV users can be expected to develop any of the problems that can result from contaminated needles. These include hepatitis, tetanus, abscesses, acquired immune deficiency syndrome (AIDS), and so on, as described for opiates in Section 6.2.8.

3. A special problem can result from the (usually inadvertent) injection of these

drugs into an artery. The resulting painful muscle and nervous tissue necrosis can necessitate amputation of the limb.

4. A major difficulty with any of the CNS depressants, including the Bz's, is *sedation*. This may result in impaired judgment and work and motor performance: these potential problems are of special importance for the longer-acting drugs, which may accumulate in the body over time. The difficulty is enhanced in the presence of liver disease or decreased albumin in the blood, but all patients should be warned to avoid activities demanding high levels of alertness and/or motor performance if they are experiencing sedation side effects. An additional problem, especially in the elderly who might already be especially sensitive to the effects of brain depressants, is the possibility of falls with a subsequent heightened risk for hip fractures.[83]

5. In the usual doses, these drugs are not likely to induce serious *cardiotoxic* symptoms in the average healthy individual—a problem especially unlikely with the Bz's, as they have less CNS brain-stem depressant activity.[54] However, all CNS depressants can suppress respirations (with the Bz's less prominent) and thus might precipitate respiratory failure in individuals with chronic obstructive lung disease.[54]

6. Serious *psychological* sequelae of moderate drug use are not likely. However, all these drugs do tend to decrease inhibitions and thus have been anecdotally reported to increase the possibility of angry outbursts.[1,41] There is also the possibility that some depressed patients will react to CNS depressants (even the Bz's) with an increase in their prior symptomatology (e.g., hostility).[1,41]

7. *Drug interactions* are a potential problem with all medications. The CNS depressants are likely to potentiate the side effects of tricyclic antidepressants and phenytoin and (through possible interference with liver metabolism) may increase blood levels of digoxin.[65,84] The actions of L-dopa may be inhibited by this class of drugs, and cimetidine may interfere with Bz metabolism and excretion.[65,85,86] Of course, the interaction between two or more CNS depressants can be severe, and an enhancement of Bz actions may be noted as long as 10 hours after an individual drinks ethanol.[65] Long-term contraceptive use can also interfere with Bz metabolism, and antacids can interfere with absorption.[87]

8. Similarly, no drug can be considered totally safe for administration during *pregnancy*. Although there is some controversy and other CNS depressants such as thalidomide are highly toxic to the fetus, there is no strong evidence of any teratogenicity for most of the currently used CNS depressants.[1,88,89] Prenatal exposure to one CNS depressant, phenobarbital, has been shown to possibly decrease testosterone in male offspring,[88] and in animals prenatal Bz's have been associated with long-term altered behavior in newborns.[90] Because this class of drugs is rarely necessary for sustaining life functioning, pregnant women should be told to avoid these medications, especially during the first trimester. This caveat probably extends to the neonatal period for women who are breast-feeding, as there is evidence that Bz's pass through the mother's milk to the baby and may be responsible for an increase in the accumulation of bilirubin.[91]

REFERENCES

1. Harvey, S. C. Hypnotics and sedatives. In A. G. Gilman, L. S. Goodman, T. W. Rall, & F. Murad (Eds.), *The Pharmacological Basis of Therapeutics* (7th ed.). New York: Macmillan, 1985, pp. 339–371.

2. Jaffe, J. H. Drug addiction and drug abuse. In A. G. Gilman, L. S. Goodman, T. W. Rall, & Murad, F. (Eds.), *The Pharmacological Basis of Therapeutics* (7th ed.). New York: Macmillan, 1985, pp. 532–581.

3. National Clearing House for Drug Abuse Information. *The CNS Depressant Withdrawal Syndrome and Its Management: An Annotated Bibliography: 1950–1983.* Rockville, Maryland: National Institute on Drug Abuse, 1975.

4. Sapira, J. D., & Cherubin, C. E. *Drug Abuse: A Guide for the Clinician.* Amsterdam: Excerpta Medica; New York: American Elsevier, 1975.

5. Covi, L., Lipman, J. H., Pattison, J. H., *et al.* Length of treatment with anxiolytic sedatives and response to their sudden withdrawal. *Acta Psychiatrica Scandinavica 49:*51–64, 1973.

6. Buston, U., Sellers, E. M., Naranjo, C. A., *et al.* Withdrawal reaction after long-term therapeutic use of benzodiazepines. *New England Journal of Medicine 315:*854–859, 1986.

7. Goodman, W. K., Charney, D. S., Price, L. H., *et al.* Ineffectiveness of clonidine in the treatment of the benzodiazepine withdrawal syndrome: Report of three cases. *American Journal of Psychiatry 143:*900–903, 1986.

8. Schneider, L. S., Syapin, P. J., & Pawluczyk, S. Seizures following triazolam withdrawal despite benzodiazepine treatment. *Journal of Clinical Psychiatry 48:*418–419, 1987.

9. Rickels, K., Case, W. G., Schweizer, E. E., *et al.* Low-dose dependence in chronic benzodiazepine users: A preliminary report on 119 patients. *Psychopharmacology 22:*407–416, 1986.

10. Campbell, R., Schaffer, C. B., & Tupin, J. Catatonia associated with glutethimide withdrawal. *Journal of Clinical Psychiatry 44:*32–33, 1983.

11. Falco, M. Methaqualone misuse: Foreign experience and United States drug control policy. *International Journal of the Addictions 11:*597–610, 1976.

12. Kay, D. C. Blackburn, A. B., Buckingham, J. A., & Karacan, I. Chapter 4: Human pharmacology of sleep. In R. I. Williams & I. Karacan (Eds.), *Pharmacology of Sleep.* New York: Wiley, 1976, pp. 419–428.

13. Schuckit, M. A. Anxiety treatment: A commonsense approach. *Postgraduate Medicine 75:*52–63, 1984.

14. Raskind, M. A., & Eisdorfer, C. When elderly patients can't sleep. *Drug Therapy,* August 1977, pp. 44–50.

15. Dement, W. C. *Some Must Watch While Others Sleep: The Portable Stanford.* Stanford, California: Stanford Alumni Association, 1972.

16. Greenblatt, D. J., & Shader, R. I. *Benzodiazepines in Clinical Practice.* New York: Raven Press, 1974.

17. Greenblatt, D. J., Harmatz, J. S., Zinny, M. A., & Shader, R. I. Effect of gradual withdrawal on the rebound sleep disorder after discontinuation of triazolam. *New England Journal of Medicine 317:*722–728, 1987.

18. Greenblatt, D. J., Shader, R. I., Franke, K., *et al.* Pharmacokinetics and bioavailability of intravenous, intramuscular, and oral lorazepam in humans. *Journal of Pharmaceutical Sciences 68:*57–63, 1979.

19. Tallman, J. F., Paul, S. M., Skolnick, P., *et al.* Receptors for the age of anxiety: Pharmacology of the benzodiazepines. *Science 207:*274–281, 1980.

20. Darragh, A., Scully, M., Lambe, R., *et al.* Investigation in man of the efficacy of a benzodiazepine antagonist, Ro 15-1788. *Lancet 1:*8–10, 1981.

21. Massotti, M., Guidotti, A., & Costa, E. Characterization of benzodiazepine and γ-aminobutyric acid recognition sites and their endogenous modulators. *Journal of Neuroscience 1:*409–418, 1981.

22. Skolnick, P., Moncada, V., Barker, J. L., et al. Pentobarbital: Dual actions to increase brain benzodiazepine receptor affinity. Science 211:1448–1450, 1981.
23. Britton, K. T., Ehlers, C. L., & Koob, G. F. Is ethanol antagonist Ro 15-4513 selective for ethanol? Science 239:648–649, 1988.
24. Schuckit, M. A. New frontiers in the treatment of anxiety. Internal Medicine (Special Issue):42–49, 1985.
25. Wheatley, D. Zopiclone: A non-benzodiazepine hypnotic controlled comparison to temazepam in insomnia. British Journal of Psychiatry 146:312–314, 1985.
26. Rickels, K. Recent advances in anxiolytic therapy. Journal of Clinical Psychiatry 42:40–44, 1981.
27. Gershon, S., & Eison, A. S. Anxiolytic profiles. Journal of Clinical Psychiatry 44:45–56, 1983.
28. Eison, A. S., & Temple, D. L. Buspirone: Review of its pharmacology and current perspectives on its mechanism of action. American Journal of Medicine 80:1–9, 1986.
29. Uhlenhuth, E. H. Discussant presentation: Buspirone: A clinical review of a new, non-benzodiazepine anxiolytic. Journal of Clinical Psychiatry 43:109–114, 1982.
30. Schweizer, E., & Rickels, K. Failure of buspirone to manage benzodiazepine withdrawal. American Journal of Psychiatry 143:1590–1592, 1986.
31. Riblet, L. A., Taylor, D. P., Eisan, M. S., & Stanton, H. C. Pharmacology and neurochemistry of buspirone. Journal of Clinical Psychiatry 43:11–15, 1982.
32. Lader, M. Psychological effects of buspirone. Journal of Clinical Psychiatry 43:62–67, 1982.
33. Moskowitz, H., & Smiley, A. Effects of chronically administered buspirone and diazepam on driving-related skills performance. Journal of Clinical Psychiatry 43:45–49, 1982.
34. Cole, J. P., Hecht-Orzack, M., Bease, B., & Bird, M. Assessment of the abuse liability of buspirone in recreational sedative users. Journal of Clinical Psychiatry 43:69, 1982.
35. Lader, M. Assessing the potential of buspirone dependence or abuse and effects of its withdrawal. American Journal of Medicine 82:20–26, 1987.
36. Roy-Byrne, P., & Katon, W. An update on treatment of the anxiety disorders. Hospital and Community Psychiatry 38:835–843, 1987.
37. Mackinnon, G. L., & Parker, W. A. Benzodiazepine withdrawal syndrome: A literature review and evaluation. American Journal of Drug and Alcohol Abuse 9:19–33, 1982.
38. Busto, U. Patterns of benzodiazepine abuse and dependence. British Journal of Addictions 81:87–94, 1986.
39. Mellinger, G. D., Balter, M. B., & Uhlenhuth, E. H. Insomnia and its treatment. Archives of General Psychiatry 42:225–232, 1985.
40. Chaplin, S. Benzodiazepine prescribing. Lancet 1:120–121, 1988.
41. Cole, J. O., Haskell, D. S., & Orzack, M. H. Problems with the benzodiazepines: An assessment of the available evidence. McLean Hospital Journal 6:46–74, 1981.
42. Blackwell, B. Benzodiazepines: Drug abuse and data abuse. Current Psychiatry Research 16:10–37, 1979.
43. Schuckit, M. Alcohol and drug interactions with antianxiety medications. American Journal of Medicine 82:27–33, 1987.
44. Cohen, S. Valium: Its use and abuse. Drug Abuse and Alcoholism Newsletter 5:1–3, San Diego: Vista Hill Foundation, 1976.
45. Nicholi, A. M. The nontherapeutic use of psychoactive drugs. New England Journal of Medicine 308:925–933, 1983.
46. Smart, R. G., Adlaf, E. M., & Goodstadt, M. S. Alcohol and other drug use among Ontario students: An update. Canadian Journal of Public Health 77:57–58, 1986.
47. Smart, R. G., Goodstadt, M. S., Adlaf, E. M., et al. Trends in the prevalence of alcohol and other drug use among Ontario students: 1977–1983. Canadian Journal of Public Health 76:157–161, 1985.
48. Brophy, J. J. Suicide attempts with psychotherapeutic drugs. Archives of General Psychiatry 17:652–657, 1967.

49. Diaz, J. Phenobarbital: Effects of long-term administration on behavior and brain of artifically reared rats. *Science 199:*90–91, 1978.
50. Regestein, Q. R., & Reich, P. Agitation observed during treatment with new hypnotic drugs. *Journal of Clinical Psychiatry 46:*280–283, 1985.
51. Schuckit, M. A., Irwin, M., & Brown, S. The history of anxiety symptoms among 171 primary alcoholics. *Journal of Studies on Alcohol* (in press).
52. Lewis, D. C., & Senay, E. C. *Treatment of Drug and Alcohol Abuse.* New York: Career Teaching Center, 1981.
53. Setter, J. G. Emergency treatment of acute barbiturate intoxication. In P. G. Bourne (Ed.), *A Treatment Manual for Acute Drug Abuse Emergencies.* Washington, D.C.: U.S. Government Printing Office, 1974, pp. 49–62.
54. Risch, S. C., Groom, G. P., & Janowsky, D. S. Interfaces of psychopharmacology and cardiology: Part II. *Journal of Clinical Psychiatry 42:*47–59, 1981.
55. *Diagnosis and Management of Reactions to Drug Abuse.* New Rochelle, New York: The Medical Letter, 1977.
56. Lorch, J. A. Haemoperfusion for acute intoxication with hypnotic drugs. *Lancet 1:*1116, 1979.
57. Allen, M. D., Greenblatt, D. K., & Lacasse, Y. Pharmacokinetic study of lorazepam overdosage. *American Journal of Psychiatry 137:*1414–1415, 1980.
58. Boldy, D. A. R., Heath, A., Ruddock, S., Vale, J. A., & Prescott, L. F. Activated charcoal for carbamazepine poisoning. *Lancet 1:*1027, 1987.
59. Editorial: Repeated oral activated charcoal in acute poisoning. *Lancet 1:*1013–1016, 1987.
60. Nutt, D., & Costello, M. Flumazenil and benzodiazepine withdrawal. *Lancet 2:*463, 1987.
61. Fraser, A. A., & Ingram, I. M. Lorazepam dependence and chronic psychosis. *British Journal of Psychiatry 147:*211, 1985.
62. McLellan, A. T., Woody, G. E., & O'Brien, C. P. Development of psychiatric illness in drug abusers. *New England Journal of Medicine 301:*1310–1314, 1979.
63. Pomara, N., Stanley, B., Block, R., *et al.* Increased sensitivity of the elderly to the central depressant effects of diazepam. *Journal of Clinical Psychiatry 46:*185–187, 1985.
64. Bergman, H., Borg, S., & Holm, L. Neuropsychological impairment and exclusive abuse of sedatives or hypnotics. *American Journal of Psychiatry 137:*215–217, 1980.
65. Scharf, M. Comparative amnestic effect of benzodiazepines. *Journal of Clinical Psychiatry 49:*134–137, 1988.
66. Raskind, M., & Eisdorfer, C. Psychopharmacology of the aged. In L. L. Simpson (Ed.), *Drug Treatment of Mental Disorders.* New York: Raven Press, 1976, pp. 123–131.
67. Ashton, H. Benzodiazepine withdrawal: Outcome in 50 patients. *British Journal of Psychiatry 82:*665–671, 1987.
68. Rickels, K., Fox, I. L., Greenblatt, D. J., *et al.* Clorazepate and lorazepam: Clinical improvement and rebound anxiety. *American Journal of Psychiatry 145:*312–317, 1988.
69. Jurgens, S. M., & Morse, R. M. Alprazolam dependence in seven patients. *American Journal of Psychiatry 145:*625–627, 1988.
70. Fyer, A. J., Liebowitz, M. R., Gorman, J. M., *et al.* Discontinuation of alprazolam treatment in panic patients. *American Journal of Psychiatry 144:*303–308, 1987.
71. Vinogradov, S. Clonidine therapy in withdrawal from high dose alprazolam. *American Journal of Psychiatry 143:*1188, 1986.
72. Stewart, R. B., Salem, R. B., & Springer, P. K. A case report of lorazepam withdrawal. *American Journal of Psychiatry 137:*1113–1114, 1980.
73. Nagy, B. R., & Dillman, C. E. Case report of unusual diazepam abstinence syndrome. *American Journal of Psychiatry 138:*694–695, 1981.
74. Preskorn, S. H., & Denner, L. J. Benzodiazepines and withdrawal psychosis. *Journal of the American Medical Association 237:*36–38, 1977.
75. Wikler, A. Diagnosis and treatment of drug dependence of the barbiturate type. *American Journal of Psychiatry 125:*758–765, 1968.

76. Smith, D. E., & Wesson, D. R. Phenobarbital technique for treatment of barbiturate dependence. *Archives of General Psychiatry 24:*56–60, 1971.
77. *Diagnosis and Management of Reactions to Drug Abuse,* New Rochelle, New York: The Medical Letter, Vol. 19(3), Feb. 1977.
78. Grant, I., Adams, K. M., & Reed, R. Subacute organic mental disorders. In I. Grant (Ed.), *Neuropsychiatric Correlates of Alcoholism.* Washington, DC: APA Press, 1986, pp. 37–60.
79. Grant, I., & Judd, L. L. Neuropsychological and EEG disturbances in polydrug users. *American Journal of Psychiatry 133*(9):1039–1042, 1976.
80. Wolkowitz, O. M., Weingartner, H., Thompson, K., & Pickar, D. Diazepam-induced amnesia: A neuropharmacological model of an "organic amnestic syndrome." *American Journal of Psychiatry 144:*25–29, 1987.
81. Kumar, R., Mac, D. S., Gabrielli, W. F., & Goodwin, D. W. Anxiolytics and memory: A comparison of lorazepam and alprazolam. *Journal of Clinical Psychiatry 48:*158–160, 1987.
82. Scharf, M. B. Anterograde amnesia with oral lorazepam. *Journal of Clinical Psychiatry 44:*362–364, 1983.
83. Ray, W. A., Griffin, M. R., Schaffner, W., *et al.* Psychotropic drug use and the risk of hip fracture. *New England Journal of Medicine 316:*363–369, 1987.
84. Castillo-Ferrando, J. R. Digoxin levels and diazepam. *Lancet 2:*368, 1980.
85. Desmond, P. V., Patwardhan, R. V., Schenker, S., *et al.* Cimetidine impairs elimination of chlordiazepoxide (Librium) in man. *Annals of Internal Medicine 93:*266–268, 1980.
86. Schuckit, M. A. Alcohol and drug interactions with antianxiety medications. *American Journal of Medicine 82:*27–34, 1987.
87. Abernethy, D. R., Greenblatt, D. J., Divoli, M., *et al.* Impairment of diazepam metabolism by low-dose estrogen-containing oral-contraceptive steroids. *New England Journal of Medicine 306:*791–792, 1982.
88. Jick, H., Holmes, L. B., Hunter, J. R., *et al.* First-trimester drug use and congenital disorders. *Journal of the American Medical Association 246:*343–346, 1981.
89. Laegried, L. Abnormalities in children exposed to benzodiazepines *in utero. Lancet 1:*108–109, 1987.
90. Kellogg, C. K., Simmons, R. D., Miller, R. K., & Ison, J. R. Prenatal exposure in rats: Long-lasting functional changes in the offspring. *Neurobehavioral Toxicology and Teratology 7:*483–488, 1985.
91. Gupta, C. Prenatal exposure to phenobarbital permanently decreases testosterone and causes reproductive dysfunction. *Science 216:*640–642, 1982.

CHAPTER 3

Alcoholism: An Introduction

3.1. INTRODUCTION

3.1.1. General Comments

Alcohol, nicotine, and caffeine are the most widely used drugs in Western civilization, alcohol being the most destructive of the three. Probably reflecting this preeminence of alcohol, there is a great deal of information available on the epidemiology, the natural history, and the treatment of alcohol-related disorders; thus alcohol is used in this text as a prototype for the discussion of other pharmacological agents. Information on alcohol is presented in three chapters: this chapter covers the pharmacology of alcohol, definitional problems surrounding this drug, the epidemiology of drinking patterns and problems, the natural history of alcoholism, and some data on etiology. Chapter 4 is an overview of treatment of acute problems. Finally, Chapter 15 offers information on rehabilitation of the alcoholic.

3.1.2. Some Definitions

3.1.2.1. General Comments

It is important at this point to note the distinction between studies of *drinking patterns* and studies of *alcoholism*. The majority of Americans drink, and a substantial minority (one third or more) of young men drink to the point of getting into temporary difficulties.[1] However, these young men usually do not go on to develop the persistent, serious alcohol-related difficulties that might be termed *alcoholism*. Therefore, the less serious problems, such as arguments with friends or missing occasional work or school because of drinking, due to their high prevalence and lack of specificity, cannot in themselves be used to predict future alcohol-related problems.[1-3] Although these difficulties are certainly experienced by almost every alcoholic early in the development of the disorder, they are seen in such a significant percentage of people who do not go on to develop alcoholism that they have little if any prognostic significance in themselves.

I diagnose to indicate prognosis and to select treatment.[4] For this purpose, the entity must be clearly defined by objective criteria that can be utilized by different clinicians in different settings; people with the syndrome must have a somewhat homogeneous, predictable course (seen in follow-up); and the disorder must not represent the prodrome of yet another diagnosis.[4,5] To be used to maximal benefit, the diagnostic criteria should have been applied to individuals randomly assigned to different treatments to determine which is the most effective and the least dangerous approach.

Unfortunately, the second edition of the *Diagnostic and Statistical Manual of Mental Disorders* (DSM-II) published by the American Psychiatric Association did not use objective terms or demonstrate any predictive validity for the syndromes outlined under alcoholism, with the result that there was a tendency to apply the labels in an inconsistent manner.[6,7] The next edition of the DSM (DSM-III) improved on the situation, presenting a definition of alcoholism requiring life problems as well as evidence of psychological or physical dependence, and further changes were made in the revised DSM-III (DSM-III-R).[6,8,9]

DSM-III lists alcohol-related states of confusion—for example, alcoholic intoxication, pathological intoxication (termed *alcohol idiosyncratic intoxication*), and alcoholic withdrawal, as well as alcoholic hallucinosis—in a manner not dissimilar from prior editions.[8] It then goes on to list some "alcoholisms," noting that both alcohol abuse (coded 305.0X) and alcohol dependence (303.9X) encompass *both* a pattern of "pathological alcohol use" (e.g., the need for daily use, repeated efforts to control, binges, alcoholic blackouts, and continuation of drinking despite the problems) *and* impairment in social or occupational functioning due to alcohol (e.g., alcohol-related violence, absence from work, legal difficulties, and arguments with significant others). The major difference between alcohol abuse and alcohol dependence is that the latter requires evidence of tolerance or a demonstration of some withdrawal symptoms after cessation of or a reduction in drinking. The prognostic implications of the specific DSM-III criteria and the benefits of differentiating between abuse and dependence have been questioned through recent data demonstrating few prognostic differences between inpatients carrying the two different diagnostic subtypes over a 1-year follow-up.[10]

In DSM-III-R, a standard set of criteria for dependence is applied to a variety of substances, requiring documentation of *problems in at least three of the following areas;* taking larger amounts of the substance over longer periods of time than intended; a desire to, but unsuccessful efforts to, cut down use of the substance; spending a great deal of time in attempting to obtain the substance and using it; evidence of frequent intoxication or withdrawal symptoms that interfere with the ability to carry out major obligations; giving up or reducing important activities; continued use of the substance despite problems; evidence of marked tolerance; evidence of characteristic withdrawal symptoms; and use of other substances at times to avoid withdrawal symptoms. This symptom pattern in at least three areas must have persisted for at least 1 month or occurred repeatedly over a longer period of time. *Psychoactive-substance abuse* of any of a variety of drugs including alcohol entails evidence of a "maladaptive pattern" of use characterized by continued use despite impairments *or* recurrent use in situations that could be considered hazardous (e.g., driving while intoxicated), with symptoms having persisted for at least 1 month or having occurred repeatedly over a longer period of time in an individual who does not otherwise meet criteria for psychoactive-substance dependence. It is of interest that the criteria originally proposed for DSM-III-R contained the rather broad definition of dependence listed above; however, reflecting a lack of evidence of prognostic implications among patients carrying abuse or dependence criteria,[10] the term "abuse" was to be dropped. Apparently, a compromise was subsequently reached whereby the term "psychoactive substance abuse" was reinserted. Whatever the reason, as applied to "alcoholism" DSM-III-R lists alcohol dependence as 303.90 and alcohol abuse as 305.00. Other alcohol-related problems listed in DSM-III-R (e.g., alcohol idiosyncratic intoxication, alcohol hallucinosis) are similar to those that appeared in DSM-III.

In general, to meet criteria for abuse or dependence on alcohol in DSM-III or DSM-III-R, an individual had to continue to use alcohol in relatively large amounts despite impairments in activities, with or without evidence of tolerance or withdrawal. Although there is little evidence to demonstrate the prognostic and treatment implications of these criteria, they are in general similar to the definition that has been used in our research over the years. The next section reviews diagnostic choices for alcoholism (including both alcohol abuse and alcohol dependence), whenever possible emphasizing data generated from longitudinal research. More limited problems associated with alcohol abuse (e.g., alcohol hallucinosis and alcohol idiosyncratic intoxication) are discussed in Section 4.2.

3.1.2.2. My Preferred Definition of Alcoholism

To be clinically useful, the diagnostic criteria must be stated in relatively objective terms, avoiding such judgments as "He drinks too much" or "I *feel* that he is becoming too psychologically dependent." There is no one best definition of alcoholism, and the different criteria overlap a great deal.[11]

1. The *quantity–frequency–variability* (QFV)[12] approach attempts to gather accurate information on drinking patterns and then to place an individual in a "deviant" category when the alcohol intake differs statistically from the average. Although this scheme has great relevance to studies of drinking patterns, its usefulness is limited by the difficulty of obtaining good information about alcohol intake because of the reticence of the individual to admit his pattern and because of his decreased memory at rapidly rising blood-alcohol levels.[13]

2. The second rubric, *psychological dependence,* is based on the occurrence of a series of subjective experiences relating drinking to such problems as stockpiling liquor, taking drinks before going to a party, and otherwise demonstrating that the individual is psychologically uncomfortable unless there is alcohol around. It is very difficult, if not impossible, to quantify this approach objectively.

3. A third diagnostic scheme, fairly widely used by physicians, centers on the occurrence of *withdrawal* or *abstinence* symptoms when an individual stops taking

alcohol.[14] However, between 85 and 95% of people experiencing withdrawal have only the more minor symptoms.[10,15] Withdrawal in this mild form can be difficult to distinguish from a hangover or a case of the flu. In any event, this definition is restrictive, as many individuals who have serious life-impairment and medical problems and who may die of an alcohol-related cause have never demonstrated obvious signs of physical withdrawal.

4. The definition that is probably most useful to clinicians, and the definition I prefer, centers on the occurrence of serious social or health *problems related to alcohol.*[4,16,17] Using this approach, each clinician can briefly review areas of life problems (e.g., work, accidents, marital problems, and arrests) with every patient—a review that takes only 3–5 minutes. Once a pattern of problems has been established through information from the patient and/or a significant other, the connection between the life difficulties and alcohol can be broached. Subsequently, the pattern of drinking and the associated quantity and frequency can be ascertained.

The research criteria note the occurrence of any major life problem related to alcohol, including a marital separation or divorce, or a record of many arrests, or physical evidence that alcohol has harmed health (e.g., a cardiomyopathy or cirrhosis), or the loss of a job or a layoff related to drinking.[18] As is true of any clinical diagnosis, the criteria must be "bent" for an individual who comes close but does not quite fit the research definition and is thus labeled a "probable" alcoholic. For instance, an individual who is self-employed and whose spouse appears to be "long-suffering and uncomplaining" and who appears to be at low risk for arrest (possibly because he either is in a powerful position or lives in a small community where he knows the police) may have many alcohol-related life problems, but may not fulfill the research diagnostic criteria. In this instance, the patient would be labeled a probable alcoholic and receive the same general treatment as the definite alcoholic, but I constantly recheck my diagnosis and recognize the lowered level of certainty in predicting the future course.

Proper diagnosis can be facilitated by understanding the effects of alcohol on various body systems. Thus, as described in Section 3.2.2, there are various patterns of laboratory results and physical signs and symptoms that, although not diagnostic, can raise the clinician's suspicion regarding the presence of alcoholism. Similarly, there is a variety of simple paper-and-pencil tests asking about alcohol-related life problems that can *help* in establishing the diagnosis.[19,20] The most widely used is the 25-item Michigan Alcohol Screening Test (MAST), as well as its shorter 10-question counterpart. Although screening tests like this can be most helpful, they do not in themselves diagnose alcoholism and cannot take the place of a clinical history carefully obtained from the patient and a relevant resource person.

3.1.2.3. Primary versus Secondary Alcoholism: Problems of Dual Diagnosis (see Figure 3.1)

To use diagnosis for prognosis and selection of treatment, it is important that one look separately at those cases that *might* be complications of other disorders

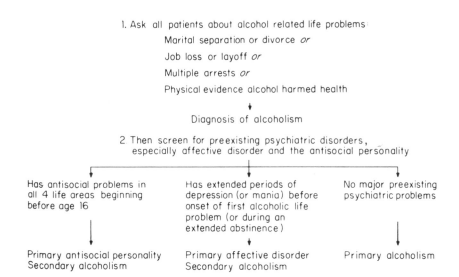

Figure 3.1. Diagnosis of alcoholism. From Schuckit.[155] Copyright 1979. Reprinted with permission of McGraw-Hill Book Company.

(secondary) and those that are more straightforward alcoholism (primary). The paradigm is similar to that used for patients with pneumonia: One case might be related to an immune deficiency; another pneumonitis might be secondary to trauma; yet another might reflect the consequences of congestive heart failure. Each exemplifies *secondary* pneumonia, the prognosis and major treatment efforts for which are dictated by the primary illness (e.g., the trauma or the heart failure).

In psychiatry or behavioral medicine, there is no single pathognomonic (diagnostic) symptom.[21−23] For instance, hallucinations and/or delusions can occur in many psychiatric disorders (e.g., affective disorders or major depressions, schizophrenia, or organic brain syndromes or major confused states), each of which has its own prognosis and most effective treatment. In a similar way, patients presenting with both repeated alcohol intoxication and serious psychotic symptomatology might either have primary alcoholism with secondary psychotic symptoms (in which case the psychoses can be expected to clear within several days to several weeks with abstinence) or might have primary schizophrenia or primary major depressive disorder of a psychotic nature with secondary alcoholism. In the latter the psychotic symptoms can be expected to persist and to respond only to proper pharmacological interventions, e.g., lithium for manic–depressive disease or antipsychotic medication for schizophrenia.[4,21−23] Thus, whether we are dealing with psychoses or alcohol problems, in order to use diagnosis for prognosis and treatment, the proper label is established by considering the constellation of symptoms and their time–course, or chronology. Psychiatric symptoms such as hallucinosis or confusion occurring *after* the onset of alcoholism or drug abuse, for instance, would be considered secondary manifestations and would be expected to clear on their own without active pharmacological intervention once abstinence is achieved.

Thus, a patient who develops alcohol abuse after the onset of another major psychiatric disorder has *secondary alcoholism,* whereas one who shows no evidence of a preexisting major psychiatric problem would be considered to have *primary alcoholism.*[17,24] It is the primary alcoholics, representing 70% or more of alcoholic patients, who can be thought of as having the "disease" alcoholism and who are most likely to fit the natural history outlined below.

On the other hand, *secondary* alcoholism can occur in the midst of almost any psychiatric picture. However, it is most likely to be seen with the antisocial personality as a secondary phenomenon, and in individuals with primary affective disorder.

Remember that the first key step in attempting to differentiate primary and secondary alcoholism is to determine whether an individual fits actual criteria for another psychiatric disorder. For instance, it is important to differentiate sadness (a temporary mood change) and major depressive disorder or to recognize the difference between someone who uses marijuana occasionally and someone who fulfills criteria for actual drug abuse or dependence. The second key step in distinguishing primary and secondary disorders is to gather the best information possible to determine the *approximate* age at which the individual *first met criteria* for each disorder. Thus, a man could have experienced sadness at age 12, started drinking at age 13, actually fulfilled criteria for primary alcoholism at age 31, and developed a secondary major depressive disorder at age 35. In this instance, the patient is likely to run the course of primary alcoholism and the depressive episode is likely to clear with abstinence alone.[23]

3.1.2.3.1. Primary Antisocial Personality Disorder (ASPD) with Secondary Alcoholism

Modifying the DSM-III-R criteria somewhat, one can define the antisocial personality or sociopath as being an individual who demonstrates antisocial life problems in *all four* of the life areas family, school, police, and peers, beginning before age 16 and before the onset of alcohol and drug abuse.[4,17,25] The sociopath runs a course of serious violence and criminal behavior, thus carrying a prognosis different from that of the primary alcoholic. Evaluations of both public and private inpatient alcoholic programs indicate that approximately 15% of male alcoholics and 5% of female alcoholics have primary antisocial personalities with secondary alcoholism.[17,22,26]

The diagnosis of definite or probable antisocial personality disorder (ASPD) can be established when a patient first enters care. The best approach focuses on determining the pattern of antisocial behaviors in several life areas before the age of 16, progressing to a discussion of antisocial problems in adulthood that are not directly related to alcohol or drug abuse. The importance of identifying the ASPD in practice relates to the prognostic information given both in the short run and over a longer period of time. While in an alcohol rehabilitation program, the ASPD subject is more likely than the average primary alcoholic to manipulate other patients against staff, stir up one staff member against another, smuggle in drugs, and demonstrate violence, and is less likely to complete the program. Therefore, these individuals frequently require a large amount of staff time, the result of which is that some programs choose to limit the number of ASPD individuals allowed at any one time within an inpatient setting or within a particular outpatient group. A longer-term consequence involves efforts to establish changes in the pattern of outcome seen among patients in any particular program or to compare the results of one program to another. Obviously, if the man with primary ASPD and secondary alcoholism has a significantly worse prognosis, this factor must be taken into consideration when comparing one program in which there is a relatively high percentage of ASPD alcoholics with another that has a lower percentage of ASPD patients.

A final note regarding treatment is in order. There is little, if any, good information about the optimal effective therapeutic mode for primary ASPD individuals. Thus, not surprisingly, the likelihood is that an alcoholic rehabilitation program will not significantly change the ASPD itself. The philosophy of treatment is that a sober ASPD individual is less likely to get into trouble and more likely to be able to adjust well to life situations than a drinking ASPD.

3.1.2.3.2. Primary Affective Disorder with Secondary Alcoholism

Disorders of mood, or affect, can entail either a serious depression or an episode of euphoria, hyperirritability, grandiosity, and disorganized thinking that is termed *mania*.[4] Because most people with primary affective disorder have depressions only (unipolar affective disorder), the major discussion here will center on depression, not mania.

Parenthetically, it is unlikely that brain-depressant intoxication or withdrawal will mimic actual mania. Therefore, an alcoholic who is not abusing brain stimulants, hallucinogens, or phencyclidine (PCP) but presents with clear-cut mania is likely to have actual bipolar manic–depressive disease as well as alcoholism. Thus, in a slight modification of the usual primary/secondary presentation, an alcoholic demonstrating mania is likely to have either two independent disorders (i.e., alcoholism and manic–depressive disease) or alcoholism that developed as a secondary complication of manic–depressive disease. In either event, in the presence of clear-cut mania, it is highly likely that short-term antipsychotic medications [such as thioridazine (Mellaril)] will be required acutely and that lithium will be required over the longer term.[4] Such a patient is an excellent example of patients with even severe alcohol-related difficulties who *require* psychiatric medications in order to function properly. Taking the lithium away from somebody with bona fide manic–depressive disease is likely to result in a severe increase in manic and/or psychotic symptoms. Thus, one important exception to the rule that an alcoholic usually does not require psychiatric medication is the patient with bipolar manic–depressive disease.

When episodes of sadness that represent a change from the person's normal level of functioning persist for at least 2 weeks, occurring throughout the day, every day, and are accompanied by changes in body functioning (e.g., insomnia, lethargy, and constipation) and changes in mind functioning (e.g., inability to concentrate, hopeless outlook for the future, and loss of interest in usual activities), the diagnosis of major depressive disorder can be made. These episodes of sadness are quite different from the normally transient grief reactions or other despondencies accompanying a loss. When the depressive episodes occur in the absence of preexisting psychiatric disorders, including alcoholism, the label of *primary affective disorder* can be assigned, with its implications for prognosis and treatment.[4]

On the other hand, serious depressions (even with associated delusions and/or hallucinations or suicidal ideation) can occur (and frequently do) in the midst of heavy drinking.[13,24,27] Primary depressive disorder can be diagnosed only if affective episodes last 2 or more weeks and interfere with life functioning *and* occur either before the onset of the first major life problem related to alcohol or during an extended period (e.g., 3+ months) of abstinence. The differential between primary affective disorder with secondary alcoholism and primary alcoholism with secondary affective disorder has important prognostic implications. The former will require antidepressants, although there is no evidence that such medications benefit the course of the usual primary alcoholic.[4,23,24]

Studies of inpatient alcoholics have shown that about 15–20% of women and 5% of men who meet the criteria for alcoholism have had affective disorder episodes either *before* their first major alcoholic life problem or during a period of 3 or more months when they were not drinking.[17,23,24,28] Such individuals would be labeled *primary affective disorder* and *secondary alcoholics*.

3.1.2.3.3. Therapeutic Implications of Differentiating Primary and Secondary Alcoholism

The treatment of alcoholic patients with primary or secondary major depressions is presented briefly in Section 15.2. Detailed discussion of the proper treatment of depressive disorders is beyond the scope of this text, but some preliminary thoughts can be offered here. The hypothetical patient who appears in an emergency room with a recent history of repeated intoxication along with complaints of severe depression *must* be carefully evaluated for suicide potential. If the patient has any combination of an actual plan of how to carry out the suicide, the means available to follow through (e.g., a gun), and a recent loss (e.g., separation from a significant individual or recent loss of a job), suicide potential should be considered very high and the situation an emergency.[29] In this situation, immediate psychiatric hospitalization in a facility that offers suicide precautions must be contemplated. This step, recognizing suicide potential and acting on the recognition, is just as important in treating individuals with primary alcoholism and secondary affective disorder as it is in treating people with the reverse. The reason is that the lifetime risk for successful suicides among alcoholics is between 10 and 15%—figures every bit as high as those for major depressive disorder.[30]

The importance of arriving at a primary psychiatric diagnosis in this hypothetical case comes in establishing the treatment plan. The probable diagnosis of primary alcoholism with secondary depressive disorder can be made by gathering a careful history from the patient and, whenever possible, from a resource person as well. In this case, it is likely that the depression will improve greatly and the suicidal ideas will disappear within several days to several weeks (or at most a month) of abstinence.[23] These individuals are *not* likely to require long-term psychiatric hospitalization and can often be transferred from a psychiatric unit to an alcohol rehabilitation program within several days to a week. The reason is that while depressions induced by brain depressants (or brain stimulants) can have symptoms similar to those of independent major depressive disorders, the intense sadness tends to be temporary and to disappear without antidepressant medication.

There are two instances in which such antidepressant medications as monoamine oxidase inhibitors [e.g., tranylcypromine (Parnate)] or tricyclic-type antidepressants [e.g., nortriptyline (Pamelor)] are needed. The first instance is the patient with documented primary major depressive disorder and secondary alcoholism; if the patient has been detoxed from alcohol and the depression still remains after 2 weeks or longer, antidepressant medication will probably be required. The second instance in which these medications may be required is a consequence of the imperfections of any diagnostic approach in psychiatry. Even when the best information is offered, perhaps 5% of patients felt to have primary alcoholism with secondary major depressive disorder still have intense and *debilitating* depressive symptoms after 2 weeks or more of abstinence. In that instance, depending on the severity of the depression and whether or not significant improvement has been observed, the persistence of intense depressive problems *could* indicate that the patient has two independent disorders—i.e., alcoholism and depressive disorder. Thus, for these approximately 5% of our patients who present with both alcoholism and depression, the failure of depressive symptoms to disappear after an appropriate period of time (perhaps 2–4 weeks) can justify a 6- to 9-month trial of antidepressant medications. The interested reader is referred to other publications for more detailed discussions of this important topic.[4,5,21,23]

3.1.2.3.4. Other Diagnoses

When careful diagnostic criteria are used,[4] alcoholism is rarely secondary to disorders other than the antisocial personality or the primary affective disorder.[21–23] A total of 10% of alcoholics demonstrate other primary diagnoses, including schizophrenia (the very slow onset of social withdrawal, hallucinations, and/or delusions that are persistent and seen during an extended abstinence[4]) or other psychiatric problems such as somatization disorder (Briquet's disease) and the anxiety disorders. In other words, these problems do not seem to occur in alcoholics more frequently than in the general population. The confusion in the literature on the relationship between alcoholism and schizophrenia[27,31,32] occurs when investigators use loose criteria for schizophrenia whereby relatively benign or transient paranoid or hallucinatory psychoses, which may accompany the heavy use of alcohol (see Section 4.2.4), are mislabeled as schizophrenia.

It is important to recognize that the comments offered here were written from the standpoint of alcohol and substance abuse programs. Thus, the data indicate that patients appearing for alcoholic or substance-abuse detoxification or rehabilitation are no more likely to have most other primary psychiatric disorders than are individuals in the general population, with the exceptions described above.[22] However, if one begins from the standpoint of a mental-health center, the picture is probably different. There is evidence that patients with bona fide primary schizophrenia may be more likely than patients in the general population to seek out and misuse drugs of abuse or to drink heavily. Because the lifetime risk for schizophrenia is only approximately 1%, there are rarely enough of these individuals to significantly impact on most alcohol treatment programs. On the other hand, because schizophrenia tends to be lifelong, the number of cases tends to increase in mental-health facilities, and staff at these facilities often have to determine what to do about the associated abuse of substance. This topic is relevant to mental-health settings because misuse of any substance, especially a brain depressant or a brain stimulant, is likely to result in a severe intensification of the schizophrenic symptoms.

It is these types of dual-diagnosis patients (e.g., with primary schizophrenia and secondary misuse of substances) who tend to "fall between the cracks" of our mental-health and substance-abuse programs. The staff in mental-health clinics often feel inadequate in dealing with substance-abuse problems and thus "hardly know where to begin" in helping the long-term schizophrenic whose symptoms are intensifying in the presence of substance abuse. The staff of alcohol and substance-abuse treatment programs have little if any experience in dealing with patients with active delusions and hallucinations and, of course, find these patients very disruptive in a group setting. In addition, many schizophrenics do not feel comfortable with the intensive confrontations that are typical of inpatient and outpatient alcohol or substance rehabilitation approaches.

Unfortunately, there is no easy answer to this dilemma. In some locales, specific "dual-diagnosis" outpatient and inpatient programs have been set up and staffed with personnel who are well-trained to handle both types of problems.[33] In our own treatment program, we have handled the problem through education of both mental-health and substance-abuse personnel. Actively psychotic schizophrenic patients in crisis are, of course, admitted to an inpatient psychiatric facility. As soon as the psychotic symptoms improve, a consultation is established with our alcohol/substance-abuse program. The goal is to have the patient begin to attend Alcoholics Anonymous (AA) and/or Narcotics or Cocaine Anonymous groups while still an inpatient in the mental-health facility. He or she is then referred to an outpatient substance-abuse group on discharge. The alcohol or substance rehabilitation staff carefully chooses the specific self-help and aftercare group to meet the needs of that particular patient—a person who usually requires a more tolerant and less intrusive group style. This approach recognizes the seriousness of the problems and accepts the absence of a perfect treatment approach, but takes advantage of existing facilities to offer the best care that can pragmatically be given.

Establishing a solid and trusting rapport between mental-health and alcohol/substance-abuse personnel is an essential step in developing a program like ours. This usually involves months of discussion and the development of a philosophy that recognizes that each appropriate patient is not only the responsibility of "the other guy," but that responsibility is to be equally shared between the two systems. The staff of each type of program recognize that chronically psychotic primary schizophrenic patients who are abusing substances are difficult to handle, treatment personnel are willing to admit their own restrictions as well as to take responsibility in their areas of expertise, and all are willing to take the extra time required to actively communicate and negotiate the optimal patient care. The *key* here is that the personnel of both types of programs (mental-health and alcohol/substance-abuse) are willing to try, communicate, and assume responsibility. All are also willing to admit that what can be offered is, while certainly imperfect, the best that is available. The longer such liaison between facilities goes on, the lower are the levels of frustration and mistrust and the greater is the amount of patient benefit that can be expected to accrue.

3.1.2.3.5. A Summary

The key to accurate labeling is to take a very careful history of the chronology of the development of psychiatric symptoms from both the patient and a resource person such as the spouse. Primary sociopathy is easily distinguished from primary alcoholism by gathering information on the extent of antisocial problems that occurred before age 16. The primary schizophrenic should demonstrate persistent and serious social withdrawal and hallucinations/delusions that occurred before the onset of serious alcohol problems and that remain throughout extended periods of abstinence.

All patients, no matter what their chief complaint, should be queried for their pattern of life problems and subsequently for the relationship of alcohol (and other drugs) to these difficulties.[22,23,34] Once a diagnosis of definite or probable alcoholism has been established, it is necessary to distinguish between the 70% of primary alcoholics and the 30% or so who have alcoholism secondary to another major preexisting psychiatric disorder. This distinction is made by asking all possible alcoholics about their pattern of life problems beginning before the age of 16, their pattern of drug-related difficulties, and the presence of any major psychiatric symptoms (e.g., serious depression or psychotic symptoms) before the onset of their first alcohol-related life problem or during an abstinent period of 3 months or longer.

3.2. PHARMACOLOGY OF ALCOHOL

3.2.1. General Comments

This widely used drug is a central nervous system (CNS) depressant that, in high enough doses, is an anesthetic. It adversely affects almost all body systems, interfering with either cell membrane functioning, intracellular respiration, or energy processing in most body cells, especially those in the CNS.[35] Even though some of the actions of alcoholic beverages are the result of their other constituents or congeners,[36] the emphasis of this chapter is on the ethanol itself.

Although the primary action of alcohol on the CNS results in depression of all activity, behavioral stimulant properties predominate at lower doses, a fact that may be related to a direct stimulant effect of alcohol or a differential depression of inhibitory neurons at relatively low blood-alcohol concentrations (BACs). The CNS depression occurs at all levels of the brain, with the first noted actions occurring in the reticular activating system and those areas most closely involved with complex functions—the cortex.[37–42]

The final level of behavioral impairment depends on the person's age, weight, sex, and prior experience with alcohol, as well as on his level of tolerance. Table 3.1 gives a rough outline of what can be expected in a nontolerant individual, with results ranging from minor impairment of motor coordination, sensation, and mood at low doses to amnesia and Stage 1 anesthesia for blood levels exceeding 300 mg alcohol/100 ml blood (300 mg%). Levels of 400–700 mg% can cause coma, respiratory failure, and death, although tolerant individuals may be awake and able to talk at blood levels exceeding 780 mg%.[41] Note that 100 mg% is equivalent to 0.1 g/100 ml. The usual drink contains about 8–10 g of absolute alcohol and (for those watching their weight) a minimum of 70 calories.[43,44]

An additional topic worthy of brief mention is the age-old search for amythistic (sobering) agents.[45] Probably the most useful data come from the demonstration

Table 3.1
Rough Correlation between Blood-Alcohol Level and Behavioral/Motor Impairment

Rising blood-alcohol level[a]	Expected effect
20–99	Impaired coordination, euphoria
100–199	Ataxia, decreased mentation, poor judgment, labile mood
200–299	Marked ataxia and slurred speech, poor judgment, labile mood, nausea and vomiting
300–399	Stage I anesthesia, memory lapse, labile mood
400 and above	Respiratory failure, coma, death

[a]mg/100 ml blood (mg % or mg/dl).

that fruit sugar (fructose) increases the rate of disappearance of ethanol from the body by 10% or more,[46] thus helping the individual sober up more rapidly. Clinical application of this finding is limited because of the possibility of resulting over-hydration and changes in the body acid–base balance. Additional interesting findings include the report that the narcotic antagonist naloxone (Narcan) might reverse alcohol-induced comas, although this effect is more likely related to a more general effect of naloxone in reversing the effects of body shock, no matter what the mechanism.[45] Additional preliminary data indicate fairly unimpressive results on the use of brain stimulants, precursors of brain neurochemicals such as L-dopa, and prostaglandin synthetase inhibitors such as ibuprofen (Nuprin) as potential sobering agents. Nonetheless, some progress has been made, and it appears likely that antagonists of specific effects of ethanol, as opposed to global antagonists with multiple actions, may indeed be revealed in coming years.[45]

3.2.2. Effects on the Body

Alcohol is a very attractive drug, as its immediate effects at moderate doses are perceived by the user as pleasant. In addition, for nonalcoholic individuals who are not taking medications and are in good physical condition, alcohol in amounts up to two drinks per day has the beneficial effects of increasing socialization, possibly stimulating the appetite, perhaps decreasing the risk of cardiovascular disease through an increase in high-density lipoproteins (HDLs), and so on.[42,44,47,48] When alcohol is taken in moderation by such individuals in good health, most pathological changes that do occur are reversible. However, as consumption increases to more than two drinks daily or when individuals who are ill drink, damage to various body systems can be more serious, and *early signs of some of these changes may give the clinician reason to increase his level of suspicion* that the patient being seen may be alcoholic. Because the physiological toxicity of alcohol has been reviewed in depth in other texts,[35,49] only a very brief review is given here.

The average alcoholic is likely to appear in the clinical setting sober, well-groomed, and with no telltale aura of alcohol. He or she will complain of any of a variety of medical and emotional problems, which must be properly diagnosed if the clinician hopes to avoid unexpected calls in the middle of the night and nonresponse to ill-advised treatments that should never have been given in the first place (e.g., sleeping pills). Thus, it is in the clinician's best interest to identify the alcoholic in order to be certain of offering maximal care at minimal risk.

Changes in body systems that can be expected in the course of alcoholism include those discussed in the following sections.

3.2.2.1. Blood Markers

The easiest and most obvious screening tests involve simple blood markers.[20] Many alcoholics have a mild elevation in uric acid, free fatty acids, a mean corpuscular volume (MCV) of approximately 95 or 100μ^3, and/or an elevation in gamma-glutamyl transferase or GGT (levels of 30–50 or more).[50,51] The first test to change is likely to be the GGT, elevations tending to occur long before other liver function tests show a rise, probably in response to the actual induction of this enzyme by ethanol. A related approach is to evaluate the pattern of 25 commonly used blood tests, which, according to one report, may be plugged into a mathematical formula to identify over 85% of alcoholics vs. controls.[52] A simpler approach has been outlined by Irwin et al.,[53] who take advantage of observations of moderate percentage increases in a limited number of laboratory tests after a baseline, abstinent test value has been established. Thus, in patients for whom baseline GGT, serum glutamic oxalacetic transaminase (SGOT), and alkaline phosphatase values have been established with abstinence (e.g., after an inpatient alcohol treatment program, following hospitalizations for any other problems), a 20% or greater increase in any one or two of these specific values correlates highly with the return to heavy drinking, even when the increase remains within the range of "normal" for a laboratory. Of course, the simple combination of the MAST score (see Section 3.1.2.2) and observation of blood tests to detect any changes can be very useful.[53,54]

3.2.2.2. Digestive System

In the digestive system, alcohol is associated with high rates of ulcer disease, as well as elevated rates of inflammation of the stomach (gastritis) or pancreas (pancreatitis), fatty liver, alcoholic hepatitis, chronic active hepatitis, and cirrhosis.[55–57] Even at low doses, alcohol disturbs the liver's sugar-producing function (gluconeogenesis) and shunts building blocks into the production of fats.[55,56,58]

Most of the problems in the liver may be secondary to the use of alcohol by liver cells as a "preferred fuel," with resultant scarcity of nicotinamide adenine dinucleotide (NAD) as a hydrogen receptor. The liver problems appear to progress from fatty liver (probably seen with repeated blood-alcohol levels of 80 mg/dl or more), to alcoholic hepatitis (probably not directly related to the fatty liver), and to subsequent cirrhosis, which may begin with early fiber deposition around the central veins, that is, central hyaline sclerosis.[59,60] Some adverse liver changes can be seen with consumption of as little as 20 g of alcohol per day in women and 40 g per day in men, although higher doses over longer periods of time are required for actual cirrhosis.[60] In reviewing this material, however, the clinician who does not specialize in treating alcoholics must remember that only 1 in 5 or so alcoholics actually presents with clinically significant cirrhosis.

3.2.2.3. Alcoholism and Cancer

Through a number of hypothesized mechanisms, alcoholics also have significantly elevated rates of cancers of the digestive tract (especially the esophagus and stomach), head and neck, and lungs.[61–63] This high risk might relate to problems from local irritation of lung or digestive tract linings, a decrease in the protective actions of mucous coverings of such linings, or a decrease in immune systems especially aimed at identifying and destroying cancer cells. The data on the increased prevalence of cancer in alcoholics remain robust even when the effects of possible dietary changes, smoking habits, and other factors are considered. While most of the increase in cancerous lesions is associated with very high levels of alcohol intake, recent data indicate that for one type of cancer, carcinoma of the breast, intake of even as little as one or two drinks per day is associated with a moderate increased risk.[64,65] In the final analysis, alcoholics or heavy drinkers must be carefully worked up for the possibility of cancer, and alcoholism must be considered as a possible additional diagnosis in patients with cancerous lesions, especially those of the head and neck, digestive tract, and lung.

3.2.2.4. Nervous System

In the nervous system, the chronic intake of alcohol results in deterioration of the peripheral nerves to both the hands and the feet (a peripheral neuropathy seen in 5–15% of alcoholics) and in temporary as well as permanent organic brain syndromes (OBSs) associated with both the direct effect of alcohol and specific vitamin deficiencies, such as the thiamine-related Wernicke–Korsakoff syndrome (seen in fewer than 5% of alcoholics).[66–70] It has been estimated that between 15 and 30% of nursing home patients with OBS are alcoholics whose alcohol-induced organicity has become permanent.[68] Additional problems associated with the CNS involve a rapidly developing permanent incoordination (cerebellar degeneration), which is seen in fewer than 1% of alcoholics, and other more dramatic but even rarer neurological disorders that can result in rapid death.[69,71] Finally, increased levels of drinking are associated with an elevated risk for hemorrhagic stroke, even when other factors such as blood pressure are controlled.[72,73]

As recognized by DSM-III-R, however, the most prevalent form of alcohol-related confusion is intoxication. Although most individuals show a clearing of clouded consciousness over a matter of hours, those with preexisting brain damage (e.g., some elderly and those with prior brain trauma) may show confusion lasting for days or weeks. Thus, alcohol must be considered a part of the differential diagnosis of all fairly rapid-onset states of confusion.[21,68]

The association between alcoholism and more permanent decreased intellectual functioning is less clear.[74] The majority of alcoholics who present for detoxification show some signs of intellectual impairment, and 40–70% may show increased brain ventricular size (possibly indicating decreased brain tissue).[75,76] Although some investigators feel that there is a correlation between increased brain ventricles and decreased functioning on psychological testing, not all agree, and it is probable that most alcoholics will recover in both parameters after months of abstinence.[75,77] The etiology of these psychological changes is not known, but it probably represents the combination of trauma, vitamin deficiencies, and a direct neurotoxic effect of alcohol on the brain.

3.2.2.5. Cardiovascular System

It has also been estimated that one quarter of alcoholics develop diseases of the heart or *cardiovascular system* as alcohol, a striated-muscle toxin, produces a heart inflammation or myocardiopathy, preclinical left ventricular abnormalities, hypertension and elevations in blood fats, including cholesterol.[35,78-80] In addition, alcohol in doses as low as one drink can decrease the cardiac output of blood and cardiac contractility in nonalcoholics with heart disease and can diminish the warning signs of pain while increasing the potential heart damage or ischemia in patients with angina.[81,82] Alcoholism must also be considered in all individuals who demonstrate mild elevations in blood pressure (e.g., 145/95), especially if the pressure appears to fluctuate with time (e.g., higher early in the week), and as little as 1 g/kg body weight per day of ethanol over 5 days can result in a significant pressure increase, especially among individuals with prior elevations in this measure.[47,81-85]

3.2.2.6. Blood Cells

Alcohol also decreases the production of all types of blood cells, with resulting large-red-blood-cell anemia (a macrocytosis, probably related to folic acid deficiency), decreased production and efficiency of white cells (probably leading to an increased predisposition toward infection), and decreased production of clotting factors and platelets (probably related to increased bruising and gastrointestinal bleeding[86-88]). There is also a decrease in thymus-derived lymphocytes, which might relate to the increased rates of cancers seen in alcoholics. The decreases in various aspects of the immune system may contribute to an increased vulnerability to tuberculosis, viral and bacterial infections, and cancers (see Section 3.2.2.3).

3.2.2.7. Body Muscle

Body muscle is also sensitive to alcohol, and an alcoholic binge can result in muscle inflammation or, in chronic abusers, muscle wasting, primarily in the shoulders and hips.

3.2.2.8. Sexual Functioning

Sexual functioning is also disturbed. Men can develop decreased sperm production and motility through the direct effects of ethanol on the testes; decreased ejaculate volume, sperm count, and sperm motility (all of which tend to improve with 3 months of abstinence)[89]; decreased production of testosterone; and impotence (through psychological mechanisms, peripheral neuropathy involving the perineal nerves, and/or the direct destruction of the testes).[90] Women can develop menstrual irregularities[91] and alcohol can affect the developing fetus—various stages of the fetal alcohol syndrome (FAS)—are described further in Section 4.2.8.2.

3.2.2.9. Other Blood Test Abnormalities

Through a variety of mechanisms, a number of other alcohol-related problems are produced. Alcohol induces a number of other blood test abnormalities, including those of liver function, glucose, blood components, creatinine phosphokinase (CPK), and uric acid.[51–54,92] An additional important problem is alcoholic ketosis, which is most likely to be seen in alcoholic patients with persistent vomiting and dehydration.[93] This clinical picture probably relates to starvation, but must be carefully distinguished from other causes of ketosis such as diabetes. It is also likely that alcohol contributes to osteoporosis, with an associated increased risk for broken bones,[94] and can have important effects on renal functioning.[95]

3.2.2.10. Driving Impairment

Any discussion of the effects of alcohol on the body would be incomplete without mention of the consequence of alcoholism that probably has the most dramatic impact on morbidity and mortality.[96] There is consistent evidence that even at a BAC as low as 15 mg/dl (i.e., approximately one drink), the ability to operate a motor vehicle is significantly impaired.[97] Similar dramatic levels of impairment have been observed with even experienced pilots operating flying simulators, and a recent study has shown impairment of piloting skills lasting 14 hours or more after BACs reached 100 mg/dl.[98] Thus, the likelihood of accidents (probably in the home and in the workplace as well as on the highways or in the skies) is significantly increased after even moderate doses of alcohol. While most first-conviction drunk drivers are not alcoholic (although they had certainly engaged in behavior dangerous to themselves as well as to those around them), it is likely that a majority of individuals who are referred from the courts to local alcohol facilities for evaluation will fit alcoholism criteria.[99] In any event, whether in alcoholics or in drivers who used poor judgment, alcohol-related motor impairment in individuals operating motor vehicles is an important part of the picture of alcohol's effects on the body.

3.2.3. Effects on Mental Processes

In addition to the physiological changes that occur with alcohol, there are a number of important emotional consequences. With modest intake, at peak or decreasing BACs most people (alcoholics and "normals") experience sadness, anxiety, irritability, and a whole host of resulting interpersonal problems.[23,24,91] At persistent higher doses, alcohol can cause almost any psychiatric symptom, including temporary pictures of intense sadness, auditory hallucinations and/or paranoia in the presence of clear thought processes (a clear sensorium), and intense anxiety. These symptoms are discussed in Sections 4.2.4, 4.2.5, and 4.2.8.1.

Insomnia can occur with simple alcohol intoxication, as this drug tends to fragment the sleep, the result being both a decrease in deep sleep stages and frequent awakenings. These problems can be expected to persist in alcoholics for 3–6 months as part of a "protracted" abstinence phase.

Another consequence of alcohol that impacts on both physical and mental functioning is the "*hangover.*" Despite the recognition of this phenomenon for hundreds of years, little systematic research has been carried out in this area. The hangover consists of a mixture of symptoms that can include headache, nausea and vomiting, thirst, decreased appetite, dizziness, fatigue, and tremor.[100,101] This is a highly prevalent phenomenon, and at least one hangover is likely to be reported in 40% or more of men age 18 or older and in 27% of women of similar age, including 5 and 1% of the two sexes, respectively, who have had an average of one or more hangovers a month during the preceding year.[102] The severity of symptoms varies greatly among individuals, but probably relates in general to the amount of alcohol consumed.[102] A number of hypothesized mechanisms for this phenomenon have been presented, including consequences of changes in vasopressin or in dopamine levels in the hypothalamus and changes in prostaglandins or in beta-adrenergic activity, as well as the possibility that these symptoms represent a mild degree of alcohol withdrawal. Other than prevention by limiting the ethanol intake, no convincing treatment approaches to this prevalent phenomenon have yet been developed.

3.2.4. Alcohol Metabolism

Alcohol is fully absorbed from the lining or membranes of the digestive tract, especially in the stomach and the proximal portion of the small intestine. Only 5–15% is excreted directly through the lungs, sweat, and urine, the remainder being metabolized in the liver at a rate of approximately one drink per hour, the equivalent of 7 g of ethanol per hour, with 1 g equaling 1 ml of 100% alcohol.[91,103] The usual route of metabolism is via the enzyme alcohol dehydrogenase (ADH), although some additional alcohol is metabolized in the liver microsomal system, as shown in

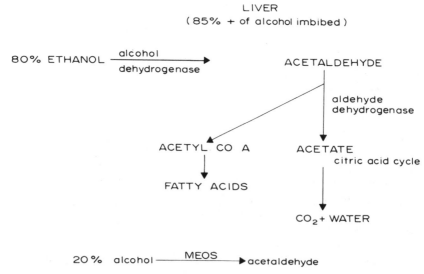

Figure 3.2. Metabolism of alcohol.[21,22] Abbreviations: (ACETYL CO A) acetyl-coenzyme A; (MEOS) microsomal ethanol-oxidizing system.

Figure 3.2. Thus, the major product of alcohol metabolism is acetaldehyde, a very toxic substance that, fortunately, is quickly metabolized to carbon dioxide and water through a variety of mechanisms.

ADH and aldehyde dehydrogenase (ALDH) are used by the body for a variety of purposes in addition to the metabolism of ethanol. Both enzymes are under genetic control, and ADH has eight or more isoenzymes in humans, each with different metabolic properties and with different patterns in various national groups.[104] ALDH possesses at least four clinically significant isoenzymes in humans, and the most physiologically active regarding acetaldehyde, ALDH–I, is absent in perhaps as many as 50% of Orientals. This finding is responsible for the higher rate of facial flushing (probably acetaldehyde-mediated) when some Oriental people drink, a finding that may be linked with the lower level of alcoholism in Orientals.[105] These brief comments are made here to give the interested reader the opportunity of reviewing other references and because these enzymes and their genetic control may have an impact on the genetic predisposition to alcoholism discussed in Section 3.5.4.

3.2.5. Tolerance and Physical Dependence

Toleration of higher doses of ethanol occurs rapidly and parallels the toleration of the depressants discussed in Section 2.1.1.3. This tolerance is both metabolic, primarily through a slight increase in both ADH activity and in the liver microsomal ethanol-oxidizing system (MEOS), and pharmacodynamic, the apparent result of a direct adaptation of CNS tissues to alcohol.[41] As is true of most drug mechanisms, behavioral factors play a role as well in the development of tolerance and physical dependence.[106] Regarding the latter, animals given a potentially lethal dose of a drug in an environment in which they have previously received sublethal drug doses are more likely to survive the drug challenge than animals with similar histories given the same dose in an environment unrelated to prior drug exposure. Cross-tolerance to other CNS-depressing drugs occurs, but it must be remembered that the concomitant administration of two or more CNS depressants may potentiate the effects of both.

Alcohol also produces a level of physical addiction that results in a withdrawal syndrome almost identical to that described for the depressants. The alcohol withdrawal syndrome is discussed in Section 4.2.6.

3.3. EPIDEMIOLOGY OF DRINKING AND ALCOHOLISM

A great many people drink, and many have minor problems, but few demonstrate a life-style centered on alcohol (i.e., alcoholism).

3.3.1. Drinking Patterns

Over two-thirds of men in Western countries drink more than just occasionally, with a male/female ratio of approximately 1.3 : 1.[43,107] The peak years with the highest percentages of drinkers and the greatest per capita consumption, are probably between 16 and 25, after which there is a decrease with age. At any stage of life, the chances of being a *drinker* (not an alcoholic) are higher for people with higher levels of education, higher socioeconomic status, and Italian or Jewish heritage.[2,107]

The average adult consumes 2.7 gallons of absolute alcohol per year, with a resultant total expenditure of many billions of dollars per year in the United States—representing almost 3% of total personal expenditures.[108] Between a quarter and a half of young men experience transient alcohol-related problems, such as arguments with friends, missing time from work, or a drunk-driving arrest.[1] These problems alone do not predict future alcoholism, and most individuals drift away from these problems with increasing age.[1,2]

A topic of great interest is young drinkers. As briefly discussed above, drinking is the "norm" in most Western societies, and adolescence is the time of learning to assume adult roles. Thus, it is not surprising that over 90% of teenagers are "drinkers" by the end of high school.[109–111] Most teenagers drink approximately two times per week, with an average intake of less than four drinks per occasion (defining a drink as 12 oz of beer, 4 oz of nonfortified wine, or 1.5 oz of 80 proof beverage).[107] On the other hand, as many as 1 in 3 high school graduates have consumed six or more drinks on at least one occasion during the preceding 3 months, including 15% of high school seniors who have consumed this amount within the last week.[112] Those young individuals who drink daily (perhaps 10% of youth by the end of high school) and/or those who demonstrate serious alcohol-related pathology are likely to have associated multiple drug problems and/or to fulfill the criteria of the antisocial personality as described in Section 3.1.2.3.[107,113]

Although 10% daily drinkers by the end of high school is an alarming statistic, this figure has not changed much over the last 10–15 years, and there is some evidence of an actual decrease in the prevalence of drinking among youth during that time period.[107,109,114] This conclusion is supported by a study of over 4200 students in 72 colleges revealing a slightly lower prevalence of drinkers in 1984–1985 than had been found 2 years earlier, as well as a 1985 survey in Canada that reported that the percentage of high school seniors who had used alcohol at least one time during the preceding 12 months rose from 92% in 1979 to 93% in 1981 and then fell to 91% by 1983.[110,115–117] These observations point out how unwise it might be to equate drinking, drinking problems, and alcoholism and demonstrate the need to view statistics on alcoholism from a longitudinal perspective.

Thus, the average person in our society is a drinker. This normal drinker's first alcohol-related experience (i.e., actually taking a drink—not just sipping from an adult's glass) tends to occur between the ages of 12 and 15, the first experience of drunkenness by the mid-teens, and, especially for males, the first temporary alcohol-related life problem at age 18–25 (e.g., missing school or work because of drinking, having an argument with a friend, driving while drunk, or being arrested once for drunk driving).[107] Regarding the latter, most individuals who have had only a single alcohol arrest do not qualify for the diagnosis of alcoholism, nor on follow-up do they demonstrate a course consistent with that disorder; however, multiple drunk-driving arrests are associated with more pervasive and persistent future problems.[118] It is probably in the late 20s to early 30s that the average drinker decreases his frequency and quantity of intake, whereas the alcoholic maintains or even increases his drinking pattern, and the resulting diagnosis is alcoholism.

3.3.2. Alcoholism

With the use of a rigorous criterion for alcoholism centering on serious life problems (see Section 3.1.2), it has been estimated that between 5 and 10% of the adult male population in the United States will demonstrate alcoholism at some time during their lives.[107] Of course, the prevalence of alcoholism varies with the severity of the criteria invoked. Using a less restrictive definition, a recent Epidemiological Catchment Area (ECA) survey demonstrated that within some population groups, as many as 20% or so of men and 10% or so of women might at some time have fulfilled such "looser" criteria for alcoholism.[11,119] Statistics generated from surveys of the general population are probably more dependable than the rates of individuals who have been diagnosed and entered treatment, because it is likely that fewer than 1 in 5 of even those men and women who meet fairly stringent alcoholic criteria have actually sought help, at least within the preceding 6 months.[120] Because of the high level of physical pathology associated with heavy drinking, 20–35% of male general medical or surgical patients are alcoholic.[107]

The highest rates of *alcoholism* are seen in men aged 30–50 years, and the rates increase with lower socioeconomic strata, with lower income and education, and among Catholics—especially French and Irish.[107,121] However, it is important to recognize that alcoholism is a problem of all socioeconomic strata, all ages, all religions, all parts of the world, and both sexes. Similar to the alcohol consumption data and as noted above, there is little consistent evidence of any marked increases in the actual rates of alcoholism between 1982 and 1985.[122]

The armed services have a reputation for high rates of alcohol problems, an observation that implies possible high rates of alcoholism.[123] These findings must be considered from the perspective that the military has a high percentage of young males (i.e., those at highest risk for alcohol-related difficulties). Indeed, once one controls for age, sex, and socioeconomic stratum, the rate of probable alcoholism (about 5–10%) and that of additional alcohol-related problems (approximately 10%) are not significantly different from those of the population in general.

Controlling for socioeconomic strata, most racial or ethnic groups show similar rates of alcoholism. Possible exceptions include low rates of alcoholism among Orientals (probably related to their high propensity for flushing and to societal norms regarding drunken behavior), low rates of persistent alcohol problems in Jews, and probable high rates in North American Indians and Eskimos.[107,124] It is not known whether these differences are related to social factors, either protecting from heavy drinking or encouraging drunkenness (for lower or higher rates, respectively), and/or genetically influenced factors.

3.4. NATURAL HISTORY OF ALCOHOLISM (see Table 3.2)

Once the diagnosis of primary alcoholism has been carefully established, it is possible to estimate the prognosis or the natural course of the disorder. The average

Table 3.2
Natural History of Primary Alcoholism

1. Age at which first drink is taken[a]	12–14
2. Age at first intoxication[a]	14–18
3. Age at which minor alcohol problem is experienced[a]	18–25
4. Usual age of onset (first major problem)	23–33
5. Usual age on entering treatment	40
6. Usual age of death	55–60
Leading cause: Heart disease	
Cancer	
Accidents	
Suicide	
7. In any year, abstinence alternates with active drinking.	
"Spontaneous remission" rate or response to nonspecific intervention	¼–⅓

[a]These ages are about the same in the general population.

primary alcoholic, male or female, demonstrates the first major alcohol-related life problem in the late 20s to early 30s, and most alcoholics present for treatment in their early 40s—after more than a decade of difficulties.[125,126] Consistent with these findings, it is likely that by age 31, approximately half of those who will fulfill the criteria for alcoholism have already done so.[125]

If alcohol problems continue, the alcoholic is likely to die 15 years earlier than the average age at death among the general population,[126,127] with the leading causes of death (in approximately decreasing order of importance) being heart disease, cancer, accidents, and suicide. These leading death causes do not include the serious disorders found at markedly higher rates in alcoholics than in the general population, such as cirrhosis, pancreatitis, and infections. As discussed in Section 3.2.2, these findings reflect the diverse organ systems affected by ethanol. Thus, in one series, over 93% of alcoholics coming in for treatment had important medical problems, including 15–25% with hypertension, ulcer disease, or chronic obstructive lung disease; approximately 10% with gastritis, epilepsy, or peripheral neuropathy; and fewer than 5% with cardiomyopathy.[128]

The course of alcoholism is a *fluctuating* one, with very few, if any, alcoholics staying persistently drunk until they die. The usual alcoholic is a blue-collar or white-collar worker who alternates periods of abstinence (and times when he is drinking very little) with periods of serious alcohol misuse. In any given month, one half of alcoholics will be abstinent, with a mean of 4 months of being dry in any 1- to 2-year period.[129] Thus, the average alcoholic has spontaneous periods of abstinence and marked decreases in drinking, which appear to alternate with times of heavy drinking.

The question of an alcoholic's returning to "controlled" or nonproblem drinking has been hotly debated.[130] The problem has centered on the definition of *controlled drinking*, with some reports including individuals drinking as many as eight drinks per day and accepting self-reports without thorough record checks or interviewing of additional relatives. However, both anecdotal information and follow-ups of groups of subjects have indicated that perhaps 1–5% of alcoholics may achieve a state, for years, of drinking low amounts of ethanol without associated problems.[131] These people are likely not to have fulfilled the more rigorous criteria for alcoholism at intake (i.e., they probably had less severe and pervasive alcohol-related problems).[125,131] Therefore, it is best to advise alcoholics that abstinence is the only relevant goal of treatment because 95% or more of alcoholics are unlikely to achieve any long period of controlled drinking; because short periods of drinking without problems are part of the natural course of most alcoholics, but usually give way to serious problems; because of the low percentage of alcoholics who can achieve stable controlled drinking; and because of the difficulties in picking out those who will be able to do this successfully.

Alcoholism is not a hopeless disorder. Not only can one expect improvement with treatment, but also there is good reason to estimate that 10–30% of alcoholics learn to abstain or to seriously limit their drinking without any exposure to a formal treatment regimen.[125,127,129,132,133] The chance of demonstrating spontaneous remission probably increases with the same factors that indicate a good prognosis for those entering treatment (e.g., having a job, living with a family, and having no police record). Anecdotally, men and women with spontaneous remission tend to name alcohol-related physical problems, changes in life-style, or spiritual experiences as having contributed to their decision to maintain abstinence.

3.5. ETIOLOGY OF ALCOHOLISM

As noted in Chapter 1, there is little space in a clinically oriented handbook to discuss etiological theories in great depth. I turn to this topic now to demonstrate both how difficult etiology is to study and how people erroneously tend to state hypotheses as fact. As we shall see, a theory that makes sense is not necessarily true, and a demonstration that Factor A is related to Factor B does not mean that the former caused the latter.

3.5.1. Psychological Theories[134]

These usually involve comparisons of alcoholics and nonalcoholics on performance on psychological tests. The approach at times neglects the possibility that the psychological attributes of alcoholics who have been drinking heavily for 10 years may be the consequence of their life-style rather than the original cause. Proponents of psychological theories may also fail to differentiate between studies of why people drink and of why people become alcoholic.

These theories include the "tension-reduction hypothesis," which states (even though most physiological evidence indicates that alcohol increases tension) that alcoholics drink in an attempt to decrease their levels of stress.[5,135] A second set of important theories centers on the premise that people begin to drink, drink abusively, or remain alcoholic because alcohol, in some way, reinforces or rewards their behavior through inducing pleasure, removing discomfort, enhancing social interactions, and fulfilling the need to feel powerful or, on the other hand, helping them to self-destruct or to abolish unpleasant memories. Studies of personality characteristics and levels of anxiety in nonalcoholic young men at high risk for the future development of alcoholism vs. controls have demonstrated few significant differences between the two groups.[136]

3.5.2. Sociocultural Theories

A second approach centers on sociocultural theories which use observations of similarities and differences among cultural groups and subgroups as they relate to drinking patterns.[137] The major importance of this approach is heuristic, and no factors that are purported to be important in the development of alcoholism in one culture have been shown to generalize to most other cultures. An example would be the statements that Jews and Italians have low rates of alcoholism *because* children are introduced to alcohol within the home setting and alcohol is used as a part of religious ceremonies—a theory that ignores the very high rate of alcoholism among the French, for whom both factors also operate.[135]

3.5.3. Biological Theories

A series of biological theories is found in the literature, including the possibility that alcoholics are seeking relief from an innate hypoglycemia, that they have allergies to alcohol or to the congeners found in alcoholic beverages, or that a differential brain responsiveness to alcohol exists in alcoholics.[135] Once again, it has not been established whether the physiological abnormalities of alcoholics were the initial cause of the heavy drinking or resulted from a life-style of relatively poor nutrition, high stress, and high doses of ethanol.

One theory, which has had a great impact in the field by developing a focus on the chemical changes in nervous-system functioning that result from alcohol, is the possibility that alcohol may produce a morphinelike substance in the brains of certain individuals that may subsequently be responsible for the level of addiction.[138,139] These substances (tetrahydropapaveroline or beta-carbolines) can be found in the condensation of acetaldehyde and brain neurotransmitters such as dopamine or serotonin in the test tube. Such observations have opened an important area of research, but it is not likely that levels of these materials capable of functioning as false neurotransmitters are actually formed in the brain after heavy drinking.[140] At present, these findings are of only theoretical interest and will require much more work before their validity can be established.

3.5.4. Genetic Factors

A series of studies has established the probable importance of genetic factors in the genesis of primary alcoholism. This disorder has been shown to run strongly *within families,* and the rate of concordance (or sameness) for alcoholism in *identical twins* may be higher than in nonidentical twins or same-sex siblings. A number of potential genetic *markers* (such as blood types) have been found to be associated with alcoholism, and some biological factors that influence the patterns of alcohol consumption in animals have been identified.[135,136] The most important information, however, comes from *separation* or adoption-type studies done in both the United States and Scandinavia, demonstrating that the children of alcoholic biological parents separated from their parents early in life and raised without knowledge of their natural parents have markedly elevated rates of alcoholism. However the children of nonalcoholics adopted into the homes of alcoholics do not show elevated rates of alcohol problems as adults.[136,141,142] The 3- to 4-fold higher risk for alcoholism in the adopted-out children of alcoholics when compared with controls was subsequently corroborated in a variety of studies of men, as well as in one study of women.[136,142−144]

Over the years since the publication of the second edition of this text, a number of laboratories have begun to search for possible markers that might be associated with an increased vulnerability to alcoholism. Most investigations have focused on sons and daughters of alcoholic fathers, studying the offspring before the alcoholism develops in hopes that differences between children of alcoholics and of controls might serve as clues to biological factors that are inherited to increase the alcoholism risk.[136,145] These investigators tend to view alcoholism as a disorder in which many specific genes place an individual at higher or lower levels of vulnerability. These genetic factors then interact with environmental factors to give a final level of risk.

Studies of sons and daughters of alcoholics have revealed several interesting potential leads. First, numerous studies have documented a decreased intensity of reaction to ethanol in sons and daughters of alcoholic fathers.[146−148] It is possible that a decreased intensity of reaction to moderate doses of alcohol could make it more difficult for some children of alcoholics to use internal feelings after drinking, to decide when it is time to stop imbibing during an evening. A second series of investigations has demonstrated that a significant subpopulation of children of alcoholics show a decreased amplitude of a brain wave thought to relate to a person's ability to identify and understand a subtle stimulus in his surroundings.[149,150] There is also evidence suggesting that children of alcoholics may differ from controls in their levels of brain waves in the alpha power range on background cortical electroencephalograms (EEGs) or in the pattern of changes in these waves after drinking,[151] a factor that could contribute to a hypothesized unique mode of reaction to ethanol in populations at high risk. These studies are mentioned to underscore the possible genetic and biological components of alcoholism, highlighting the high risk for alcoholism experienced by children of alcoholics as well as the hope that future studies might markedly enhance our abilities to prevent alcoholism before it begins and to more adequately treat it once it develops.[136,148]

Thus, the best data to date indicate that alcoholism is a genetically influenced disorder with a rate of heritability (i.e., the chance of inheriting the disorder) similar to that expected for diabetes or peptic ulcer disease. The mechanism of predisposition may be different from the vulnerability to affective disorder, antisocial personality disorder, and most other psychiatric syndromes.[23,152–154] These findings may have great importance in helping to elucidate the psychological, social, and cultural factors that impact on the genesis of alcoholism. It may now be possible to prospectively study groups of individuals at high risk for alcoholism and to identify the factors that determine whether the predisposition is expressed and to identify other causative factors.

REFERENCES

1. Cahalan, D. *Problem Drinkers*. San Francisco: Jossey-Bass, 1970.
2. Fillmore, K. M., & Midanik, L. Chronicity of drinking problems among men: A longitudinal study. *Journal of Studies on Alcohol 45:*228–236, 1984.
3. Schuckit, M. A. Alcohol and alcoholism. In E. Braunwald, K. J. Isselbacher, R. G. Petersdorf, *et al.* (Eds.), *Harrison's Principles of Internal Medicine* (11th ed.). New York: McGraw-Hill, 1986, pp. 2106–2110.
4. Goodwin, D. W., & Guze, S. B. *Psychiatric Diagnosis* (4th ed.). New York: Oxford University Press, 1988.
5. Schuckit, M. A. Anxiety treatment: A commonsense approach. *Postgraduate Medicine 75:*52–63, 1984.
6. Rounsaville, B. A field trial of DSM III-R psychoactive substance dependence disorders. *American Journal of Psychiatry 144:*351–355, 1987.
7. Schuckit, M. A. Drug classes and problems. *Drug Abuse and Alcoholism Newsletter* 17(1): 1–4, 1988.
8. *Diagnostic and Statistical Manual of Mental Disorders* (3rd ed.). Washington, D.C.: American Psychiatric Press, 1980.
9. American Psychiatric Association: *Diagnostic Criteria from the DSM III-R*. Washington, D.C.: American Psychiatric Press, 1987.
10. Schuckit, M. A., Zisook, S., & Mortola, J. Clinical implications of DSM-III diagnoses of alcohol abuse and alcohol dependence. *American Journal of Psychiatry 142:*1403–1408, 1985.
11. Boyd, J., Weissman, M., Thompson, W., & Myers, J. Different definitions of alcoholism. *American Journal of Psychiatry 140:*1309–1313, 1983.
12. Cahalan, D. A multivariate analysis of correlates of drinking-related problems in a community study. *Social Problems 17:*234–247, 1969.
13. Goodwin, D. W., Crane, J., & Guze, S. B. Loss of short term memory as a predictor of the alcoholic blackout. *Nature 227:*201, 1970.
14. Sellers, E. M., & Kalant, H. Alcohol intoxication and withdrawal. *New England Journal of Medicine 294:*757–762, 1976.
15. Victor, M. Treatment of alcoholic intoxication and the withdrawal syndrome. *Psychosomatic Medicine 28:*636–649, 1966.
16. Criteria Committee, National Council of Alcoholism, Criteria for the diagnosis of alcoholism. *American Journal of Psychiatry 129:*127–135, 1972.
17. Schuckit, M. A. Alcoholism and sociopathy: Diagnostic confusion. *Quarterly Journal of Studies on Alcoholism 34:*157–164, 1973.
18. Schuckit, M. A., Pitts, F. N., Reich, T., *et al.* Two types of alcoholism in women. *Archives of General Psychiatry 20:*301–306, 1969.
19. Heglund, J., & Vieweg, B. The Michigan Alcoholism Screening Test. *Journal of Operational Psychiatry 15:*55–65, 1984.

20. Schuckit, M. A., & Irwin, M. Diagnosis of alcoholism. In M. Geokas (Ed.), *Medical Clinics of North America* 72:1133–1153, 1988.

21. Schuckit, M. A. Alcoholism and other psychiatric disorders. *Hospital and Community Psychiatry* 34:1022–1027, 1983.

22. Schuckit, M. A. The clinical implications of primary diagnostic groups among alcoholics. *Archives of General Psychiatry* 42:1043–1049, 1985.

23. Schuckit, M. A. Genetic and clinical implications of alcoholism and affective disorder. *American Journal of Psychiatry* 143:140–147, 1986.

24. Schuckit, M. A. A study of alcoholics with secondary depression. *American Journal of Psychiatry* 140:711–714, 1983.

25. Robins, L. N. Sturdy childhood predictors of adult antisocial behaviour: Replications from longitudinal studies. *Psychological Medicine* 8:611–622, 1978.

26. Schuckit, M. A., & Winokur, G. A short-term follow-up of women alcoholics. *Diseases of the Nervous System* 33:672–678, 1972.

27. Brown, S. A., & Schuckit, M. A. Changes in depression among abstinent alcoholics. *Journal of Studies on Alcohol* 49:412–417, 1988.

28. Powell, B. J., Read, M. R., Penick, E. C., *et al.* Primary and secondary depression in alcoholic men: An important distinction? *Journal of Clinical Psychiatry* 48:98–101, 1987.

29. Hawton, K. Assessment of suicide risk. *British Journal of Psychiatry* 150:145–153, 1987.

30. Beck, A., Steer, R., & Trexler, L. Alcohol abuse and eventual suicide. *Journal of Studies on Alcohol* (in press).

31. Blankfield, A.: The position of psychiatry in alcohol dependence. *Drug and Alcohol Dependence* 19:259–264, 1987.

32. Hellerstein, D., & Meehan, B. Outpatient gtoup therapy for schizophrenics with substance abuse. *American Journal of Psychiatry* 144:1337–1339, 1987.

33. Kofoed, L., Kania, J., Walsh, T., & Atkinson, R. M. Outpatient treatment of patients with substance abuse and coexisting psychiatric disorders. *American Journal of Psychiatry* 143:867–872, 1986.

34. Rounsaville, B. J., Dolinsky, Z. S., Babor, T. F., & Meyer, R. E. Psychopathology as a predictor of treatment outcome of alcoholics. *Archives of General Psychiatry* 44:505–513, 1987.

35. Secretary of Health and Human Services: Sixth Special Report to the U.S. Congress on Alcohol and Health. Rockville, Maryland: United States Department of Health and Human Services, ADAMHA, DHHS Pub. (ADM) 87-1519, 1987.

36. Gavaler, J. S., Rosenblum, E. R., Van Thiel, D. H., *et al.* Biologically active phytoestrogens are present in bourbon. *Alcoholism: Clinical and Experimental Research* 11:399–406, 1987.

37. Mello, N. K., & Griffiths, R. R. Alcoholism and drug abuse: An overview. In H. Y. Meltzer (Ed.), *Psychopharmacology: The Third Generation of Progress.* New York: Raven Press, 1987, pp. 1511–1514.

38. Naranjo, C. A., Sellers, E. M., & Lawrin, M. O. Modulation of ethanol intake by serotonin uptake inhibitors. *Journal of Clinical Psychiatry* 47:16–22, 1986.

39. Lawrin, M., Naranjo, C., & Sellers, E. Identification and testing of new drugs. *Psychopharmacology* 22:1020–1025, 1986.

40. Friedman, M. J., Krstulovic, A. M., Severinghaus, J. M., & Brown, S. J. Altered conversion of tryptophan to kynurenine in newly abstinent alcoholics. *Biological Psychiatry* 23:89–93, 1988.

41. Jaffe, J. H. Drug addiction and drug abuse. In A. G. Gilman, L. S. Goodman, T. W. Rall, & F. Murad (Eds.), *The Pharmacological Basis of Therapeutics* (7th ed.). New York: Macmillan, 1985, pp. 532–581.

42. Borg, S., Liljeberg, P., & Mossberg, D. Alcohol consumption, dependence, and central norepinephrine metabolism in humans. In J. Engel & L. Oreland (Eds.), *Brain Reward Systems and Abuse.* New York: Raven Press, 1987, pp. 181–185.

43. Royal College of General Practitioners. Alcohol—A balanced view. *Journal of the Royal College of General Practitioners,* pp. 1–25, 1986.
44. Baum-Raicker, C. The health benefits of moderate alcohol consumption: A review of the literature. *Drug and Alcohol Dependence 15:*207–227, 1985.
45. Liskow, B. I., & Goodwin, D. W. Pharmacological treatment of alcohol intoxication, withdrawal and dependence: A critical review. *Journal of Studies on Alcohol 48:*356–370, 1987.
46. Iber, F. L. Evaluation of an oral solution to accelerate alcoholism detoxification. *Alcoholism: Clinical and Experimental Research 11:*305–311, 1987.
47. Criqui, M. H. Alcohol consumption, blood pressure, lipids, and cardiovascular mortality. *Alcoholism: Clinical and Experimental Research 10:*564–569, 1986.
48. Burr, M. L., Fehily, A. M., Butland, B. K., *et al.* Alcohol and high-density-lipoprotein cholesterol: A randomized controlled trial. *British Journal of Nutrition 56:*81–86, 1986.
49. Schmidt, W., & Popham, R. E. The role of drinking and smoking in mortality from cancer and other causes in male alcoholics. *Cancer 47:*1031–1041, 1981.
50. Lumeng, L. New diagnostic markers of alcohol abuse. *Hepatology 6:*742–745, 1986.
51. Weill, J., Schellenberg, F., LeGoff, A., & Bernard, J. The decrease of GGT during abstinence. *Alcohol 5:*1–3, 1988.
52. Ryback, R. S., Eckhardt, M. J., & Pautler, C. P. Biochemical and hematological correlates of alcoholism. *Research Communications in Chemical Pathology and Pharmacology 27:*533–550, 1980.
53. Irwin, M., Baird, S., Smith, T. L., & Schuckit, M. A. Use of laboratory tests to monitor heavy drinking. *American Journal of Psychiatry 145:*595–599, 1988.
54. Cyr, M., & Wartman, S. The effectiveness of routine screening questions in alcoholism. *Journal of the American Medical Association 259:*51–54, 1988.
55. Lieber, C. S. Alcohol and the liver: 1984 update. *Hepatology 4:*1243–1260, 1984.
56. Orrego, H., Blake, J. E., Blendis, L. M., *et al.* Long-term treatment of alcoholic liver disease with propylthiouracil. *New England Journal of Medicine 317:*1421–1427, 1987.
57. Hayashida, M., Alterman, A. I., McLellan, A. T., *et al.* Is inpatient medical alcohol detoxification justified? Paper presented at the Meeting of the Committee on Problems of Drug Dependence, Philadelphia, May 6, 1987.
58. Norton, R., Batey, R., Dwyer, T., & MacMahon, S. Alcohol consumption and the risk of alcohol-related cirrhosis in women. *British Medical Journal 295:*80–82, 1987.
59. Nouchi, T., Worner, T. M., Sato, S., & Lieber, C. S. Serum procollagen type III N-terminal peptides and laminin P1 peptide in alcoholic liver disease. *Alcoholism: Clinical and Experimental Research 11:*287–291, 1987.
60. Frank, D., & Raicht, R. F. Alcohol-induced liver disease. *Alcoholism: Clinical and Experimental Research 9:*66–82, 1985.
61. Young, T. B., Folrd, C. M., & Brandenburg, J. H. An epidemiologic study of oral cancer in a statewide network. *American Journal of Otolaryngology 7:*200–208, 1986.
62. Lieber, C. S., Garro, A., Leo, M. A., & Worner, T. Alcohol and cancer. *Hepatology 6:*1005–1019, 1986.
63. Wu, A. H., Paganini-Hill, A., Ross, R. K., & Henderson, B. E. Alcohol, physical activity and other risk factors for colorectal cancer: A prospective study. *British Journal on Cancer 55:*687–694, 1987.
64. Schatzkin, A., Jones, Y., Hoover, R. N., *et al.* Alcohol consumption and breast cancer in the epidemiologic follow-up study of the first national health and nutrition examination survey. *New England Journal of Medicine 316:*1169–1173, 1987.
65. Editorial: Does alcohol cause breast cancer? *Lancet 1:*1311, 1985.
66. Victor, M., Adams, R. D., & Collins, G. H. *The Wernicke–Korsakoff Syndrome: A Clinical and Pathological Study of 245 Patients, 82 with Post-Mortem Examinations.* Philadelphia: Davis, 1971.

67. Harper, C., Kril, J., & Daly, J. Are we drinking our neurones away? *British Medical Journal* *294:*534–536, 1987.

68. Eckardt, M. J. & Martin, P. R. Clinical assessment of cognition in alcoholism. *Alcoholism: Clinical and Experimental Research 10:*123–127, 1986.

69. Estrin, W. J. Alcoholic cerebellar degeneration is not a dose-dependent phenomenon. *Alcoholism: Clinical and Experimental Research 11:*372–375, 1987.

70. Grant, I. Alcohol and the brain: Neuropsychological correlates. *Journal of Consulting and Clinical Psychology 55:*310–324, 1987.

71. Kissin, B., & Begleiter, H. (Eds.). *The Biology of Alcoholism, Vol. 3: Clinical Pathology.* New York: Plenum Press, 1971.

72. Donahue, R. P., Abbott, R. D., Reed, D. M., & Yano, K. Alcohol and hemorrhagic stroke. *Journal of the American Medical Association 255:*2311–2314, 1986.

73. Gill, J. S., Zezulka, A. V., Shipley, M. J., *et al.* Stroke and alcohol consumption. *New England Journal of Medicine 315:*1041–1046, 1986.

74. Bowden, S. C. Brain impairment in social drinkers? No cause for concern. *Alcoholism: Clinical and Experimental Research 11:*407–410, 1987.

75. Pfefferbaum, A., Rosenbloom, M., Crusan, K., Jernigan, T. L. Brain CT changes in alcoholics: Effects of age and alcohol consumption. *Alcoholism: Clinical and Experimental Research 12:*81–87, 1988.

76. Jacobson, R. Female alcoholics: A controlled CT brain scan and clinical study. *British Journal of Addiction 81:*661–669, 1986.

77. Parsons, O. Intellectual impairment in alcoholics. *Acta Medica Scandanavica 17:* (Suppl.) 33–46, 1987.

78. Greenspan, A. J., & Schaal, S. F. The "holiday heart": Electrophysiologic studies of alcohol effects in alcoholics. *Annals of Internal Medicine 98:*135–139, 1983.

79. Klatsky, A. L., Friedman, G. D. & Siegelaub, M. S. Alcohol and mortality: A ten-year Kaiser–Permanente experience. *Annals of Internal Medicine 95:*139–145, 1981.

80. Dancy, M., Leech, G., Bland, J. M., *et al.* Preclinical left ventricular abnormalities in alcoholics are independent of nutritional status, cirrhosis, and cigarette smoking. *Lancet 1:*1122–1123, 1985.

81. Horwitz, L. D. Alcohol and heart disease. *Journal of the American Medical Association 232:*959–960, 1975.

82. Lang, R. M., Borow, M. M., Neumann, A., & Feldman, T. Adverse cardiac effects of acute alcohol ingestion in young adults. *Annals of Internal Medicine 102:*742–747, 1985.

83. Saunders, J. B. Alcohol: An important cause of hypertension. *British Medical Journal 294:*1045–1046, 1987.

84. Rosengren, A., Wilhelmsen, L., Pennert, K., *et al.* Alcoholic intemperance, coronary heart disease and mortality in middle-aged Swedish men. *Acta Medica Scandinavica 222:*201–213, 1987.

85. Malhotra, M., Mathur, D., Menta, S. R., & Khandelwal, P. D. Pressor effects of alcohol in normotensive and hypertensive subjects. *Lancet 2:*584–586, 1985.

86. Savage, D., & Lindenbaum, J. Anemia in alcoholics. *Medicine (Baltimore) 65:*322–338, 1986.

87. MacGregor, R. R. Alcohol and immune defense. *Journal of the American Medical Association 256:*1474–1479, 1986.

88. Watson, R. R., Mohs, M. E., Eskelson, L., *et al.* Identification of alcohol abuse and alcoholism with biological parameters. *Alcoholism: Clinical and Experimental Research 10:*364–385, 1986.

89. Brzek, A. Alcohol and male fertility (preliminary report). *Andrologia 19:*32–36, 1987.

90. Irwin, M., Dreyfus, E., Baird, S., *et al.* Testosterone in chronic alcoholic men. *British Journal of Addictions 83:*949–953, 1988.

91. Mendelson, J. H., & Mello, N. K. Biologic concomitants of alcoholism. *New England Journal of Medicine 301:*912–921, 1979.

92. Connelly, D. M., Harries, E. H. L., & Taberner, P. V. Differential effects of ethanol on the

plasma glucose of non-alcoholic light and heavy social drinkers. *Alcohol and Alcoholism 22:23–29*, 1987.

93. Fulop, M., Ben-Ezra, J., & Bock, J. Alcoholic ketosis. *Alcoholism: Clinical and Experimental Research 10:610–615*, 1986.

94. Bikle, D. D., Genant, H. K., Cann, D., *et al.* Bone disease in alcohol abuse. *Annals of Internal Medicine 103:42–48*, 1985.

95. Eiser, A. R. The effects of alcohol on renal function and excretion. *Alcoholism: Clinical and Experimental Research 11:127–138*, 1987.

96. Colquitt, M., Fielding, P., & Cronan, J. F. Drunk drivers and medical and social injury. *New England Journal of Medicine 317:1262–1266*, 1987.

97. Moskowitz, H., Burns, M. M., & Williams, A. F. Skills performance at low blood alcohol levels. *Journal of Studies on Alcohol 46:482–485*, 1985.

98. Yesavage, J. A., & Leirer, V. O. Hangover effects on aircraft pilots 14 hours after alcohol ingestion: A preliminary report. *American Journal of Psychiatry 143:1546–1550*, 1986.

99. Miller, B. A., Whitney, R., & Washousky, R. Alcoholism diagnoses for convicted drinking drivers referred for alcoholism evaluation. *Alcoholism: Clinical and Experimental Research 10:651–656*, 1986.

100. Boglin, R. M., Nostrant, T. T., & Young, M. J. Propranolol for the treatment of the alcoholic hangover. *American Journal of Drug and Alcohol Abuse 13:175–180*, 1987.

101. Smith, C. M. Symptoms of intoxication and hangovers perceived to modify subsequent alcoholic beverage consumption. Paper presented at the Meeting of the Committee on Problems of Drug Dependence, Philadelphia, June 14–19, 1987.

102. Bouden, S., Walton, N., & Walsh, K. The hangover hypothesis. *Alcoholism: Clinical and Experimental Research 12:25–29*, 1988.

103. Lieber, C. S. Interactions of alcohol and nutrition: Introduction to a symposium. *Alcoholism: Clinical and Experimental Research 7:2–4*, 1983.

104. Schuckit, M. A. Biochemical markers of a predisposition to alcoholism. In S. B. Rosalki (Ed.), *Clinical Biochemistry of Alcoholism*. Edinburgh: Churchill Livingstone, 1983, pp. 20–50.

105. Suwaki, H., & Ohara, H. Alcohol-induced facial flushing and drinking behavior in Japanese men. *Journal of Studies on Alcohol 46:196–198*, 1985.

106. Wanger, J. R. Ethanol tolerance in the rat is learned. *Science 213:575–578*, 1981.

107. Schuckit, M. A. Chapter 1: Overview: Epidemiology of alcoholism. In M. A. Schuckit (Ed.), *Alcohol Patterns and Problems*. New Brunswick, New Jersey: Rutgers University Press, 1985, pp. 1–42.

108. Hilton, M. E., & Clark, W. B. Changes in American drinking patterns and problems, 1967–1984. *Journal of Studies on Alcohol 48:515–522*, 1987.

109. Editorial: National survey finds continuing decline in use of illicit drugs by high school seniors. *Hospital and Community Psychiatry 36:1011*, 1985.

110. Smart, R. G., Goodstadt, M. S., Adlaf, E. M., *et al.* Trends in the prevalence of alcohol and other drug use among Ontario students: 1977–1983. *Canadian Journal of Public Health 76:157–161*, 1985.

111. Engs, R. C., & Hanson, D. J. College students' drinking patterns and problems. In J. S. Sherwood (Ed.), *Alcohol Policies and Practices on College and University Campuses, Vol. 7: NASPA Monograph Series*, National Association of Student Personnel Administrators, 1987, pp. 57–68.

112. Wiggins, J. A., & Wiggins, B. B. Drinking at a Southern university: Its description and correlates. *Journal of Studies on Alcohol 48:319–324*, 1987.

113. Kandel, D. B., Davies, M., Karus, D., & Yamaguchi, K. The consequences in young adulthood of adolescent drug involvement. *Archives of General Psychiatry 43:746–654*, 1986.

114. Johnson, L. P., Bachman, J. G., & O'Malley, P. M. Drugs and tne nation's high school students. In G. G. Nahos & H. C. Frede (Eds.), *Drug Abuse in the Modern World*. New York: Pergamon Press, 1981, pp. 87–98.

115. Hanson, D. J., & Engs, R. C. College students' drinking problems: 1982–1985. *Psychological Reports 58:*276–278, 1986.
116. Smart, R. G., & Adlaf, E. M. Patterns of drug use among adolescents: The past decade. *Social Science Medicine 23:*717–719, 1986.
117. Smart, R. G., & Mann, R. E. Large decreases in alcohol-related problems following a slight reduction in alcohol consumption in Ontario 1975–1983. *British Journal of Addiction 82:*285–291, 1987.
118. Swenson, P. R., Struckman-Johnson, D. L., Ellingstad, V. S., *et al.* Results of a longitudinal evaluation of court-mandated DWI treatment programs in Phoenix, Arizona. *Journal of Studies on Alcohol 42:*642–653, 1981.
119. Robins, L. N., Helzer, J. E., Weissman, M. M., *et al.* Lifetime prevalence of specific psychiatric disorders in three sites. *Archives of General Psychiatry 41:*949–958, 1984.
120. Kamerow, D. B., Pincus, H. A., & Macdonald, D. I. Alcohol abuse, other drug abuse, and mental disorders in medical practice. *Journal of the American Medical Association 255:*2054–2057, 1986.
121. Blazer, D., Crowell, B. A., & George, L. K. Alcohol abuse and dependence in the rural south. *Archives of General Psychiatry 44:*736–740, 1987.
122. Eagles, J. M., & Besson, J. A. O. Changes in the incidence of alcohol-related problems in northeast Scotland, 1974–1982. *British Journal of Psychiatry 147:*39–43, 1985.
123. Armor, D. J., Orvis, B. R., Carpenter-Huffman, P., & Polich, J. M. *The Control of Alcohol Problems in the U.S. Air Force.* Santa Monica, California: Rand, 1981.
124. Schaefer, J. M. Firewater myths revisited. *Journal of Studies on Alcohol 42:*99–117, 1981.
125. Vaillant, G. E. Natural history of male alcoholism. *Archives of General Psychiatry 39:*127–133, 1982.
126. Editorial: Dying for a drink? *Lancet 2:*1249, 1987.
127. Tuchfeld, B. S. Spontaneous remission in alcoholics: Empirical observations and theoretical implications. *Journal of Studies on Alcohol 42:*626–641, 1981.
128. Ashley, M. J. The physical disease characteristics of inpatient alcoholics. *Journal of Studies on Alcohol 42:*1–11, 1981.
129. Ludwig, A. M. On and off the wagon. *Quarterly Journal of Studies on Alcohol 33:*91–96, 1972.
130. Pendery, M. L. Matlzman, I. M., & West, L. J. Controlled drinking by alcoholics? Refutation of a major affirmative study. *Science 217:*169–175, 1981.
131. Helzer, J., Robins, L., Taylor, J., *et al.* The extent of long-term moderate drinking among alcoholics. *New England Journal of Medicine 312:*1678–1682, 1985.
132. Ludwig, A. M. Cognitive processes associated with ''spontaneous'' recovery from alcoholism. *Journal of Studies on Alcohol 46:*53–58, 1985.
133. Drew, L. R. H. Alcoholism as a self-limiting disease. *Quarterly Journal of Studies on Alcohol 29:*956–967, 1968.
134. Blane, H., & Leonard, K. *Psychological Theories of Drinking and Alcoholism.* New York: Guilford Press, 1987.
135. Schuckit, M. A. Etiologic theories on alcoholism. In N. Estes and E. Heinemann (Eds.), *Alcoholism.* St. Louis: C. V. Mosby, 1986, pp. 15–30.
136. Schuckit, M. A. Biomedical and genetic markers of alcoholism. In H. W. Geodde and D. P. Agarwal (Eds.). New York, Pergamon Press (in press).
137. Heath, D. B. Anthropology and alcohol studies: Current issues. *Annual Review of Anthropology 16:*99–120, 1987.
138. Sjoquist, B. Brain salsolinol levels in alcoholism. *Lancet 1:*675–676, 1982.
139. Bloom, F., Barchas, J., Sandler, M., & Usden, E. (Eds.). *Beta-carbolines and Tetrahydroisoquinolines.* New York: Alan R. Liss, 1982.
140. Korsten, M. A., Matsuzaki, S., Feinman, L., & Lieber, C. S. High blood acetaldehyde levels after ethanol administration: Difference between alcoholic and nonalcoholic subjects. *New England Journal of Medicine 292:*386–389, 1975.
141. Gurling, H. M. D., Phil, M., Grant, S., & Dangl, J. The genetic and cultural transmission of

alcohol use, alcoholism, cigarette smoking and coffee drinking: A review and an example using a log linear cultural transmission model. *British Journal of Addiction 80:*269–272, 1985.

142. Goodwin, D. W. Alcoholism and genetics. *Archives of General Psychiatry 42:*171–174, 1985.

143. Schuckit, M. A. A search for biological markers in alcoholism: Application to psychiatric research. In R. M. Rose & J. Barren (Eds.), *Alcoholism: Origins and Outcome.* New York: Raven Press, 1988, pp. 143–156.

144. Schuckit, M. A. Reactions to alcohol in sons of alcoholics and controls. *Alcoholism: Clinical and Experimental Research 12:*465–470, 1988.

145. Schuckit, M. A. Biological vulnerability to alcoholism. *Journal of Consulting and Clinical Psychology 55:*301–309, 1987.

146. Lex, B., Lukas, S., Greenwald, N., & Mendelson, J. Alcohol-induced changes in body sway in women at risk for alcoholism. *Journal of Studies on Alcohol 49:*346–356, 1988.

147. Schuckit, M. A., & Gold, E. O. A simultaneous evaluation of multiple markers of ethanol/placebo challenges in sons of alcoholics and controls. *Archives of General Psychiatry 45:*211–216, 1988.

148. Schuckit, M. A. Progress in the search for genetic markers of an alcoholism risk. In S. Parvez, Y. Burov, H. Ollat, & H. Parvez (Eds.), *Progress in Alcohol Research, Vol. 2: Alcohol and Behavior: Basic and Clinical Aspects.* Amsterdam, Holland: VNU Science Press (in press).

149. Begleiter, H., Porjesz, B., & Bihari, B.: Auditory brainstem potentials in sons of alcoholic fathers. *Alcoholism: Clinical and Experimental Research 11:*477, 1987.

150. Schuckit, M. A., Gold, E. O., Croot, K., & Finn, P. P300 latency after ethanol ingestion in sons of alcoholics and controls. *Biological Psychiatry 24:*310–315, 1988.

151. Ehlers, C., & Schuckit, M. A. EEG changes after ethanol in sons of alcoholics and controls. *Journal of Studies on Alcohol* (in press).

152. Drake, R. E., & Vaillant, G. E. Predicting alcoholism and personality disorder in a 33-year longitudinal study of children of alcoholics. *British Journal of Addiction 83:*799–808, 1988.

153. Hesselbrock, V. M., Hesselbrock, M. N., & Stabenau, J. R. Alcoholism in men patients subtyped by family history and antisocial personality. *Journal of Studies on Alcohol 46:*59–64, 1985.

154. Tabakoff, B., Hoffman, P. L., Lee, J. M., *et al.* Differences in platelet enzyme activity between alcoholics and nonalcoholics. *New England Journal of Medicine 318:*134–139, 1988.

155. Schuckit, M. A. Treatment of alcoholism in office and outpatient settings. In J. H. Mendelson & N. K. Mello (Eds.), *Diagnosis and Treatment of Alcoholism.* New York: McGraw-Hill, 1979, pp. 295–324.

Alcoholism: Acute Treatment

4.1. INTRODUCTION

Alcohol is the most commonly abused substance creating serious medical and psychological problems. I present here an overview of *emergency problems,* but the extensive discussion of rehabilitation that serves as a prototype for the rehabilitation of substance abusers is discussed in general until Chapter 15.

4.1.1. Identifying the Alcoholic

The "obvious" alcoholic who gets drunk and calls in the middle of the night or who has signs of cirrhosis represents a minority of individuals with alcoholism. The usual alcohol abusing patient is a middle-class family man or homemaker presenting with complaints of insomnia, sadness, nervousness, or interpersonal problems. Because 5–10% of adult men develop alcoholism (the rate for women being approximately one third of that) and the rate of alcohol problems in medical and surgical inpatients may be over 25%, it is important to consider alcoholism a part of the differential diagnosis for every individual.[1] The index of suspicion should be even higher for those with some of the more typical medical problems, including high blood pressure, ulcer disease, elevated uric acid, a macrocytosis, a high gamma-glutamyl transferase (GGT), or any fluctuating medical condition that is otherwise difficult to explain (see Section 3.2.2).

Therefore, I take the two or three minutes necessary to query *every* patient about alcohol-related life problems. I begin by asking about *general* areas of difficulty, including such questions as: "How are things going with your [spouse]?" "Have you had any accidents since I last saw you?" "How are things going on the job?" "Have you had any arrests or traffic tickets?" If there is a general life problem, I then try to determine what role, if any, alcohol may have played in that problem, and I go on to questions about the quantity and frequency of drinking. If the patient appears evasive or if I have any further doubts, I interview the spouse privately.

4.1.2. Obtaining a History

Once I have established either a definite or a probable diagnosis of alcoholism, I must determine whether or not there are any preexisting primary psychiatric disorders (as outlined in Figure 3.1 and discussed in depth in Section 3.1.2.3). Thus, I first do a brief review of antisocial problems early in life, including such questions as: "How did you do in school?" "What was the highest grade you completed?" "Did you ever run away from home overnight before you were 16?" "Did you have any police record prior to age 16?" "When you were in junior high school or high school, did you get in a lot of fights and did you ever use a weapon in a fight?" Next, I ask about any depression that has occurred all day, every day, for periods of at least 2 weeks or that has been associated with the body and mind changes described in Section 3.1.2.3. If these depressive episodes have occurred, I then determine whether they existed prior to the first major alcohol-related life problem or occurred during a time when the individual had been abstinent for at least 3 months.

These steps are well worth my time, as complex and perplexing medical and psychological problems associated with alcoholism can be very confusing and can lead to serious complications through improper diagnosis and treatment. I can practice good preventive medicine and save myself a number of middle-of-the-night calls into the emergency room by maintaining a high level of suspicion of alcoholism.

4.2. EMERGENCY PROBLEMS

The most frequent emergency problems for alcoholics involve toxic reactions and accidents. Almost 8% of all emergency room patients have alcohol problems as part of their mode of presentation, rates that increase to 33% for accident victims.[2] Recognition of the presence of alcohol (whether alcoholism is involved or not) is important, as this drug alters the patient's reactions to emergency procedures.

4.2.1. Panic Reactions (Possibly 303.00 or 292.89 in DSM-III-R) (see Section 1.6.1)

4.2.1.1. Clinical Picture

Because alcohol is a depressant drug, acute intoxication rarely involves acute panic. However, as discussed in Section 4.2.6, the signs and symptoms of alcoholic withdrawal do not actually end on Day 4 or 5; the problems, including anxiety, are likely to be observed for a number of months. In this condition of protracted abstinence, the patient can demonstrate irritability, restlessness, hyperventilation, insomnia, and distractability, problems that will likely diminish as the period of abstinence lengthens.[3-8] Thus, almost any form of increased anxiety, ranging from panic to general nervousness, can be seen for 3–12 months after cessation of drinking. It does not seem appropriate that the diagnosis of a major anxiety syndrome be considered in this situation, because the anxiety is not likely to have been observed before the alcohol-related life problems and is likely to disappear or at least improve greatly with time alone.

4.2.1.2. Treatment

After taking an electrocardiogram (EKG), doing a physical examination, and evaluating to rule out acute withdrawal, the cornerstone of treatment is reassurance and education. The symptoms respond to behavioral approaches, including relaxation training, exercise, and biofeedback.[9] Of course, I refer these patients for alcohol counseling.

4.2.2. Flashbacks

Flashbacks are not noted with alcohol.

4.2.3. Toxic Reactions (see Sections 1.6.3, 2.2.3, 6.2.3, and 14.4)

Toxic reactions to alcohol are usually the result of the narrow range between the anesthetic and the lethal doses of this drug, or they reflect the potentiating interaction seen between alcohol and other central nervous system (CNS) depressants (see Section 13.2.3).

4.2.3.1. Clinical Picture

The overdose from alcohol results from CNS depression to the point of respiratory and circulatory failure. The danger is heightened when alcohol is taken in combination with other CNS-depressing drugs, such as any of the hypnotics or antianxiety drugs, but it can also occur with drugs of other classes, such as the opiates. The clinical picture of an ethanol overdose is basically similar to that described for the depressants in Section 2.2.3.

4.2.3.1.1. History

The patient usually presents smelling of alcohol with a history of a recent ingestion of high doses of alcohol, perhaps accompanied by other CNS depressants, such as sleeping pills [e.g., the barbiturates or flurazepam (Dalmane)] or the antianxiety drugs [e.g., chlordiazepoxide (Librium) or diazepam (Valium)]. If no history can be obtained directly from the patient, a friend or relative might supply the relevant information, or there may be obvious evidence of drug ingestion (e.g., empty bottles).

4.2.3.1.2. Physical Signs and Symptoms

These are identical to the physical manifestations reported for other CNS depressants in Section 2.2.3. Basically, the patient presents with depressed functioning of the CNS and changed vital signs, including a slow pulse, a lowered respiratory rate, and a low blood pressure.

4.2.3.1.3. Psychological State

This also resembles the picture described for the other CNS depressants in Section 2.2.3, including signs of severe intoxication (i.e., the person is very drunk) along with confusion and irritability of mood.

4.2.3.1.4. Relevant Laboratory Data

The diagnosis, resting with the history and the physical examination, is aided by the toxicological screen (10 cc blood or 50 ml urine) for both alcohol and other CNS depressants. The remaining laboratory tests are those necessary to properly exclude other causes of stupor (e.g., low glucose) and to monitor the physical status (e.g., blood counts and, if the patient is very stuporous, blood gases, as shown in Table 1.5).

4.2.3.2. Treatment

A fatal toxic reaction has been reported with blood-alcohol levels as low as 350 mg% in nontolerant individuals.[10] The treatment procedures follow those outlined for CNS depressants in Section 2.2.3.2, but there are a few differences:

1. Treatment involves carrying out the necessary emergency procedures to guarantee adequate ventilation, circulation, and control of shock; making a careful evaluation to rule out ancillary medical problems, such as electrolyte disturbances, cardiac disorders, associated infections, and subdural hematomas; and then establishing general supportive measures while the body metabolizes the alcohol.

2. Some investigators report that oral or intravenous (IV) fructose can enhance the rate of ethanol metabolism by 10–25%.[11,12] The mechanism is probably via an increased rate of reoxidation of the hydrogen receptor nicotinamide adenine dinucleotide (NAD) so that more is available for ethanol. However, oral administration of fructose can result in abdominal colic, and IV use may contribute to lactic acidosis. Therefore, this approach is rarely used in clinical situations.

3. If you suspect that opiates were also ingested, naloxone (Narcan) [0.4 mg, intramuscular (IM) or IV] should be given. If, as outlined in Section 6.2.3.2 (item 8), the patient does not respond to two doses given within ½ hour, it is almost certain that opiates were not part of the respiratory and cardiac depression. There is some anecdotal evidence that symptoms of shock accompanying alcohol toxic reactions uncomplicated by opiate misuse may themselves respond to 0.4 mg of naloxone IV, which can be repeated twice in 10 minutes. However, laboratory experiments have failed to confirm these findings in animals or humans.[13]

4.2.4. Psychosis and Depression (e.g., 291.30 in DSM-III-R) (see Sections 1.6.4, 2.2.4, and 5.2.4)

4.2.4.1. Clinical Picture

The chronic ingestion of alcohol can cause suspiciousness that can progress to the point of frank paranoid delusions, that is, *alcoholic paranoia*. Similarly, alcohol can cause persistent hallucinations, usually voices accusing the patient of being a bad person or a homosexual (although at times the hallucinations can be visual or tactile), an example of *alcoholic hallucinosis*. Both pictures can develop in the midst of a drinking bout, occur in an otherwise clear sensorium [i.e., there is no organic brain syndrome (OBS)], begin during alcoholic withdrawal, or have an onset within several weeks of the cessation of drinking. Both run a course of complete recovery within several days to several weeks if no further drinking occurs.[14,15] Clinically, the syndrome resembles the stimulant-induced psychosis (see Section 5.2.4) and psychoses associated with other depressant drugs (see Section 2.2.4). It is not a form of schizophrenia, as there is no increased family history of that disorder in these individuals, and there is no evidence that alcoholic paranoia or hallucinosis progresses to schizophrenia.[16]

As noted in Section 3.1.2.3, alcohol can induce serious states of depression in alcoholics or nonalcoholics. This depression looks cross-sectionally identical to the major affective disorders and can include a high suicide risk.[15-18] However, primary alcoholism with secondary depression is likely to show a clearing of the depressed mood after several days or weeks of abstinence without active treatment, whereas primary affective disorder may require intervention with antidepressants or (for manic–depressive disease) lithium.

In addition, states of violence are frequently associated with alcohol intoxication. An individual with a history of violence unrelated to alcohol may demonstrate severe aggression as he becomes tired, agitated, and perhaps hypoglycemic in the midst of heavy drinking. Thus alcohol is associated with crimes of violence, although many such violent individuals are probably antisocial personalities and/or drug abusers who are also using alcohol abusively. One specific form of alcohol-related violence, pathological intoxication or alcohol idiosyncratic reaction, is discussed in Section 4.2.8.1.

4.2.4.2. Treatment

1. If the patient has no insight into his delusions or hallucinations (i.e., believes that they are real), he should be hospitalized so that he will be protected from acting out his delusions.

2. Treatment should be aimed at giving the patient insight and at evaluating and treating any medical problems associated with his heavy intake of alcohol.

3. Although any psychotic picture is likely to clear spontaneously within a few days or several weeks, an antipsychotic agent like haloperidol (Haldol) at 1–5 mg per day (but up to 20 mg each day, if needed) by mouth, or IM if needed, may help keep the patient comfortable until the psychosis clears. There is no indication for continued use of these drugs, and they should be stopped within 2 weeks. If the patient has demonstrated delusions and/or hallucinations before the onset of heavy drinking or has a history of persistence of the psychosis despite abstinence, the diagnosis of primary schizophrenia with secondary alcohol problems should be entertained and antipsychotic medications continued.[15,16]

4.2.5. Organic Brain Syndrome (e.g., 291.00, 291.10, and 291.20 in DSM-III-R) (see Sections 1.6.5 and 2.2.5)

4.2.5.1. Clinical Picture

Alcohol can cause mental confusion and clouding of consciousness through the direct effects of the drug, alcohol-related vitamin deficiencies, and indirect consequences of alcohol intake, such as trauma and metabolic disturbances. Therefore, states of serious confusion can be seen during alcohol intoxication, during withdrawal from alcohol, as a complication of vitamin deficiency (e.g., thiamine), as the result of trauma (e.g., a subdural hematoma), and probably as the result of many years of heavy drinking.[15] The latter is probably the result of a combination of factors, including the direct toxic effect of ethanol on neurons.

4.2.5.1.1. Direct Effects of Alcohol

1. *Acute and subacute*[19]: At relatively low doses (i.e., one or two drinks), judgment and performance are impaired, but at blood-alcohol levels in excess of 150 mg%, a picture of confusion and disorientation occurs for most nontolerant people. The OBS can be seen at even lower doses for the elderly and for individuals with preexisting brain disorders, such as those with prior head trauma and subsequent unconsciousness. The course is *usually* relatively benign, and a clearing of confusion occurs as blood-alcohol levels decrease. However, in the elderly and those with prior brain damage, the state of confusion may last for days or longer, and alcohol intoxication may thus be an important part of the differential diagnosis of acute-onset confusion.

2. *Chronic* heavy doses of alcohol are associated with a number of organic pictures, some of which may be permanent. As noted previously, 15–30% of nursing home patients with chronic OBS have histories of alcoholism. This OBS may result in part from the deleterious effects of alcohol on nerve cells, but it is also probably the combined result of alcohol, vitamin deficiencies, and trauma. A number of studies have corroborated the direct toxic effects of ethanol on neurons even when other aspects of nutrition are controlled.[20] The clinical picture and the treatment would be similar to those for vitamin-related organicities, as discussed in the next section.

4.2.5.1.2. Vitamin Deficiencies

In the presence of alcohol, the body does not absorb thiamine adequately and uses what thiamine there is at a faster rate. This fact may be of great importance, especially to individuals with inefficient thiamine-dependent enzymes.[21,22] The result is a syndrome consisting of a mixture of neurological problems, such as ataxia, nystagmus, and the paralysis of certain ocular muscles, which characterize *Wernicke's syndrome,* and psychological symptoms, such as markedly decreased recent memory, confusion, and a tendency to make up stories to fill in memory deficits (confabulation), known as *Korsakoff's syndrome.* The Wernicke–Korsakoff syndrome (or variations thereof) runs an unpredictable course, with a tendency toward rapid and complete improvement of most neurological signs with the administration of adequate thiamine, but with a slower resolution of the mental clouding and a possibly permanent OBS.[23,24]

4.2.5.1.3. Other Causes of Organicity in Alcoholics

Any individual presenting with confusion, disorientation, and decreased intellectual functioning should receive a thorough evaluation for trauma (and resultant subdural hematomas), infections, and metabolic abnormalities (especially glucose, magnesium, and potassium problems). Regarding glucose, alcohol interferes with gluconeogenesis (sugar production) as well as with the actions of insulin and may cause pancreatic damage; thus, alcoholics may show hyper- or, more frequently, hypoglycemia when they enter treatment. These problems tend to revert toward normal after several weeks of abstinence.

4.2.5.2. Treatment

1. The cornerstone of treatment is finding and treating the physical causes (e.g., infection, electrolyte abnormalities, and consequences of trauma).

2. All patients should receive thiamine in doses of 100 mg IM daily for at least 3 days, followed by oral multiple-vitamin preparations. Persisting signs of confusion—especially when difficulties with recent memory are out of proportion to those expected from the global mental status and/or when confusion is associated with neurological problems such as a VIth-cranial-nerve palsy—should be met with continued thiamine for 2 months or longer, as the Wernicke–Korsakoff syndrome may continue to improve over a long period of time.[23]

3. Patients should be given good general nutrition and lots of opportunity to rest.

4. Although improvement in the level of organic impairment is to be expected, the mental confusion may clear slowly, and it may not be possible to establish the exact degree of permanent intellectual deterioration for several months.

4.2.6. Alcoholic Withdrawal (e.g., 291.80 and 291.00 in DSM-III-R) (see Sections 1.6.6, 2.2.6, and 6.2.6)

4.2.6.1. Clinical Picture

This is an example of the *depressant withdrawal syndrome* and is similar to that which results from the other CNS depressants, as discussed in Section 2.2.6. Figure 4.1 outlines a simple approach to the symptomatology expected during withdrawal.

4.2.6.1.1. History

Some withdrawal symptoms, usually mild in nature, can be expected in most alcoholics who have been drinking daily. The intensity of the symptoms is difficult to predict with certainty, but the common pattern described in this section may be helpful.

The alcoholic may present with a clear history of alcohol abuse, but more often he comes to the physician with a variety of psychological or physical complaints, as described in Section 4.1.1. It is wise to have a high index of suspicion for possible alcoholic withdrawal in all new patients, especially for those who present with any of the more obvious stigmata of alcoholism, ranging from a high MCV (see Table 1.5) to liver failure, cancer of the esophagus, or cancer of the head and neck. When a patient presents with any of the physical problems often associated with alco-

Symptoms   Treatment

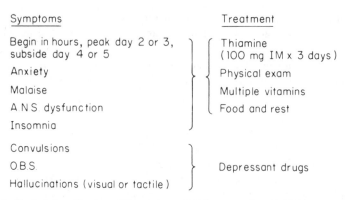

Begin in hours, peak day 2 or 3,   Thiamine
subside day 4 or 5   (100 mg IM x 3 days)

Anxiety   Physical exam

Malaise   Multiple vitamins

A.N.S dysfunction   Food and rest

Insomnia

Convulsions

O.B.S.   Depressant drugs

Hallucinations (visual or tactile)

Figure 4.1. Alcohol detoxification. Abbreviations: (IM) intramuscular; (A.N.S.) autonomic nervous system; (O.B.S.) organic brain syndrome. From Schuckit.[71] Copyright 1979. Reprinted with permission of the McGraw-Hill Book Company.

holism or demonstrates a tremor and gives a history of alcohol misuse, the possibility of withdrawal must be carefully considered.

4.2.6.1.2. Physical Signs and Symptoms

Some 95% of alcoholics never evidence severe signs of withdrawal.[1] Several recent studies have documented the incidence of various types of symptoms among consecutive series of male and female alcoholics entering treatment. These evaluations, showing the predominance of mild physical symptoms, revealed that approximately one half or more of patients may evidence some level of autonomic nervous system (ANS) dysfunction, including sweating, an increase in heart rate, increases in respiratory rate, and mild elevations in temperature.[25,26] Also seen in half or more were signs of increased deep tendon reflex activity and tremor. Gastrointestinal (GI) symptoms including anorexia or nausea and vomiting were seen in one third to one half, while emotional complaints including sadness and psychosomatic symptoms were seen in 75% or more.[25]

The most common of the more severe, rarer alcohol withdrawal symptoms are hallucinations and grand mal seizures, seen in, respectively, only 5 and 1–4% of a consecutive series of alcoholic inpatients in the two surveys.[25,26] In fact, full-blown delirium tremens (DTs), characterized by severe ANS dysfunction, confusion, and the possible concomitance of seizures, is reported for fewer than 1% of patients, with some studies indicating an incidence of less than 0.1%, or 1 in 1000 patients.[25,27,28] Consistent with this information is the recently reported mortality rate of less than 1 in 500 patients during alcoholic withdrawal.[29]

Because alcohol is a brain depressant with a relatively short half-life, the acute and usually mild withdrawal syndrome begins within 12 hours or less of the decrease in blood-alcohol levels; symptoms are likely to peak in intensity by 48–72 hours and are usually greatly reduced by 4–5 days. While it is this primary withdrawal syndrome that is the focus of treatment, it is also important to recognize that, as discussed in Section 4.2.1., mild levels of anxiety, insomnia, and perhaps ANS dysfunction (secondary abstinence) are likely to continue for many months. Although the etiology of alcoholic withdrawal is not totally understood, it has been definitely established that it depends on the direct effects of alcohol.[28] However, the severity of the symptoms also may relate to the level of acidosis reached or to either direct or indirect disturbances in the electrolytes, including magnesium.

4.2.6.1.3. Psychological State

This is as dramatic as the physical problems and consists of nervousness, a feeling of decreased self-worth, and a high drive to continue drinking. For the 5% or so mentioned above, it can include an obvious OBS or hallucinations.

4.2.6.1.4. Relevant Laboratory Tests

There are no laboratory tests that are pathognomonic for alcoholic withdrawal. For an individual entering an abstinence syndrome, however, it is necessary to rule out all serious physical problems. Thus, it is important to perform an adequate neurological examination, to determine the cardiac status through an EKG, and to do any of the relevant laboratory procedures outlined in Table 1.5. Abnormalities in liver and kidney function, as well as in glucose levels, should be monitored throughout withdrawal. They can be expected to return to normal within a week in most individuals, unless there has been serious permanent damage to the relevant organs.

4.2.6.2. Treatment

The treatment of acute withdrawal is dictated by the probable etiological mechanisms as well as the usual symptomatology. The number of variations in therapeutic approaches reflects the relatively mild nature of most withdrawal syndromes as well as the need to balance cost and efficacy. While the comments offered below are based on clinical trials whenever possible, the relatively large number of therapeutic evaluations for alcoholic withdrawal since 1954 includes only a small percentage (about one third) that incorporate random controls, and even these more sophisticated studies often had important deficiencies.[29]

Treatment for alcoholic withdrawal can be artibrarily divided into the steps described in Sections 4.2.6.2.1–4.2.6.2.6.

4.2.6.2.1. Physical Examination

In recognition of the increased risk for medical problems among alcoholics, a thorough physical examination is an essential first step in the treatment of alcoholic withdrawal. Special emphasis must be placed on searching for evidence of cardiac arrhythmias or heart failure, the possibility of upper or lower GI bleeding; infections, including pneumonias; problems with liver failure or associated ascites; or neurological impairment, including peripheral neuropathies.

In alcoholics who otherwise appear relatively healthy, dehydration is relatively uncommon, and there is evidence that overhydration may exist.[30] Therefore, in the absence of severe or prolonged vomiting, bleeding, or significant failure of other systems, oral fluids, not IV infusions, should be used.

4.2.6.2.2. Vitamins and Minerals

Alcohol is absorbed primarily from the proximal small intestine, the site of absorption of many vitamins. Because of direct interference with absorption as well as increased excretion of these nutrients, even apparently well-nourished alcoholics are assumed to be possibly deficient in folic acid, thiamine, and possibly niacin. In the absence of stigmata of severe vitamin deficiencies, these problems are usually easily corrected with oral multiple vitamins given for a period of weeks, making sure that folic acid and thiamine are included.

There is also a need to at least consider administration of multiple vitamins that contain minerals as well. For example, in the presence of alcoholism, a relatively mild zinc deficiency can develop with associated decreased sexual functioning, decreased night vision, altered protein metabolism, diarrhea, skin lesions, and a decrease in mental functioning.[31] It has also been reported that some alcoholics might develop deficiencies in magnesium and others might present with decreased body stores of vitamin D.[32,33] However as discussed in the next section, it is not clear that there is a need for more supplementation than can be offered with multiple vitamins.

4.2.6.2.3. Nonpharmacological Approaches to Treating Withdrawal

All detoxification programs offer numerous general supports. These include a physical evaluation and reality-orientation techniques for patients showing mild levels of confusion, as well as the opportunity for sleep and adequate nutrition.[26,34] Taking advantage of the usual mild nature of the withdrawal syndrome and the probable rapid recovery, a number of programs have evaluated the response of patients treated with these general supports alone, without additional medications. Estimates from various programs indicate that 75% or more of detoxification patients improve markedly with this "social model" or "nonmedicinal" treatment regimen.[34−36]

Of course, with treatment limited to these general supports, some physiological symptoms of withdrawal are likely to appear, but the patient's level of comfort can still improve. Not all patients will do well, however. In one series of 1024 patients, 8% had to be referred to an emergency room from a social-model detoxification center, including 2.5% of the total who required inpatient admission.[26] Other studies indicate that the combined risk for convulsions, confusion, and hallucinations requiring some intense intervention is about 5% of alcoholics.[36]

Treatment personnel and legislators are thus faced with some choices. Social-model treatment approaches that do not use medications can save a great deal of money. This comes from the decreased need for physicians and nurses, the savings on the cost of medications, the possible shorter inpatient stay, and the absence of drug side effects for patients.[26] To be optimally effective, however, these programs need close medical backup so that patients who demonstrate medical problems, severe confusion, or convulsions can be properly treated and evaluated. It is also important that no matter what the basic approach, all patients be given a physical examination.

4.2.6.2.4. Medications for the General Treatment of Withdrawal

Medications are used to decrease overall symptoms (especially ANS dysfunction), increase levels of comfort, and decrease the risk for convulsions and DTs. The treatments discussed in this section assume that the patient has not already developed severe levels of confusion and agitation, because, unfortunately, a pharmacological therapy for DTs has not been fully established.

Theoretically, brain-depressant withdrawal syndromes occur because physical addiction has developed and the drug was decreased too quickly. Thus, reinstitution of the specific drug of abuse or any drug with cross-tolerance (e.g., other brain depressants) should help ameliorate symptoms. There are indications that any brain depressant, including barbiturates, chloral hydrate, paraldehyde, and the benzodiazepines, can help alcoholics during withdrawal. If they all work, the choice rests mostly with considerations of safety.

Almost all reviews of alcoholic withdrawal agree that the optimal medicinal treatment utilizes the *benzodiazepines* (Bz's).[37] Bz's are less likely to cause neurotoxicity when injected IM, less likely to cause severe decreases in respiratory rate or hypotension, and can be administered without causing discomfort to other patients through a disagreeable smell. Even with the use of rigorous evaluation criteria,[29] the Bz's are the only medications consistently demonstrated by controlled trials to be superior to placebo in treating alcoholic withdrawal. As a result, when the clinician decides that pharmacological therapies should be added to general supportive care, the treatment of choice is a Bz.

Within this class of medications, one can select either a longer-acting drug, such as diazepam (Valium) or chlordiazepoxide (Librium), or a shorter-acting Bz such as oxazepam (Serax) or lorazepam (Ativan). An asset of the longer-acting drugs in their relatively smooth withdrawal, because, reflecting the long half-life, drug blood levels decrease slowly over time. Therefore, it is not necessary to be certain that medications are administered every 4 hours, and it is likely that drugs can be decreased rapidly after the first 24–48 hours. The dangers of the longer-acting drugs, however, include the problem of exaggerated drug accumulation in individuals with clinically significant liver impairment and the probability that if the clinician is not careful, the buildup of the drug can cause severe lethargy, drowsiness, and ataxia.[38] On the other hand, the shorter-acting drugs, while safer in severe liver disease and less likely to accumulate, have their own problems in that doses must be given every 4 hours for fear that falling Bz blood levels might add to the preexisting alcoholic withdrawal syndrome and even precipitate seizures.

The recommended compromise takes advantage of the assets and liabilities of both long-acting and short-acting drugs. Short-acting Bz's should be reserved for patients with evidence of actual liver failure or those in whom cognition is severely impaired at the time therapy is begun. For the average alcoholic going through withdrawal, longer-acting drugs should be used, the needed dose being determined on Day 1 and then decreased by 20% of the Day 1 dose with each subsequent 24 hours—i.e. stopping the drug by Day 4 or 5. In addition to the rapid tapering of drugs, an important safeguard is to skip the dose when the patient is lethargic or asleep.

For example, chlordiazepoxide can be begun as 25 mg by mouth [PO (Latin *per os*)] (this drug is not well absorbed IM) given four times a day (QID), with an additional 25-mg dose on Day 1 if needed because of increased tremor or other signs of ANS dysfunction. This establishes the dose on Day 1, which is then subsequently cut to zero over the next 4–5 days. Sellers and colleagues offer a similar approach using diazepam.[38] In their approach, Day 1 symptoms are treated with 20 mg of diazepam by mouth every 2 hours up to a maximum of 100 mg. This dosage is subsequently decreased by 25–50% over the following several days.[38,39]

While fewer data are available, other authors have suggested *alternative possible medicinal approaches* to treating alcoholic withdrawal. The most promising of these approaches are directed specifically at the ANS dysfunction and include the alpha-adrenergic agonists such as clonidine (Catapres) or lofexidine or beta-blockers such as propranolol (Inderol) and atenolol (Tenormin). The beta-blockers decrease symptoms of tremor, fast heart rate, and hypertension, but probably do little to address the anxiety and drug craving or the propensity to seizures.[40] These drugs have the additional problem of possibly masking withdrawal symptoms that might be monitored in an attempt to avoid seizures or DTs.[41] The profile of effects for alpha-adrenergic agonists during alcoholic withdrawal is similar, with good evidence for control of blood pressure and other ANS functions, but fewer data supporting effects on sleep, craving, or the propensity to seizures.[42-44] Despite the drawbacks, these two groups of drugs, as well as some others, deserve further evaluation as possible treatments for the alcoholic withdrawal syndrome.[40,45]

The same optimism cannot be expressed for a variety of other drugs that have been proposed for the treatment of alcoholic withdrawal. Antipsychotic medications (or major tranquilizers) such as haloperidol (Haldol) and chlorpromazine (Thorazine) could theoretically help produce sedation, but their mechanisms of action are not hypothesized to directly affect withdrawal symptoms. These drugs also carry the potential problem of increasing the risk for seizures, and there is no evidence that their routine use in alcoholic withdrawal is effective or that the benefits are greater than the potential dangers, which include acute and chronic movement disorders.[46] A second, somewhat related drug, hydroxyzine (Atarax), has also been suggested for the treatment of withdrawal, but this medication has been shown by at least one controlled trial to be less effective and more likely to be associated with DTs or convulsions than are the Bz's.[47,48] A number of other agents have been suggested, including several antidepressants, with no evidence of efficacy.[49]

Finally, the 1–4% prevalence of seizures during withdrawal raises the question of whether anticonvulsant medications should be added to the Bz's. While more research is required, the data to date do not indicate that anticonvulsants are needed for the treatment of the average alcoholic going through withdrawal, except for patients with evidence of an independent seizure disorder.[38] Neither observations of animal withdrawal seizures nor human clinical trials support the probability that phenytoin (Dilantin) adds significant seizure protection above that given by adequate treatment with Bz's alone.[37,38,50–53] Nor is there evidence to date to justify the addition of carbamazepine (Tegretol) or valproic acid, and controlled studies do not support the need for magnesium sulfate in addition to a Bz.[54,55]

In summary, the pharmacological treatments of choice for alcoholic withdrawal are the Bz's. Preliminary data support the possible usefulness of alpha-adrenergic agonists and beta-blockers, but more studies are required before these drugs will be prescribed in clinical situations. To date, no other drugs are justified in routine alcoholic withdrawal treatment.

4.2.6.2.5. Optimal Setting for the Treatment of Mild to Moderate Withdrawal

Common sense dictates that the most thorough physical examination, greatest opportunity for close observation, and largest number of treatment options are provided by supervision of withdrawal in an inpatient treatment setting. On the other hand, the rising cost of inpatient care would result in a rapid consumption of the limited monies available for treatment if all alcoholics were detoxified in a hospital. Because of the usual mild nature of the withdrawal syndrome, many public administrators and legislators have opted to establish a series of levels of care ranging from outpatient to "social-model" detoxification facilities to inpatient care when needed.

Feldman *et al.* were among the first to recommend outpatient detoxification.[56,57] As described more recently by several authors [56,57], the plan calls for a careful physical examination and gathering of a past history to exclude individuals with signs of impending severe withdrawal, histories of severe withdrawal seizures in the past, or those with medical or psychiatric symptoms that might impair their ability to function outside the hospital. The latter include severe and suicidal depression, confusion, and evidence of psychotic symptoms without insight. In our own outpatient setting, the remaining individuals—or preferably their "significant others"—are given a 1- to 2-day supply of a Bz for the alcoholic (e.g., four to six 25-mg tablets of chlordiazepoxide), and the patient is offered the opportunity of spending part of the day at the rehabilitation center as an outpatient (perhaps participating in lectures or groups) and asked to return daily over the next 3–5 days for a readjustment of medications and brief physical evaluation centering on ANS functioning. He is warned to visit the emergency room if symptoms of withdrawal rapidly escalate, and a drug dose is to be omitted if the patient is sleepy or lethargic.

Social-model detoxification centers incorporate much of the same philosophy, but offer greater day and night supervision. In a setting of this type, patients are screened for medical problems, those severely ill are referred to an emergency room or an inpatient program for any needed Bz's and other self-medications, and all participants are given good nutrition, vitamins, and a place to sleep. The general atmosphere is one of reassurance, and patients are encouraged to stay for 3 or 4 days. In all settings, it is important to introduce patients to the available rehabilitation programs.

4.2.6.2.6. Treatment of Delirium Tremens (DTs)

The literature is not clear on the optimal treatment for full-blown DTs.[58] Fortunately, this serious medical syndrome, characterized by severe confusion and agitation (i.e., delirium) along with hallucinations and delusions (which can be seen in any type of delirium) and ANS dysfunction, is relatively rare. The first and potentially most important step in treatment is to carry out a thorough physical examination, because the stresses of DTs added to a preexisting medical problem can have lethal consequences. The second step in care involves the usual general supportive measures (using IV fluids carefully if there is objective evidence of dehydration) as well as the prescription of multiple vitamins including thiamine and folic acid as described in Section 4.2.6.2.2.

Finally, the optimal pharmacological treatment of this syndrome has not been established, and it is not clear that any medication will shorten the usual 3- to 5-day course. Some clinicians recommend using Bz's, sometimes in high doses (e.g., 200 mg or more of chlordiazepoxide per day) to control behavior, with the major goal of theoretically decreasing the number of individuals who will develop seizures while sedating patients so that they are less dangerous to themselves and to those around them. Other clinicians, fearing the possible excessive sedation and hypotension that could be expected with the high levels of Bz's that can be required for DTs, recommend antipsychotic drugs such as haloperidol (Haldol). This group of medications might actually lower the seizure threshold and, at least theoretically, would have no major direct effect on CNS-depressant withdrawal syndromes, but can be used in doses titrated to decrease agitation, wandering about the ward, and threats to other patients. It is hoped that future years will bring careful and deliberate studies of DTs so that more specific treatment guidelines can be offered.

4.2.7. Medical Problems

The deleterious effects of alcohol on alcoholics are so ubiquitous that it is impossible to discuss adequately all the resulting medical conditions in this short handbook. One is faced with recognition of the complications described in Section 3.2.2.

It is also important to consider alcohol-induced complications in *nonalcoholics* with chronic disorders. Examples include the increased chance of bleeding in individuals with ulcer disease, respiratory depression in people with emphysema, the adverse effects of alcohol on the livers of people with infectious hepatitis, the interference with normal pancreatic functioning in those who already have pancreatitis, the deterioration in sugar metabolism that might adversely affect diabetics, and the impairment of cardiac functioning in individuals with heart disease.[2,59]

Alcohol also adversely affects the metabolism and the efficacy of a wide variety of medications, including potentiation of the adverse effects of analgesics, adverse interactions with antidepressants, and interference with the proper actions of all psychotropic medications.[15,60] The problems extend to antihypertensive drugs, as alcohol may potentiate orthostatic drops in blood pressure, and to hypoglycemic agents and anticoagulants because of the induction of liver metabolic enzymes.

4.2.8. Other Problems

4.2.8.1. Alcohol Idiosyncratic Intoxication (291.40 in DSM-III-R)

4.2.8.1.1. Clinical Picture

This syndrome (which is probably both overdiagnosed and understudied) consists of the development of violent behavior at low doses of alcohol, usually followed by exhaustion and amnesia for the episode.[61,62] Although this diagnosis may be included as part of a legal defense for individuals who commit violent acts under the influence of ethanol, it is a relatively rare phenomenon and is seen primarily in individuals with evidence of organic brain damage.

4.2.8.1.2. Treatment

Although no specific treatment regimen has been worked out, there are a number of commonsense suggestions.

1. The patient should be evaluated for a CNS epileptic focus, especially temporal-lobe epilepsy.

2. Treatment in the midst of an episode is symptomatic and involves firm attempts to control behavior, such as using antipsychotics [such as haloperidol (e.g., 5 mg IM)], which may be repeated in 1 hour, if necessary.

3. All patients with this picture should be warned to abstain from drinking or at least to avoid alcohol when they are tired, hungry, or under stress. They should be told that they are legally responsible for violent acts committed after voluntarily imbibing ethanol.

4.2.8.2. Fetal Alcohol Syndrome (FAS)

4.2.8.2.1. Clinical Picture

This syndrome consists of a combination of any of a number of components, including multiple spontaneous abortions; a baby with a low birth weight for gestational stage (a smaller size that is never "caught up"); malformations in facial structure, including shortened palpebral fissures, a flattened bridge of the nose, and an absent philtrum; ventricular septal defects of the heart; malformations of the hands and feet (especially syndactyly); and levels of mental retardation that may be mild or moderately severe. Problems in behavior and learning are also likely to persist at least into later childhood.[63,64] The amount of ethanol involved, the timing of the drinking, the possible role of associated nutritional deficiencies, and other aspects of the clinical situation required to produce the fetal alcohol syndrome (FAS) are unknown.[65,66]

The exact role of alcohol in producing specific impairment in the developing fetus has not been conclusively proved, nor is it certain whether alcohol's effect on sperm from alcoholic fathers contributes to these phenomena.[67,68] However, the information available to date favors either a direct or an indirect role of alcohol in problems in fetal development.[69] First, there is ample evidence, described in Section 3.2.2, that alcohol is capable of causing bodily damage in almost all systems, including the heart, the muscles, and the nervous system. Second, ethanol and acetaldehyde [the first breakdown product of ethanol (see Section 3.2.4)] readily cross to the fetus. Third, the developing baby does not have efficient alcohol- or acetaldehyde-metabolizing systems, and the result is that these substances are likely to stay with the baby over an extended period of time.[70] Thus, the clinical observations of the possibility of an FAS along with this theoretical information are enough to convince most prudent parents that it is unwise for pregnant women to drink excessively, and as is true of all substances, it is probably safest for them to take no alcohol at all.

4.2.8.2.2. Treatment

The only treatment is prevention. Women should be advised not to drink at any time during pregnancy or, if they must drink, to keep their alcohol intake as low as possible.

REFERENCES

1. Schuckit, M. A. Overview: Epidemiology of alcoholism. In M. A. Schuckit (Ed.), *Alcohol Patterns and Problems*. New Brunswick, New Jersey: Rutgers University Press, 1985, pp. 1–41.
2. Schuckit, M. A. Alcohol and alcoholism: An introduction for the health care specialist. *Emergency Product News 8(5):*26–30, 1976.
3. De Soto, D. B., O'Donnell, W. E., Allred, L. J., & Lopes, C. E. Symptomatology in alcoholics at various stages of abstinence. *Alcoholism: Clinical and Experimental Research 9:*505–512, 1985.
4. Roelofs, S. M. F. J. Hyperventilation, anxiety, craving for alcohol: A subacute alcohol withdrawal syndrome. *Alcohol 2:*501–505, 1985.
5. Wellman, M. The late withdrawal symptoms of alcohol addiction. *Canadian Medical Association Journal 70:*526–529, 1954.
6. Vaillant, G. E., & Milofsky, E. The etiology of alcoholism: A prospective viewpoint. *American Psychology 37:*494–504, 1982.
7. Schuckit, M. A., Irwin, M., & Brown, S. The history of anxiety symptoms among 171 primary alcoholics. *Journal of Studies on Alcohol* (in press).
8. Liljeberg, P., Mossberg, D., & Borg, S. Clinical conditions and central noradrenergic activity in alcoholics during longterm abstinence. Paper presented at the International Society for Biomedical Research on Alcoholism Annual Meeting, Helsinki, June 10, 1986.

9. Schuckit, M. A. Anxiety treatment: A commonsense approach. *Postgraduate Medicine 75:*52–63, 1984.

10. Perper, J. A. Sudden, unexpected death in alcoholics. *Alcohol Health and Research World, Fall:*18–24, 1975.

11. Lowenstein, L. M., Simone, R., Boulter, P., *et al.* Effect of fructose on alcohol concentrations in the blood in man. *Journal of the American Medical Association 213:*1899–1902, 1970.

12. Von Wartburg, J.-P. Comparison of alcohol metabolism in humans and animals. In K. Eriksson, J. D. Sinclair, & K. Kiianmaa (Eds.), *Animal Models in Alcohol Research,* London: Academic Press, 1980.

13. Levine, A. S., Hess, S., & Morley, J. E. Alcohol and the opiate receptor. *Alcoholism: Clinical and Experimental Research 7:*83–84, 1983.

14. Victor, M., & Hope, J. M. The phenomenon of auditory hallucinations in chronic alcoholism: A critical evaluation of the status of alcoholic hallucinosis. *Archives of General Psychiatry 126:*451–481, 1955.

15. Schuckit, M. A. Alcoholism and other psychiatric disorders. *Hospital and Community Psychiatry 34:*1022–1027, 1983.

16. Schuckit, M. A. The history of psychotic symptoms in alcoholics. *Journal of Clinical Psychiatry 43:*53–57, 1982.

17. Schuckit, M. A. Genetic and clinical implications of alcoholism and affective disorder. *American Journal of Psychiatry 143:*140–147, 1986.

18. Frances, R. J., Franklin, J., & Flavin, D. K. Suicide and alcoholism. *American Journal of Drug and Alcohol Abuse 13:*327–341, 1987.

19. Grant, I., Reed, R., & Adams, K. M. Diagnosis of intermediate-duration and subacute organic mental disorders in abstinent alcoholics. *Journal of Clinical Psychiatry 48:*319–323, 1987.

20. Hughes, T. P., & Jackson, J. B. C. Neuronal loss in hippocampus induced by prolonged ethanol consumption in rats. *Science 209:*711–713, 1980.

21. Blass, J. P., & Gibson, C. E. Abnormality of a thiamine-requiring enzyme in patients with Wernicke–Korsakoff syndrome. *New England Journal of Medicine 297:*1367–1370, 1977.

22. Mukherjee, A. B., Svoronos, S., Ghazanfari, A., *et al.* Transketolase abnormality in cultured fibroblasts from familial chronic alcoholic men and their male offspring. *Journal of Clinical Investigations 79:*1039–1043, 1987.

23. Victor, M., Adams, R. D., & Collins, G. H. *The Wernicke–Korsakoff Syndrome.* Philadelphia: Davis, 1971.

24. Parsons, O. A., Butters, N., & Nathan, P. E. *Neuropsychology of Alcoholism.* New York: Guilford Press, 1987.

25. Olbrich, R. Alcohol withdrawal states and the need for treatment. *British Journal of Psychiatry 134:*466–469, 1979.

26. Whitfield, C. L., Thompson, G., & Lamb, A. Detoxification of 1,024 alcoholic patients without psychoactive drugs. *Journal of the American Medical Association 239:*1409–1410, 1978.

27. Cheshdedjiev, P., & Atanassov, V. Prophylaxis of the actue psychotic complications in chronic alcoholic cases and the role of the withdrawal syndrome in their genesis. *Alcoholism 8:*107–109, 1972.

28. Ng, S. K., Hauser, A., Burst, J. C., *et al.* Alcohol consumption and withdrawal in new-onset seizures. *New England Journal of Medicine 319:*666–673, 1988.

29. Moskowitz, G., Chaimers, T. C., & Sacks, H. S. Deficiencies of clinical trials of alcohol withdrawal. *Alcoholism: Clinical and Experimental Research 7:*42–46, 1983.

30. Knott, D. H., & Beard, J. D. A diuretic approach to acute withdrawal from alcohol. *Southern Medical Journal 62:*485–488, 1969.

31. McClain, C. J., Antonow, D. R., Cohen, D. A., & Shedlofsky, S. I. Zinc metabolism in alcoholic liver disease. *Alcoholism: Clinical and Experimental Research 10:*582–589, 1986.

32. Flink, E. B. Magnesium deficiency in alcoholism. *Alcoholism: Clinical and Experimental Research 10:*590–594, 1986.

33. Gascon-Barre, M. Influence of chronic ethanol consumption on the metabolism and action of vitamin D. *Journal of the American College of Nutrition 4:*565–574, 1985.

34. Naranjo, C. A., Sellers, E. M., & Chater, M. Nonpharmacologic intervention in acute alcohol withdrawal. *Clinical Pharmacology and Therapeutics 34*:814–819, 1983.
35. Talbott, G. D. Treatment of the alcohol withdrawal syndrome: A new approach. *Maryland State Medical Journal 25*:30–32, 1976.
36. Shaw, J. M., Kliesar, G. S., & Sellers, E. M. Development of optimal treatment tactics for alcohol withdrawal: Assessment and effectiveness of supportive care. *Journal of Clinical Psychopharmacology 1*:382–389, 1981.
37. Liskow, B. I., & Goodwin, D. W. Pharmacological treatment of alcohol intoxication, withdrawal, and dependence: A critical review. *Journal of Studies on Alcohol 48*:356–370, 1987.
38. Sellers, E. M., & Naranjo, C. A. New strategies for the treatment of alcohol withdrawal. *Psychopharmacology Bulletin 22*:88–92, 1986.
39. Sellers, E. M., & Kalant, H. Drug therapy: Alcohol intoxication and withdrawal. *New England Journal of Medicine 294*:757–762, 1978.
40. Kraus, M. I., Gottleib, L. D., & Horwitz, R. I. Randomized clinical trial of atenolol in patients with alcohol withdrawal. *New England Journal of Medicine 313*:905–909, 1985.
41. Zechnich, R. J. Beta blockers can obscure diagnosis of delirium tremens. *Lancet 1*:1071–1072, 1982.
42. Baumgartner, G. R., & Rowen, R. C. Clonidine vs. chlordiazepoxide in the management of acute alcohol withdrawal syndrome. *Archives of Internal Medicine 147*:1223–1226, 1987.
43. Schuckit, M. Clonidine and the treatment of withdrawal. *Drug Abuse and Alcoholism Newsletter 17*(3):1–4, 1988.
44. Nutt, D., Glue, P., Molyneux, S., & Clark, E. α-2-Adenoceptor function in alcohol withdrawal: A pilot study of the effects of IV clonidine in alcoholics and normals. *Alcoholism: Clinical and Experimental Research 12*:14–18, 1988.
45. Sellers, E. M., & Naranjo, C. A. Strategies for improving the treatment of alcohol withdrawal. In C. A. Naranjo & E. M. Sellers (Eds.), *Research Advances in New Pharmacological Treatments for Alcoholism*. New York: Elsevier, 1985, pp. 157–170.
46. Palestine, M. L., & Alatoree, E. Control of acute alcohol withdrawal symptoms: A comparative study of haloperidol and chlordiazepoxide. *Current Therapeutic Research, Clinical and Experimental 20*:289–299, 1976.
47. Wilbur, R., & Kilik, F. A. Anticonvulsant drugs in alcohol withdrawal: Use of phenytoin, primidone, carbamazepine, valproic acid, and the sedative anticonvulsants. *American Journal of Hospital Pharmacology 38*:1138–1143, 1981.
48. Dilts, D. L., Keleher, D. L., & Hoge, G. Hydroxyzine in the treatment of alcohol withdrawal. *American Journal of Psychiatry 134*:92–93, 1977.
49. Solorzano, L., Keller, J., & Kaplan, H. L. Selectivity of drug action in ethanol withdrawal. Paper presented at the American Society of Clinical Pharmacology and Therapeutics Annual Meeting, New York, April 4, 1984.
50. Sellers, E. M., Naranjo, C. A., & Harrison, M. Diazepam loading: Simplified treatment of alcohol withdrawal. *Clinical Pharmacology and Therapeutics 34*:822–826, 1983.
51. Devenyi, P., & Harrison, M. L. Prevention of alcohol withdrawal seizures with oral diazepam loading. *Canadian Medical Association Journal 132*:798–800, 1985.
52. Donat, D. J., Kaplan, H. L., & Sellers, E. M. Phenytoin is not needed in ethanol withdrawal. Paper presented at the American Society for Clinical Pharmacology and Therapeutics Annual Meeting, New York, April 4, 1984.
53. Sandor, P., Sellers, E. M., & Dumbrell, M. Effect of short- and long-term alcohol use on phenytoin kinetics in chronic alcoholics. *Clinical Pharmacology and Therapeutics 30*:390–397, 1981.
54. Butler, D., & Messiha, F. S. Alcohol withdrawal and carbamazepine. *Alcohol 3*:113–129, 1986.
55. Wilson, A., & Vulcano, B. A double-blind, placebo-controlled trial of magnesium sulfate in the ethanol withdrawal syndrome. *Alcoholism: Clinical and Experimental Research 8*:542–545, 1984.
56. Alterman, A. Hayashida, M., & O'Brien, C. Treatment response and safety of ambulatory medical detoxification. *Journal of Studies of Alcohol 49*:160–166, 1988.

57. Webb, M., & Unwin, A. The outcome of outpatient withdrawal from alcohol. *British Journal of Addiction 83:*929–934, 1988.
58. Nordstrom, G., & Bergland, M. Delirium tremens. *Journal of Studies of Alcohol 49:*178–185, 1988.
59. Criqui, M. H. Alcohol consumption, blood pressure, lipids, and cardiovascular mortality. *Alcoholism: Clinical and Experimental Research 10:*564–569, 1986.
60. Ciraulo, D. A., Barnhill, J. G., Boxenbaum, H. G., & Jaffe, J. H. Antidepressant pharmacokinetics in alcoholics. Paper presented at the American Psychiatric Association Annual Meeting, Washington, D.C., May 5, 1986.
61. Coid, J. Mania à potu: A critical review of pathological intoxication. *Psychological Medicine 9:*709–719, 1979.
62. Maletzky, B. M. The diagnosis of pathological intoxication. *Journal of Studies on Alcohol 37(9):*1215–1228, 1976.
63. Streissguth, A. P., Barr, H. M., Sampson, P. D., J. C., et al. Attention, distraction and reaction time at age 7 years and prenatal alcohol exposure. *Neurobehavioral Toxicology and Teratology 8:*717–725, 1986.
64. Morrow-Tlucak, M., & Ernhart, D. B. Maternal prenatal substance use and behavior at age 3 years. *Alcoholism: Clinical and Experimental Research 11:*225, 1987.
65. United States Department of Health and Human Services. *Sixth Special Report on Alcohol and Health.* Rockville, Maryland: DHHS Publication (ADM) 87-1519, 1987, pp. 80–96.
66. Little, R., & Sing, C. Father's drinking and infant birth weigtt. *Teratology 36:*59–65, 1987.
67. Friedler, G.: Paternal exposure to opioids and ethanol: Effects on offspring. Paper presented at the Committee on Problems of Drug Dependence 49th Annual Meeting, Philadelphia, June 14–18, 1987.
68. Abel, E. L., & Moore, C. Effects of paternal alcohol consumption in mice. *Alcoholism: Clinical and Experimental Research 11:*533–535, 1987.
69. Pierce, D. R., & West, J. R. Blood alcohol concentration: A critical factor for producing fetal alcohol effects. *Alcohol 3:*269–272, 1986.
70. Schuckit, M. A. Acetaldehyde and alcoholism: Methodology. In V. Hesselbrock, E. Shaskan, & R. Meyer (Eds.), *Biological and Genetic Markers of Alcoholism.* Washington, D.C.: National Institute on Alcohol Abuse and Alcoholism, U.S. Government Printing Office, 1984, pp. 23–48.
71. Schuckit, M. A. Inpatient and residential treatments of alcoholism. In J. H. Mendelson & N. K. Mello (Eds.), *Diagnosis and Treatment of Alcoholism.* New York: McGraw-Hill, 1979, pp. 325–354.

Stimulants—Including Cocaine

5.1. INTRODUCTION

Stimulants are widely prescribed and greatly misused medications that have very limited bona fide medical uses. It is important that the clinician know these drugs well, as their misuse can mimic a variety of medical and psychiatric syndromes.

Nonmedicinal use of stimulants has occurred for many centuries, beginning even before the discovery of coca leaves by natives of the Andes in their effort to decrease hunger and fatigue.[1,2] Cocaine itself was first isolated in Germany in 1857, and its local anesthetic properties were applied in ophthalmology in the 1880s.[3,4] Amphetamine was first synthesized in 1887, and its clinical properties were recognized in about 1930, but until the mid-1950s or early 1960s, stimulants were felt to be generally safe. These claims were made despite evidence of the widespread misuse of cocaine in Germany after World War I[5] and epidemics of the misuse of stimulants in Japan after World War II.[6-8]

5.1.1. Pharmacology (see Section 11.7.2 and Chapter 12)

5.1.1.1. General Characteristics and Background

The stimulants encompass a variety of drugs, including all forms of cocaine and amphetamines (some of which are listed in Table 5.1), that share the ability to stimulate the central nervous system (CNS) at many levels.[4] I will limit this discussion to those substances that are the most clinically important, avoiding other stimulants (such as strychnine) that are not usually abused. Two other important stimulants, nicotine and caffeine, are consumed in large amounts, but because of their relatively low potency, they are reserved for separate discussion in Chapter 12. Other more "exotic" drugs with marked stimulant properties are used in specific areas of the world and can produce the patterns of problems typical of stimulants in general. An example is khat, a stimulant used in leaf form in North Africa and Yemen and reported to be capable of inducing psychoses.[9,10]

In preparing this third edition, I considered allotting a separate chapter to cocaine. This reflects the epidemiological data cited below demonstrating that in its

Table 5.1
Some Commonly Abused Stimulants

Generic name	Trade name
Amphetamine	Benzedrine
Benzphetamine	Didrex
Caffeine	—
Chlorphentermine	Pre-Sate
Cocaine	—
Dextroamphetamine	Dexedrine
Diethylpropion	Tenuate, Tepanil
Fenfluramine	Pondimin[a]
Methamphetamine	Desoxyn, Fetamin
Methylphenidate	Ritalin
Phenmetrazine	Preludin
Phentermine	Ionamin, Wilpo

[a]This drug may be less likely to be reinforcing, as it has not been shown to be self-administered in animals.[33]

various forms, cocaine was one of the "fad" drugs of the last decade. While efforts are made to highlight information on this important substance in this chapter on stimulants, the clinical patterns of problems and the relevant treatment approaches are almost identical for cocaine and other stimulants such as amphetamines. Thus, a separate chapter on cocaine would have resulted in an unacceptable amount of interchapter redundancy.

As a group, the stimulants, including cocaine, work at least in part by causing the release of neurotransmitters (chemicals that stimulate neighboring neurons), such as norepinephrine (NE), from nerve cells. Some, in addition, mimic the functions of transmitters like NE through a direct effect on the nerve cells themselves.

The effects of cocaine occur through a variety of mechanisms, including the blocking of initiation or conduction of peripheral nerve impulses (contributing to its local anesthetic effect), direct stimulation of the CNS, and blockade of catecholamine uptake (NE more than epinephrine) at nerve terminals.[11,12] The acute effects of cocaine also produce a decrease in the reuptake of dopamine (DA) into the cells, with a resulting increase in the amount of DA in the synapse—the space between neurons. In other experiments, such changes in DA are associated with self-stimulatory behavior, repetitive stereotyped actions, hyperactivity, a decrease in appetite, and sexual excitation in animals.[11] It is likely that acute effects on DA are temporary and that subsequent cell feedback mechanisms actually result in a net decrease in this substance, even after relatively short periods of time. Also, there is evidence that receptors particularly sensitive to cocaine might be associated with DA-uptake inhibition.[13] Cocaine is also thought to affect the levels of another brain neurotransmitter, serotonin, with actions that appear to contribute to a decrease in this substance and its most prominent metabolite.[11,14]

Cocaine is sold "on the street" as an impure powder, most frequently being "cut" or expanded with glucose, lactose, and mannitol, with a resulting cocaine purity level of somewhere between 0 and 17% in the average street sample. Cocaine is well absorbed through all modes of administration,[12] but it is most often injected intravenously (IV) or "snorted" [intranasally (IN)]. For snorting, powder is arranged on a glass in thin lines, 3–5 cm long, each with approximately 25 mg of the active substance, which is then inhaled into the nostrils through a straw or rolled paper.[4] The "average" dose used by the usual nontolerant person is between 20 and 100 mg.[23]

Recently, the drug has been smoked on tobacco, although such use is inefficient, as cocaine sulfate has a melting point of almost 200°C.[15] As a result, cocaine "freebase" has been developed to lower the melting point to 98°C for use sprinkled over tobacco or smoked in special pipes. The freebase is produced by adding a strong base (e.g., buffered ammonia) to an aqueous solution of cocaine and then extracting the alkaline freebase precipitate.[16]

Similar changes in the salt structure have resulted in a crystallized form of cocaine known on the streets as "crack" or "rock." The relatively low melting point and the ready solubility of this form in water as well as the "new marketing techniques associated with its relatively novel form" appear to have contributed to the widespread use of this form of cocaine.[17] On the other hand, the predominant actions of cocaine are similar, no matter what the salt form. Thus, the same pattern of problems is likely to appear with "crack" or "rock" as is likely to be seen with "freebase" or other forms of cocaine, although due to the rapid onset and intense effects with smoking, crack may be particularly likely to precipitate psychoses.[18]

The blood levels of this CNS stimulant are fairly similar whether it is taken IV or IN, smoked, or taken orally,[19] although the half-life may differ with the different routes. Through most modes of administration, the peak blood levels develop rapidly (within 5–30 minutes). Most of the drug disappears over 2 hours (a half-life of approximately 1 hour), although some activity persists for 4 hours or longer.[20,21] The longest-lasting effects are probably seen after IN ingestion, as the active drug appears to remain in the nasal mucosa for 3 hours or longer, probably reflecting local constriction of the blood vessels.[21] The actual amount ingested varies with the purity of the preparation, but a cigarette can contain as much as 300 mg.[22] Most of the active drug is metabolized in the liver, but some is acted on by plasma esterases, and a small amount is excreted unchanged in the urine.[3,12] Cocaine does not disappear rapidly from the body, and traces are likely to be found in urine samples for 3 days or longer.[23]

Because of the high cost of coke on the streets, a number of cocaine "substitutes" (not truly related to cocaine itself) have been developed.[24,25] Some (e.g., "iceberg" and "snort") contain benzocaine and/or procaine, whereas others contain about 75 mg of caffeine (e.g., "cocaine snuff," "coca snow," and "incense") or other mild stimulants (e.g., "zoom"). The effects of these drugs would be expected to resemble those of caffeine, and the reader is referred to Chapter 12 for further information.

5.1.1.2. Predominant Effects

The most obvious actions of stimulants are on the CNS, the peripheral nervous system (outside the CNS), and the cardiovascular system. Clinically, the drugs cause euphoria, decrease fatigue and the need for sleep, may increase feelings of sexuality, interfere with normal sleep patterns, decrease appetite, increase energy, and tend to decrease the level of distractibility in children.[4] It would seem likely that the impairment of judgment and the psychological changes seen with stimulants might also pose problems in the operation of motor vehicles, although such problems have been difficult to document.[26,27]

Physically, the drugs produce a tremor of the hands, restlessness, and a rapid heart rate. Most of the substances have actions similar to those of amphetamine, although methamphetamine (Desoxyn) has fewer cardiac effects (especially at low doses) and methylphenidate (Ritalin) and phenmetrazine (Preludin) have lower levels of potency.[4] Cocaine is quite potent, having effects similar to those of IV amphetamine.[4,12,28]

If we use cocaine as an example, it is possible to look more closely at the predominant effects. The CNS actions show a biphasic response, lower doses tending to improve motor performance but higher doses causing a deterioration, with subsequent severe tremors and even convulsions.[3,12] Additional CNS effects include nausea and possible emesis, dilated pupils, and an increase in body temperature, probably reflecting both direct actions on the brain and indirect actions through muscle contractions.[12] Regarding the muscles, there is no evidence that cocaine produces an increase in strength, but there is a decrease in fatigue, probably mediated through CNS effects.[12] The cardiovascular results are also biphasic, smaller doses tending to produce a decrease in heart rate via actions on the vagus nerve, but higher doses producing both an increased heart rate and vasoconstriction, with a resulting elevation in blood pressure.[3,12] The actions on the heart may produce arrhythmias both directly through the effects of the drug and indirectly through catecholamine release.[12]

5.1.1.3. Tolerance and Dependence

5.1.1.3.1. Tolerance

Tolerance to stimulant drugs develops within hours to days. It is the result of *metabolic* tolerance [an alteration in drug distribution and metabolism perhaps related to increased acidity of the body (acidosis) or an increased rate of metabolism], *pharmacodynamic* tolerance (as exemplified by toleration of injections of up to 1 g of methamphetamine IV every 2 hours), and behavioral tolerance.[4,12,28] An additional example of pharmacodynamic tolerance is the demonstration that even when constant cocaine blood levels are maintained through an IV infusion, the euphoric effects tend to rapidly disappear, while the feelings of anxiety and heightened levels of energy remain throughout a 4-hour experiment.[29]

The topic of tolerance is especially important in relation to cocaine, for which a very rapid development of acute tolerance is noted. For example, both the euphoric and the cardiovascular manifestations of the substance diminish much more rapidly than the plasma levels.[4,30] The magnitude of the final level of tolerance may be quite large, as it has been reported that humans have taken up to 10 g of cocaine a day and monkeys have self-administered, after several days, doses that would have produced convulsions and cardiorespiratory complications in naive animals.[30,31] Although the metabolic tolerance noted for cocaine is high (the plasma half-life has been reported to decrease from 93 to 48 minutes with repeated administration in animals), pharmacodynamic and *behavioral* tolerance are also shown to be important.[30]

On the other hand, an important phenomenon of *reverse tolerance* can also be noted, demonstrating once again that drug actions vary with drug history and clinical circumstances. Some individuals show an increasing effect of repeated doses of the medications, perhaps related to a CNS process similar to enhanced cellular sensitivity or kindling.[32] Although there is a cross-tolerance between most of the stimulant drugs, it is not known whether it generalizes to cocaine.[4,12]

5.1.1.3.2. Physical Dependence

We are used to thinking of withdrawal symptoms as they relate to depressant and opiate drugs, expecting individuals to show anxiety, anorexia, loss of appetite, sleeplessness, and so on. As a result, there was a debate about whether actual physical withdrawal can be expected with stimulants. This debate was reflected in DSM-III, which did not list stimulant withdrawal.[33] However, most investigators and clinicians feel that such a syndrome exists. This syndrome is described in detail in Section 5.2.6.

5.1.1.4. Purported Medical Uses

This section and Table 5.2 are included to reinforce the fact that despite the claim that stimulants are effective for many medical disorders, in most instances the

Table 5.2
Purported Medical Uses of Stimulants

Use	Comment
Narcolepsy	A *rare* disorder that responds to other REM-supressing drugs as well.
Attention deficit disorder with hyperactivity	Very much overdiagnosed. Responds to stimulants or antidepressants.
Obesity	Stimulants result in *temporary relief.* Dangers far outweigh assets.
Fatigue	Rule out medical diseases or depression. Stimulants do not work.
Depression	Stimulants can make the picture worse.
Dysmenorrhea	No proven usefulness.

potential benefit *does not* outweigh the potential harm. This is true, at least in part, because of the rapid development of tolerance to stimulants, which seriously limits their ability to maintain a level of clinical usefulness.

Problems for which stimulants have been prescribed include those described in the following sections.

5.1.1.4.1. Narcolepsy

This disorder—characterized by falling asleep without warning, through the development of rapid-eye-movement (REM) or "dream-type" sleep at any time of the day or night—is associated with falling attacks (catalepsy). Stimulants can both modify and prevent attacks,[4] in part by decreasing REM sleep. However, narcolepsy may be a very rare disorder and should be diagnosed only with brain-wave or electroencephalographic (EEG) studies, and other REM-decreasing drugs are available, including most of the antidepressants. Stimulants should be used very carefully, if at all, for this disorder.

5.1.1.4.2. Attention Deficit Disorder with Hyperactivity (ADD-H)

This syndrome of children, and perhaps adults, is characterized by a short attention span and an inability to sit quietly, with resultant difficulty in learning, and may be associated with signs of minimal brain damage.[34] However, hyperactivity is a common reaction to stress in childhood, and the diagnosis should not rest solely with the rapid evolution of a symptom of overactivity, especially when it occurs in relationship to a life problem.[35] ADD-H, which appears before age 6, becomes much more incapacitating once school begins. For a person with a bona fide ADD-H, stimulants have been shown to be effective in decreasing symptomatology and in increasing the ability to learn. In addition, carefully prescribed medication does not predispose the child to go on to drug abuse.[35] This is probably the only disorder for which stimulants are the primary drug of choice, but alternate modes of pharmacotherapy, including antidepressants, are available.[36]

5.1.1.4.3. Obesity

Stimulants do decrease the appetite, but only temporarily, with activity lasting *at most* 3 or 4 weeks.[37] In almost all controlled investigations, weight lost while on stimulants reappears within a relatively short period of time after the drug is stopped. Thus, considering the abuse potential of these drugs, their use in weight reduction is contraindicated.

5.1.1.4.4. Other Problems

The stimulants have also been used for *fatigue, depression, menstrual pain* or *dysmenorrhea,* and some *neurological disorders.* Controlled studies have demonstrated that the drugs are not effective for these problems, and their potential dangers outweigh their usefulness.

5.1.2. Epidemiology and Patterns of Abuse

Enough stimulants are manufactured legally to give 50 doses each year to every man, woman, and child in the United States, with an estimated half of this amount finding its way into illegal channels.[38] This availability, when added to that of the drugs that enter the country illegally (e.g., cocaine) and other drugs coming from illegal manufacturing sources, allows for high levels of stimulant abuse.

Although the stimulants are extremely dangerous, their stimulating and euphoria-producing properties make them very appealing drugs. It has been estimated, for example, that in the late 1970s and early 1980s the major limiting factors in the abuse of cocaine in the United States were its high cost and limited availability. These drugs produce great levels of morbidity, with 15% of patients admitted to metropolitan psychiatric hospitals having traces of amphetamine in their urine.[6]

Precise figures on the pattern of abuse of stimulants including cocaine are not available, but these drugs are taken by members of all social strata. In recent years, much information has been published in professional journals as well as in the public press about the pattern of use of these substances. To minimize confusion in looking at this information, it is important to recognize that some data relate to whether an individual has ever used the substance, some describe use over the preceding 30 days (i.e., a measure of current involvement), while others present information on stimulant-related problems. Regarding stimulants in general, the marked increase in use of these substances observed during the 1970s and discussed in the second edition seems to have leveled off. For amphetamines, a series of surveys in Ontario, Canada, in 1979 showed that 9% of high school seniors had used these drugs at least once *over the preceding 12 months,* figures that increased to 23% by 1983, but then plateaued.[39,40] This general trend was corroborated in the United States, where about 20% of high school seniors had used amphetamines *at least once* at the time of the survey in 1982, with similar figures for young adults in general in 1983.[41,42]

A similar and equally impressive "fad" for increases and then leveling off in use of *cocaine* has also been reported in the 1970s and on into the early 1980s. As reported by the Canadian group, 4.1% of students in grades 7 to 13 had used cocaine in the early 1980s, with only a modest increase to 4.8% by 1985.[43] Focusing on high school seniors' current use (within the 30 days preceding the survey), the Canadian figures were 4% in 1979, 3% in 1981, and 4% to 5% in 1983,[39] figures similar to the United States use rate of 7% in 1985.[44-46]

Like abusers of CNS depressants, abusers of stimulants other than cocaine can be rather simplistically divided into those more middle-class individuals who obtain the drug on prescription from one or more physicians (medical abusers) and the predominantly young population who primarily misuse drugs obtained from street suppliers or friends (street abusers). Either group may use a given drug either singly or in an attempt to modify the effect of other substances, usually CNS depressants as described in Chapter 13. Stimulants also appear to be used more and more in middle-class social settings as part of an attempt to increase a party "high."

5.1.2.1. Medical Abusers

Medical abusers usually begin using the medications to reduce weight, to treat fatigue or menstrual cramps, to study for exams, or to aid in long-distance drives. The patient may get all the drug from one physician, attempting to obtain multiple or refillable prescriptions, or may receive simultaneous supplies from a variety of medical resources. In this setting, anecdotally, abuse tends to begin with a slow escalation of the dose, perhaps in response to the sadness, fatigue, and increased appetite that are seen when tolerance develops. Attempts to stop the medication result in fatigue and an increased need for sleep (hypersomnia), leading, in turn, to drug-dose escalation.

A related pattern of social abuse is seen in students, individuals working odd hours, truck drivers, and other people with abnormal sleep cycles or the need to get a big job done in a short period of time without much sleep. Under these circumstances, fatigue and depression secondary to the use of the stimulants are almost certain to develop, and some individuals also demonstrate paranoia, emotional lability, and even violence.

5.1.2.2. Street Abusers

The street abuser is attempting to achieve an altered state of consciousness by taking oral, IV, or inhaled drugs. In one pattern, the person chronically misuses the drug either singly or in combination with depressant medications. In another mode, the person initiates repeated periods of "runs" of amphetamines or cocaine,[47] taking the drug around the clock for 2–4 days. Problems with withdrawal and psychosis can occur with any method of drug administration and pattern, but are most likely to be seen with the IV method during a "run."

5.1.3. Establishing the Diagnosis

Any substance that so thoroughly mimics other medical and psychiatric emergencies and that is so readily available both on prescription and "on the street" must be considered part of the differential diagnosis in most psychiatric emergency room situations. As with the other drugs of abuse, one must have a high index of suspicion or the diagnosis will be missed.[1,35] Because it is important to gather a careful history from both the patient and any available resource person about the use of stimulant drugs, I ask each patient about his pattern of prescription and illegal drug-taking. I ask specifically about stimulants when an individual presents with any of the following problems:[48]

1. A restless, hyperalert state
2. An anxietylike attack (usually nervousness plus a rapid pulse)
3. A high level of emotional lability or irritability
4. Aggressive or violent outbursts
5. Paranoia or increased levels of suspiciousness[49]

6. Hallucinations, especially auditory or tactile (touch)
7. Confusion or an organic brain syndrome
8. Depression
9. Lethargy
10. Any evidence of IV drug use, such as needle marks or skin abscesses
11. Abnormalities in the nasal lining or mucosa such as might be expected with inhaling stimulants
12. Worn down teeth (from tooth grinding while intoxicated)

Also, in an emergency room, any individual presenting with *dilated pupils, increased heart rate, dry mouth, increased reflexes, elevated temperature, sweating* or *behavioral abnormalities* should be considered a possible stimulant-drug misuser. Under such circumstances, or if there is a hint of stimulants from either the patient or the family, it is a good idea to take blood or urine for a toxicological screen.

5.2. EMERGENCY PROBLEMS

Drug-induced psychiatric disturbances are probably more prevalent among abusers of CNS stimulants than among the users of any other type of drug.[48,50] The difficulties can include maniclike states, serious psychoses resembling schizophrenia, depressions almost identical to major affective disorders (especially during withdrawal), and panic states. These all tend to be transitory and disappear over a period of hours or days when the drug is stopped. The most frequently seen clinical problems associated with stimulant abuse are the panic reaction (frequently presenting as "pseudo-heart attack"), a temporary psychosis, and medical problems.[3,51] While DSM III-R lists cocaine and amphetamine problems separately, the clinical patterns are so similar that the two drugs are discussed together here.

5.2.1. Panic Reactions (e.g., 305.60 and 292.89 in DSM-III-R)

5.2.1.1. Clinical Picture (see Sections 1.6.1, 7.2.1, 8.2.1, and 14.2)

Stimulant drugs can give rise to at least two related forms of panic. In the first instance, the individual, even when taking stimulants in relatively "normal" doses, can experience a rapid heart rate, palpitations, anxiety, nervousness, and hyperventilation [the last resulting in altered blood carbon dioxide (CO_2) levels]. The subsequent chest pains, in combination with anxiety and palpitations as well as shortness of breath, can give the individual the feeling that he is having a heart attack.[1,52]

The second rather classic picture relates to the psychological anxiety and nervousness that can be associated with stimulants. In such instances, the individual may "panic," feeling that he is losing control or going crazy.

5.2.1.2. Treatment

Treatment involves careful evaluation to rule out medical or psychiatric disorders, reassurance, and time.

1. The patient should be evaluated for bona fide medical illness, including the possibility of a heart attack or hyperthyroidism.
2. A careful history should be taken to rule out preexisting psychiatric disorders, especially panic disorder or affective disorder.[48,53]
3. Blood (10 cc) should be drawn or a urine sample taken (50 ml) for toxicological tests.
4. If the first two points are negative, the patient should be told that his reaction is a result of the drug and that the effects should wear off over the next 2–4 hours.
5. The patient should be reassured that he will recover totally.
6. Of course, if stimulant misuse is a regular occurrence for the patient, he should be referred for evaluation and counseling to an outpatient drug treatment program or an interested health professional.
7. Medications should be used sparingly, if at all. If needed, the antianxiety drugs [e.g., chlordiazepoxide (Librium), 10–25 mg by mouth, repeated several times in 30–60 minutes, if necessary] may be helpful.

5.2.2. Flashbacks

The relatively short length of action and the rapid metabolism of stimulants do not make them conducive to the development of flashbacks.

5.2.3. Toxic Reactions (see Sections 2.2.3, 4.2.3, 6.2.3, and 14.4)

5.2.3.1. Clinical Picture

5.2.3.1.1. History

The patient may have any sociocultural background. He or she could be an athlete or a member of the culture on the "street" where abuse may be oral or IV; may have a high-risk job (e.g., may be a truck driver or a student at exam time); or may have a history of some "medical" use of stimulants. The clinical picture may develop within minutes (e.g., with IV use or snorting) or more slowly over hours to days, as with oral use in cross-country truck drivers. Anecdotal evidence indicates that there was an increase in stimulant-related deaths of as much as 3-fold during the early 1980s,[54] perhaps reflecting an increase in street-drug purity, an increase in doses self-administered by individuals, or an actual increase in the number of people taking these drugs.

5.2.3.1.2. Physical Signs and Symptoms

Evidence of sympathetic nervous system overactivity dominates the clinical picture for toxic reactions of all stimulants, including cocaine.[7,23,55] Thus, the patient presents with a rapid pulse, an increased respiratory rate, and an elevated body temperature. At high levels of overdose, the picture progresses to *grand mal convulsions,* markedly elevated blood pressure, and a very high body temperature, up to 41°C rectally—all of which can lead to cardiovascular shock.[54,56-58] It has been estimated that between 100 and 200 mg of dextroamphetamine (Dexedrine) and similar doses of cocaine can be lethal in a nontolerant individual, but chronic users may tolerate 1 g or more, and the use of up to 10 g of cocaine/day has been reported.[3,28,30] Blood levels in potentially lethal overdoses can vary 10- to 100-fold, making this a highly unpredictable and dangerous syndrome.[57,58]

Death is often related to a strokelike CNS vascular picture, cardiac arrhythmias, or the high body temperature and is likely to be associated with muscle rigidity, delirium, and agitation.[54,59,60] There may also be signs of IV drug use (e.g., needle marks or abscesses) or, if the patient takes the drug nasally, an inflammation of the nasal mucous membranes or, with cocaine, a destruction of all or part of the nasal septum.

5.2.3.1.3. Psychological State

Taken in excessive doses, stimulants produce restlessness, dizziness, loquaciousness, irritability, and insomnia. These may be associated with headache, palpitations, and the physical signs and symptoms listed in Section 5.2.3.1.2. As the dose increases, toxic behavioral signs develop, including a high level of suspiciousness, repetitive stereotyped behaviors, bruxism (grinding of the teeth), stereotypy (repetitive touching and picking at various objects and parts of the body), and the repetitious dismantling of mechanical objects, such as clocks.[12,51]

5.2.3.1.4. Relevant Laboratory Tests

With the exception of a toxicological screen and the usual vital-sign changes expected with stimulants, there are rarely dramatic laboratory test results.

5.2.3.2. Treatment

The treatment chosen will depend on the clinical condition of the patient at the time he comes for treatment.

1. Emergency care to ensure a clear *airway, circulatory* stability, and treatment of *shock* should be carried out as described in Sections 2.2.3.2, 4.2.3.2, 6.2.3.2, and 14.4.3.1.
2. For an *oral overdose,* gastric lavage should be carried out through either a nasogastric tube (for a conscious patient) or after intubation (for a comatose patient).
3. *Elevated body temperature* must be controlled, with all fevers above 102°F orally being treated with cold water, ice packs, or, at higher temperatures, a hypothermic blanket (see also item 7).
4. *Repeated seizures* should be treated with doses of IV diazepam (Valium) of from 5 to 20 mg injected *very slowly* over a minute and repeated in 15–

20 minutes as needed. In this instance, intubation should be strongly considered, as IV diazepam could result in laryngospasm or apnea.

5. A major elevation in *blood pressure* (e.g., a diastolic pressure of over 120 mm) lasting for over 15 minutes requires the usual medical regimen for malignant hypertension, which may include a phentolamine (Regitine) IV drip of 2–5 mg given over 5–10 minutes. Failure to treat this symptom vigorously could result in CNS hemorrhage.

6. To help *excretion* of the stimulant, the urine should be acidified with ammonium chloride with the goal of obtaining a urinary pH below 6.6. This usually requires 500 mg orally every 3–4 hours.[60]

7. *Hyperthermia* and marked *agitation* can be treated with a dopamine-blocking agent such as haloperidol (Haldol), beginning with doses of 5 mg orally per day, but the dose might have to be a good deal higher for some individuals.[60,61] An alternate drug is chlorpromazine (Thorazine) in doses of 25–50 mg intramuscularly (IM) or orally, to be repeated in 30–60 minutes, if needed, but in this instance, one must be especially careful to avoid precipitating an anticholinergic crisis (see Section 11.9.1) or a severe drop in blood pressure.[57] This danger, once again, underscores my preference for avoiding medications unless absolutely needed.

8. Patients rarely require dialysis, even though most of these drugs would respond to such measures if needed (see Section 14.4.3.2).

9. For cocaine (and possibly other stimulants as well), propranalol (Inderal), 1 mg/min IV up to 5–8 mg total, might help control blood pressure, pulse, and respiratory effects,[62] but not all authors agree.[60]

10. Blood and urine should be drawn for baseline studies and toxicological tests, which will help you rule out the concomitant use of other medications.

11. Once the patient begins to recover or if the overdose was not medically very serious, he should be placed in a quiet room with a minimal amount of stimulation.

12. Treatment of unintentional overdoses in children requires basically the same approach.[63]

5.2.4. Psychosis or Delusional Disorder (292.11 for cocaine and other stimulants in DSM-III-R) (see Sections 1.6.4, 2.2.4, and 4.2.4)

The stimulant-induced psychosis gives a temporary but potentially dramatic picture. The clinical state can be seen with *all* the major stimulants, including methylphenidate, pemoline, the amphetamines, prescription (and some nonprescription) weight-reducing products, and cocaine.[51,64] The specific mechanisms responsible for the psychosis are not known, but it would seem likely that alterations in DA and perhaps NE could contribute, as could experiences with other drugs, and possibly behavioral conditioning.[65] Whatever the important factors, it is most likely that psychoses will be observed after ingestion of the more potent drugs such as methamphetamine or cocaine.

5.2.4.1. Clinical Picture

A high level of suspiciousness and paranoid delusions in a *clear sensorium* (the patient is alert and oriented) developing after an individual takes stimulants is called an amphetamine, cocaine, or *stimulant psychosis*.[6,47,49–51,59] This picture usually develops gradually with chronic abuse, although it can be seen acutely with one very large amphetamine dose. The psychosis has been noted in normal volunteers when 10 mg of dextroamphetamine was given in slowly escalating doses, as well as after acute infusions over 4 hours,[49,66] and pictures resembling human psychoses have been seen in animals after the administration of stimulants.[67–69] The paranoia is usually associated with hallucinations, either auditory or tactile (the individual feels things crawling on him), but it can also be seen with visual hallucinations or illusions and is usually accompanied by a very labile mood.[51,59] This picture often contains repetitive compulsive behavior.

The paranoid delusions can be very frightening to the patient. There is usually little or no insight or understanding, and the suspiciousness has been known to result in unprovoked violence to the point of murder.[70] For instance, it has been reported that in the midst of the epidemic of amphetamine abuse in Japan, 30 of the 60 convicted murder cases in a 2-month period were related to the abuse of amphetamines.

With cessation of the stimulants, the psychosis usually clears within days to a week, the hallucinations disappearing first and the delusions later.[7,51] This is followed by increased sleep (often accompanied by disturbing dreams) and a depression that may last 2 weeks or longer. It has been reported that as many as 10% of patients originally presenting with amphetamine or stimulant psychosis might have some residual symptoms for up to 1 year or more. However, this persistence of symptoms is usually hypothesized to represent a triggering or uncovering of a preexisting psychotic state or a marked vulnerability to psychotic disorders such as schizophrenia.[7,8,71] Another important attribute of this clinical picture is that those individuals who have demonstrated dramatic psychoses while abusing stimulants in the past are probably the ones most likely to show similar pictures if they should return to stimulant drugs.[7,8]

The psychosis mimics an acute schizophrenic picture or mania. However, schizophrenia, as defined by Goodwin and Guze,[53] has a relatively slow onset and is usually associated with a stable, somewhat bland mood; also, a schizophrenic rarely shows abnormal physical findings. On the other hand, a physical evaluation of the amphetamine psychotic can reveal severe weight loss, excoriations (from scratching at nonexistent bugs), needle marks, and elevated blood pressure, heart rate, and temperature.[59] These physical findings are quite variable, and their absence does not rule out amphetamine psychosis.

The cocaine psychosis (basically identical to that of the other major stimulants) has been noted for many years, having been thoroughly described by Freud.[22,47] There is probably a progression from ''snow lights'' (seeing colored lights when cocaine is administered) to hallucinations of geometrical forms and on to tactile hallucinations. Frank visual and/or auditory hallucinations are most likely to occur in psychologically vulnerable individuals, in those taking the drug for an extended period of time, or in those taking relatively high doses.[22,47]

Hallucinations are reported by only a minority of stimulant abusers, with 15% relating histories of visual hallucinations, 13% tactile, 7% olfactory (usually of an unpleasant nature), 4% auditory, and 4% gustatory in one series.[22,47] An important part of the sensory change involves a perception that bugs are crawling under the skin, or formication (a term derived from the latin word for "ant").[22,47] It is worthy of note that any of the stimulants can produce serious paranoid delusions without insight and either with or without accompanying hallucinations. In dealing with these patients, it is important to recognize that no matter how prominent their hallucinations, this is *not* schizophrenia and is likely to clear relatively quickly even if no antipsychotic medications are used.[72]

5.2.4.2. Treatment

Treatment of the stimulant psychosis is relatively straightforward, as, even without active therapy, the pathological picture tends to disappear within days to a week.[12,51]

1. If the individual is out of contact with reality, it is best to hospitalize him.
2. The patient should be carefully screened for any signs of serious physical pathology, as psychotic symptoms can be part of an overdose. A discussion of the treatment of the overdose is given in Section 5.2.3.2.
3. Vital signs must be carefully recorded, and elevated blood pressures, especially those over 120 diastolic, should be treated with drugs such as phentolamine (Regitine) in doses of 2–5 mg given over 5–10 minutes. Special care must be given to avoid precipitating hypotension.
4. In evaluating the clinical picture, consider the possibility that the individual may have also been abusing a depressant, and check for signs of depressant withdrawal.
5. In general, the patient should be placed in a quiet, nonthreatening atmosphere and should be treated with the general precautions one would extend to any paranoid patient (e.g., do not perform any procedures without thorough explanation, do not touch the patient without permission, and avoid any rapid movements in the patient's presence).[59]
6. The treatment personnel should assume an appearance of self-confidence, but the possibility of delusionally provoked or wholly unprovoked assaultive behavior should be noted.
7. As is true in a toxic reaction, it is possible that the administration of ammonium chloride (500 mg every 3–4 hours) to acidify the urine might help cut the psychosis short.[59]
8. A careful history of preexisting psychoses, especially schizophrenia or a serious manic or depressive disorder, should be taken from the patient and available resource people.

9. Although my preference is to avoid medications, if behavior cannot otherwise be controlled, drugs can be considered[74]:

   a. Some authors recommend chlorpromazine (Thorazine) in doses of 50–150 mg by mouth or 25–50 mg IM, to be repeated up to four times a day, if needed, with special care to avoid anticholinergic problems or hypotension.[28,61] I avoid this drug, as it tends to increase the half-life of amphetamine.[61]

   b. Others recommend the use of haloperidol (Haldol) in doses beginning with 5 mg/day up to 20 mg daily given orally or IM.[61] As would be true of chlorpromazine, the drug need be given for only 3–4 days. The clinical usefulness of antipsychotic medications such as haloperidol is underscored by the probability that this drug can actually block the development of stimulant psychoses in experimental situations.[7,8] However, it must be remembered that stimulant abusers probably appear for care with altered levels of DA sensitivity, and there are anecdotal reports that they might be especially likely to develop severe stiffness or dystonia or to increase the use of stimulants when given this drug.[72,73]

   c. Some authors recommend the use of diazepam (Valium) in doses of 10–30 mg orally or 10–20 mg IM to control anxiety or overactivity.[74] However, I feel that there is no place for CNS-depressant drugs in treating the amphetamine psychosis, and they may increase the risk of violence.[61]

10. Patients should be referred after discharge to a drug treatment center to help them deal with their drug problems and to rule out the existence of other psychiatric disorders.

5.2.5. Organic Brain Syndrome or Delirium (292.81 in DSM III-R for cocaine and other stimulants)

Confusion and disorientation can develop when an individual takes so much of the drug that his normal mental processes are disturbed.

5.2.5.1. Clinical Picture (see section 1.6.5)

The organicity tends to be a transient problem consisting of any of the following symptoms: confusion, disorientation, hallucinations, delusions, paranoia, loose association of ideas, and behavioral problems of bruxism and repeated touching or stereotypic behavior.[7,12] It should be noted that the stimulants may cause cerebrovascular changes when taken chronically, and there are reports of increased rates of cerebral hemorrhage, subarachnoid bleeding, subdural hematomas, and vascular lesions resembling periarteritis nodosa in stimulant misusers.[50] There is also some *anecdotal* evidence that abusers of amphetamines and other stimulant drugs demonstrate a potentially permanent decrease in mentation and concentration, and there is good evidence that some neuropsychological deficits can be seen for weeks and even up to 3 months of abstinence.[75,76] Thus, the abuse of stimulant drugs should be considered a part of the differential diagnosis of any individual who presents with signs of CNS organicity, and it is important that one carefully evaluate the neurological functioning of all stimulant abusers seen in practice.

5.2.5.2. Treatment

1. Because the organicity tends to be transient, the general approach is to give supportive care following the guidelines offered in Section 5.2.4.2.
2. However, one must be certain to carry out an adequate neurological examination to rule out all the possible causes of an OBS, including a focal CNS lesion or intracranial bleeding.
3. One can roughly estimate the prognosis by determining which, if any, preexisting psychiatric disorder is present or if evidence of brain malfunctioning was present before the onset of the drug-induced problem.

5.2.6. Withdrawal (292.0 in DSM-III-R for cocaine and other stimulants)

5.2.6.1. Clinical Picture

5.2.6.1.1. History

Depending on the type of abuse involved (e.g., "street" vs. medical), the patient may give an obvious history of drug abuse, or a great deal of probing and gathering information from friends and relatives may be required to establish the accurate diagnosis. The withdrawal may begin insidiously, with the patient having no idea why he is depressed, lethargic, or irritable, or it may have a more dramatic onset.

5.2.6.1.2. Physical Signs and Symptoms

For cocaine, amphetamines, and other CNS stimulants, there is usually no specific physical pathology present, other than the usual type of medical problems seen in any abuser. The withdrawal syndrome can begin while the individual continues to take stimulants as tolerance develops, and it may include a variety of nonspecific muscular aches and pains.[12]

5.2.6.1.3. Psychological State

The clinical syndrome for withdrawal has been thought to divide into a series of phases.[77-79] In this scheme, during the first 9 hours to 14 days, the "crash" is characterized by intense craving and cocaine-seeking behavior. In this early phase, the cocaine or stimulant abuser experiences intense agitation, feelings of depression, and a decrease in appetite that then give way to fatigue with associated insomnia, continued depression, and a decrease in craving, all of which result in a final experience of exhaustion, a rebound in appetite, and a need to sleep. This most acute phase is then followed over the next 1–10 weeks by "withdrawal." Early in this second phase, sleep patterns begin to normalize, feelings of cocaine craving are relatively low, and the mood is fairly normal, but this soon progresses into a recurrence of fatigue, anxiety, and associated anhedonia. This is hypothesized to be followed by an indefinite period of time during which there is improvement in mood and ability to enjoy experiences, but also craving and a desire to return to the drug—topics further explored in the discussion of stimulant rehabilitation in Section 15.4.

5.2.6.1.4. Relevant Laboratory Tests

There are no specific laboratory tests that will help here. Of course, all IV drug abusers should be screened for possible hepatitis (e.g., the liver function tests listed in Table 1.5) and signs of occult infection (a WBC as listed in Table 1.5), and they should be given a good neurological examination. A toxicological screen may be helpful, but the signs of withdrawal might not appear until the stimulant drugs have been metabolized.

5.2.6.2. Treatment

Treatment is simply addressing the *symptoms,* as the major acute syndrome tends to dissipate within days on its own (except for the depression and lethargy, which may remain for several months). Many clinicians prefer to carry out withdrawal in an inpatient setting in order to offer maximal support. However, it is also possible to use a series of decreasing frequencies of hospital visits as an outpatient (e.g., three times the first week, then two or three times the second week, then one or two times the third week—decreasing over 21 days), offering some of the general supports outlined below.

1. The patient must be given a careful neurological and physical examination.
2. The possibility of the concomitant abuse of other drugs, especially depressants, must be considered. Blood and urine samples should be sent for toxicological screening, and the patient should be carefully queried about other drug use.
3. A careful history of the drug-abuse pattern and prior psychiatric disorders must be obtained.
4. The patient should be placed in quiet surroundings and allowed to sleep.[59]
5. If the patient is markedly despondent, (temporary) suicide precautions should be considered.
6. Although, once again, I prefer to avoid medications, some authors suggest that many of the symptoms associated with stimulant (especially cocaine) withdrawal might relate to a depletion of brain dopamine (DA) in cocaine-abusing patients.[80,81] Recent clinical trials have suggested that cocaine abusers who are prescribed between 0.625 and 2.5 mg of the DA agonist bromocriptine (Parodyl) per day in divided doses have a significant diminu-

tion of depression, sleep disturbance, and loss of energy and are likely to report reduced craving for cocaine. This open trial (i.e., there were no double-blind controls) indicated that bromocriptine could be successfully stopped after several weeks of treatment.[80] It must be stressed, however, that until careful double-blind trials are carried out, DA-boosting drugs such as bromocriptine should be considered experimental and not be used in the usual clinical settings.[81] Other drugs of potential importance in cocaine and stimulant drug rehabilitation are discussed in Section 15.4.

7. In general, allowing the person several days to recover and having him sleep and eat as much as he needs will usually result in the diminution of all symptoms.

5.2.7. Medical Problems

The medical problems associated with overdose were described in Section 5.2.3. Additional problems that must be considered are as follows:

1. Complications from the use of contaminated needles include endocarditis, tetanus, hepatitis, emboli, abscesses, acquired immune deficiency syndrome (AIDS), and so on (see Section 6.2.8).[82]
2. Apparent signs of a stroke can accompany the strong contraction of blood vessels caused by stimulants.
3. A related phenomenon occurs in those individuals who sniff cocaine. The constriction of blood vessels in the nasal mucosa can be so severe that the nasal septum is destroyed.[3,23,83]
4. Another problem after snorting or smoking coke is possible aspiration subsequent to laryngeal or pharyngeal anesthesia.[3]
5. Pulmonary problems can also develop after smoking stimulants, including cocaine. These range from local irritation such as bronchitis through possible decreases in actual pulmonary diffusion abilities.[83]
6. The elevated blood pressure that can accompany the use of stimulant drugs can cause an intracranial hemorrhage.
7. As briefly noted in Section 5.2.3, the rapid intake of any of these drugs, especially cocaine or methamphetamine, results in a rapid onset of an increased heart rate and can actually result in cardiac fibrillation, respiratory arrest, and death.[83] An associated phenomenon that occurs as a consequence of the stimulation of the heart as well as the spasms in cardiac blood vessels is the possibility of a myocardial infarction or heart attack, with numerous cases documented in otherwise healthy young adults.[84,85] These potentially lethal cardiac complications appear to be unpredictable and are likely to occur in both naive and regular stimulant abusers.
8. Cocaine and other brain stimulants are also likely to cross the placenta to the fetus. The result can be a decrease in the delivery of oxygen as well as

the direct effects of the stimulant on the fetus resulting in small-vessel and cardiac changes similar to those reported above.[86] It appears that cocaine abuse during pregnancy might result in a significant increase in spontaneous abortions, premature labor, and abruptio placenta as well as in infants born with an apparent (temporary) diminished response to the environment.[87,88]

9. The stereotyped behavior during intoxication can include bruxism (grinding of the teeth), which can wear down the teeth and cause dental difficulties.

10. A variety of skin problems, including scratches (secondary to delusions about bugs in the skin) and skin ulcers, can be noted.

REFERENCES

1. Gawin, F., & Ellinwood, E. Cocaine and other stimulants. *New England Journal of Medicine 318:*1173–1182, 1988.
2. Kleber, H. Cocaine abuse and its treatment. *Journal of Clinical Psychiatry 49(Supplement):*1–38, 1988.
3. Schuckit, M. Cocaine: An update. *Drug Abuse and Alcoholism Newsletter 17*(15):1–4, 1988.
4. Jaffe, J. H. Drug addiction and drug abuse. In A. G. Gilman, L. S. Goodman, T. W. Rall, & F. Murad (Eds.), *The Pharmacological Basis of Therapeutics* (7th ed.). New York: Macmillan, 1985, pp. 532–581.
5. Spitz, H. I., & Rosecan, J. S. (Eds.). *Cocaine Abuse: New Directions in Treatment and Research.* New York, Brunner/Mazel, 1987.
6. Ellinwood, E. H., Jr. Amphetamine psychosis: Individuals, settings, and sequences. In E. H. Ellinwood & S. Cohen (Eds.), *Current Concepts on Amphetamine Abuse.* Rockville, Maryland: National Institute of Mental Health, 1970, pp. 143–157.
7. Sato, M. Acute exacerbation of methamphetamine psychosis and lasting dopaminergic supersensitivity—A clinical survey. Paper presented at the American College of Neuropsychopharmacology Annual Meeting, Maui, Hawaii, December 10, 1985.
8. Sato, M., Chen, C. C., Akiyama, S., & Otsuki, S. Acute exacerbation of paranoid psychotic state after long-term abstinence in patients with previous methamphetamine psychosis. *Biological Psychiatry 18:*429–440, 1983.
9. Crichlow, S. Khat-induced paranoid psychosis. *British Journal of Psychiatry 150:*247–249, 1987.
10. Mayberry, J., Morgan, G., & Perkin, E. Khat-induced schizophreniform psychosis in the United Kingdom. *Lancet 1:*455, 1984.
11. Kozel, N. H., & Adams, E. H. *Cocaine Use in America: Epidemiologic and Clinical Perspectives.* Rockville, Maryland: Department of Health and Human Services, NIDA Research Monograph 61, 1985, pp. 130–150.
12. Franz, D. N. Central nervous system stimulants. In A. G. Gilman, L. S. Goodman, T. W. Rall, & F. Murad (Eds.), *The Pharmacological Basis of Therapeutics* (7th ed.). New York: Macmillan, 1985, pp. 582–588.
13. Ritz, M. C., Lamb, R. J., Goldberg, S. R., & Kuhar, M. J. Cocaine receptors on dopamine transporters are related to self-administration of cocaine. *Science 237:*1219–1223, 1987.
14. Angrist, B., Corwin, J., Bartlik, B., & Cooper, T. Early pharmacokinetics and clinical effects of oral D-amphetamine in normal subjects. *Biological Psychiatry 22:*1357–1368, 1987.
15. Brower, K. J., Blow, F. C., & Beresford, T. P. Forms of cocaine and psychiatric symptoms. *Lancet 1:*50, 1988.
16. Wesson, D. R., & Smith, D. E. Low dose benzodiazepine withdrawal syndrome: Receptor site mediated. *Newsletter: California Society for the Treatment of Alcoholism and Other Drug Dependencies 9:*1–4, Jan./Feb. 1982.

17. Editorial: Crack. *Lancet 2:*1061, 1987.
18. Honer, W. G., Gewirtz, G., & Turey, M. Psychosis and violence in cocaine smokers. *Lancet 2:*451–452, 1987.
19. VanDyke, C., Jatlow, P., Ungerer, J., *et al.* Oral cocaine: Plasma concentrations and central effects. *Science 200:*211–213, 1978.
20. Javaid, J. I. Cocaine plasma concentration: Relation to physiological and subjective effects in humans. *Science 202:*227–228, 1978.
21. VanDyke, C., Barash, P. G., Jatlow, P., *et al.* Cocaine: Plasma concentrations after intranasal application in man. *Science 191:*859–861, 1976.
22. Siegel, R. K. Cocaine smoking. *New England Journal of Medicine 300:*373, 1979.
23. Grabowski, J., & Dworkin, S. I. Cocaine: An overview of current issues. *International Journal of the Addictions 20:*1065–1088, 1985.
24. Siegel, R. K. Cocaine substitutes. *New England Journal of Medicine 302:*817, 1980.
25. Wesson, D. R., & Morgan, J. P. Stimulant look-alikes. *Newsletter: California Society for the Treatment of Alcoholism and Other Drug Dependencies 9:*1–4, Oct. 1982.
26. Hurst, P. M. Amphetamines and driving. *Alcohol, Drugs, and Driving 3:*13–17, 1987.
27. Byck, R. The effects of cocaine on complex performance in humans. *Alcohol, Drugs and Driving 3:*9–11, 1987.
28. Paul, S. M., Hulihan-Giblin, B., Skolnick, P., *et al.* (+)-Amphetamine binding to rat hypo-thalamus: Relation to anorexic potency of phenylethylamines. *Science 218:*487–489, 1982.
29. Sherer, M., Kumor, K., DeBorja, J., *et al.* Psychiatric effects of four-hour infusions of cocaine. Paper presented at the American Psychiatric Association Annual Meeting, Washington, D.C., May 13, 1986.
30. Woolverton, W. L., Kandel, D., & Schuster, C. R. Tolerance and cross-tolerance to cocaine and d-amphetamine. *Journal of Pharmacological Therapy 205:*525–535, 1979.
31. Matsuzaki, M., Spingler, P. J., Misra, A. L., *et al.* Cocaine: Tolerance to its convulsant and cardiorespiratory stimulating effects in the monkey. *Life Sciences 19:*193–204, 1976.
32. Post, R. M., & Kopanda, R. T. Cocaine, kindling and psychosis. *American Journal of Psychiatry 133:*627–634, 1976.
33. American Psychiatric Association. *Diagnostic Criteria from the DSM III-R.* Washington, D.C., American Psychiatric Press, 1987.
34. Wender, P. H. Minimal brain dysfunction: An overview. In M. A. Lipton, A. DiMascio, & K. F. Killam (Eds.), *Psychopharmacology: A Generation of Progress.* New York: Raven Press, 1978, pp. 312–321.
35. Schuckit, M., Petrich, J., & Chiles, J. Hyperactivity: Diagnostic confusion. *Journal of Nervous and Mental Disease 166:*79–87, 1978.
36. Gomez, R. L., Janowsky, D., Zetin, M., *et al.* Adult psychiatric diagnosis and symptoms compati-ble with the hyperactive child syndrome: A retrospective study. *Journal of Clinical Psychiatry 42:*389–394, 1981.
37. Douglas, J. G., Preston, P. G., Haslett, C., *et al.* Long-term efficacy of fenfluramine in treatment of obesity. *Lancet 1:*384–486, 1983.
38. Angrist, B. M., & Gershon, S. Psychiatric sequelae of amphetamine use. In R. I. Shader (Ed.), *Psychiatric Complications of Medical Drugs.* New York: Raven Press, 1972, pp. 23–35.
39. Smart, R. G., Goodstadt, M. S., Adlaf, E. M., & Sheppard, M. A. Trends in the prevalence of alcohol and other drug use among Ontario students: 1977–1983. *Canadian Journal of Public Health 76:*157–161, 1985.
40. Smart, R. G., & Adlaf, E. M. Patterns of drug use among adolescents: The past decade. *Social Science Medicine 23:*717–719, 1986.
41. Nicholi, A. M. The nontherapeutic use of psychoactive drugs. *New England Journal of Medicine 308:*925–933, 1983.
42. Editorial: National survey finds continuing decline in use of illicit drugs by high school seniors. *Hospital and Community Psychiatry 36:*1011, 1985.
43. Smart, R. G., Adlaf, E. M., & Goodstadt, M. S. Alcohol and other drug use among Ontario students: An update. *Canadian Journal of Public Health 77:*57–58, 1986.

44. Editorial: Epidemiology of drug usage. *Lancet 1:*147, 1985.
45. Kandel, D. B., & Logan, J. A. Patterns of drug use from adolescent to young adulthood: Periods of risk for initiation, continued use, and discontinuation. *American Journal of Public Health 74:*660–666, 1984.
46. White, H. R. Longitudinal patterns of cocaine use among adolescents. *American Journal of Drug and Alcohol Abuse 14:*1–15, 1988.
47. Siegel, R. K. Cocaine hallucinations. *American Journal of Psychiatry 135:*309–314, 1978.
48. Schuckit, M. A. Alcoholism and other psychiatric disorders. *Hospital and Community Psychiatry 34:*1022–1027, 1983.
49. Angrist, B. M., & Gershon, S. The phenomenology of experimentally-induced amphetamine psychosis—Preliminary observations. *Biological Psychiatry 2:*95–107, 1970.
50. McLellan, A. T., Woody, G. E., & O'Brien, C. P. Development of psychiatric illness in drug abusers. *New England Journal of Medicine 301:*1310–1314, 1979.
51. Segal, D. S., & Schuckit, M. A. Animal models of stimulant-induced psychosis. In I. Creese (Ed.), *Stimulants: Neurochemical, Behavioral, and Clinical Perspectives.* New York: Raven Press, 1982, pp. 131–168.
52. Aronson, T. A., & Craig, T. J. Cocaine precipitation of panic disorder. *American Journal of Psychiatry 143:*643–645, 1986.
53. Goodwin, D. W., & Guze, S. B. *Psychiatric Diagnosis* (4th ed.). New York: Oxford University Press, 1988.
54. Kosten, T. R., & Kleber, H. D. Sudden death in cocaine abusers: Relation to neuroleptic malignant syndrome. *Lancet 1:*1198, 1987.
55. Fischman, M. W. Cocaine and the amphetamines. In H. Y. Meltzer (Ed.), *Psychopharmacology: The Third Generation of Progress.* New York: Raven Press, 1987, pp. 1543–1554.
56. Gold, M. S. 800-COCAINE: Survey of 500 callers. Paper presented at the Biological Psychiatry Annual Meeting, Chicago, May 5, 1986.
57. Smart, R. G., & Anglin, L. Do we know the lethal dose of cocaine? *Journal of Forensic Sciences 32:*303–312, 1987.
58. Wetli, C. V., & Fisbain, D. A. Cocaine-induced psychosis and sudden death in recreational cocaine users. *Journal of Forensic Sciences 30:*873–880, 1985.
59. Kosten, T., & Kleber, H. Rapid death during cocaine abuse. *American Journal of Drug and Alcohol Abuse 14:*335–346, 1988.
60. Catravas, J. D., Waters, I. W., Walz, M. A., *et al.* Antidotes for cocaine poisoning. *New England Journal of Medicine 301:*1238, 1977.
61. Angrist, M. D., Less, H. K., & Gershon, S. The antagonism of amphetamine-induced symptomatology by a neuroleptic. *American Journal of Psychiatry 131:*817–821, 1974.
62. Rappolt, R. T. Propranolol in cocaine toxicity. *Lancet 2:*640–641, 1976.
63. Espelin, D. E., & Done, A. K. Amphetamine poisoning: Effectiveness of chlorpromazine. *New England Journal of Medicine 278:*1361–1365, 1978.
64. Sternback, H. Pemoline-induced mania. *Biological Psychiatry 16:*987–989, 1981.
65. Ando, K., Hironaka, N., & Yanagita, T. Psychotic manifestations in amphetamine abuse—Experimental study on the mechanisms of psychotic recurrence. *Psychopharmacology Bulletin 22:*763–768, 1986.
66. Sherer, M., Kumor, K., Golden, R., & Jaffe, J. Continuous infusion of cocaine—A model for cocaine psychosis? Paper presented at the Society of Biological Psychiatry Annual Meeting, Washington, D.C., May 10, 1986.
67. Nielsen, E. B., & Lyon, M. Behavioral alterations during prolonged low level continuous amphetamine administration in a monkey family group (*Cercopithecus aethiops*). *Biological Psychiatry 17:*423–435, 1982.
68. Griffith, J. D., Cavanaugh, J. H., & Oates, J. A. Psychosis induced by the administration of D--amphetamine to human volunteers. In D. H. Efron (Ed.), *Psychotomimetic Drugs.* New York: Raven Press, 1970.
69. Bell, D. S. The experimental reproduction of amphetamine psychosis. *Archives of General Psychiatry 29:*35–40, 1973.

70. Ellinwood, E. H., Jr. Assault and homicide associated with amphetamine abuse. *American Journal of Psychiatry 127:*1170–1176, 1971.

71. Perkins, K. A., Simpson, J. C., & Tsuang, M. T. Ten-year follow-up of drug abusers with acute or chronic psychosis. *Hospital and Community Psychiatry 37:*481–484, 1986.

72. Roberts, D. Self-increased–self-administration of cocaine following haloperidol. *Pharmacology, Biochemistry and Behavior 26:*37–43, 1987.

73. Kumor, K., Sherer, M., & Jaffe, J. Haloperidol-induced dystonia in cocaine addicts. *Lancet 2:*1341–1342, 1986.

74. Dimijian, G. G. Differential diagnosis of emergency drug reactions. In P. G. Bourne (Ed.). *A Treatment Manual for Acute Drug Abuse Emergencies.* Washington, D.C.: U.S. Government Printing Office, 1974, pp. 1–7.

75. Grant, I., Mohns, L., Miller, M., & Reitan, R. M. A neuropsychological study of polydrug users. *Archives of General Psychiatry 33:*973–978, 1976.

76. Grant, I., Adams, K. M., Carlin, A. S., *et al.* Organic impairment in polydrug users: Risk factors. *American Journal of Psychiatry 135:*178–184, 1978.

77. Gawin, F. H., & Kleber, H. D. Neuroendocrine findings in chronic cocaine abusers: A preliminary report. *British Journal of Psychiatry 147:*569–573, 1985.

78. Weiss, R. D., Mirin, S. M., Michael, J. L., & Sollogub, A. C. Psychopathology in chronic cocaine abusers. *American Journal of Drug and Alcohol Abuse 12:*17–129, 1986.

79. Gawin, F. H., & Kleber, H. D. Abstinence symptomatology and psychiatric diagnosis in cocaine abusers. *Archives of General Psychiatry 43:*107–113, 1986.

80. Roehrich, H., Dackis, C. A., & Gold, M. S. Bromocriptine. *Medicinal Research Reviews 7:*243–269, 1987.

81. Gutierrez-Esteinou, R. Interactions of bromocriptine with cocaine. *American Journal of Psychiatry 145:*1173, 1988.

82. Curran, J. W., Jaffe, H. W., Hardy, A. M., *et al.* Epidemiology of HIV infection and AIDS in the United States. *Science 239:*610–616, 1988.

83. American Psychiatric Association, Committee on Drug Abuse. Position statement on psychoactive substance use and dependence: Update on marijuana and cocaine. *American Journal of Psychiatry 144:*698, 1987.

84. Schachne, J. S., Roberts, B. H., & Thompson, P. D. Coronary-artery spasm with myocardial infarction: Association with cocaine use. *New England Journal of Medicine 310:*1665–1666, 1984.

85. Isner, J. M., Estes, N. A. M., Thompson, P. D., *et al.* Acute cardiac events temporally related to cocaine abuse. *New England Journal of Medicine 315:*1438–1443, 1986.

86. Woods, J. R., Plessinger, M. A., & Clark, K. E. Effect of cocaine on uterine blood flow and fetal oxygenation. *Journal of the American Medical Association 257:*957–961, 1987.

87. Chasnoff, I. J., Burns, W. J., Schnoll, S. H., & Burns, K. A. Cocaine use in pregnancy. *New England Journal of Medicine 313:*666–669, 1985.

88. Smith, C. G., & Asch, R. H. Drug abuse and reproduction. *Fertility and Sterility 48:*355–373, 1987.

Opiates and Other Analgesics

6.1. INTRODUCTION

This chapter is concerned with those pain-killing drugs (analgesics) that are most likely to be misused, ranging from propoxyphene (Darvon) through the synthetic, opiatelike drugs to the major opiates, including morphine and heroin. The generalizations made here apply to almost all prescription painkillers, with the exception of the newer prescription antiinflammatory medications. The material might also be relevant to the newer opiate-type drugs, including the mixed agonist–antagonist butorphanol (Stadol or Borphanol), which is similar to buprenorphene and nalbuphene, as well as fentanyl (Sublimaze). Most of these newer medications have not yet met the test of time to determine their actual propensity to develop adverse reactions, including addiction.[1,2]

Of course, many opiates are useful and medically important drugs. Even heroin, which is rapidly converted to morphine in the body, has potent pain–killing properties.[3] As a group, however, these drugs are liable to misuse.

Historically, the widespread opiate abuse observed in Europe and the United States at the turn of the century was the result of morphine and related compounds purchased legally, primarily by middle-class women.[4–6] The preponderance of medical abusers of opiates continued until the drugs were placed under legal control in the early 1900s, after which the "street" misuse of these substances began, primarily in young men from poor areas. Since the mid-1960s, however, abuse of these substances has spread once again to the middle class, where the drugs are obtained through both physicians and the "black market."

6.1.1. Pharmacology (see Section 11.5 for over-the-counter analgesics)

6.1.1.1. General Characteristics

The major opiates include natural substances, such as opium, morphine, and codeine; semisynthetic drugs produced by minor chemical alterations in the basic poppy products [e.g., heroin, hydromorphone (Dilaudid), and oxycodone (Percodan)]; and synthetic analgesics, such as propoxyphene (Darvon) and meperidine

118

Table 6.1
Opiate Analgesics

Drug type	Generic name	Trade name
Analgesics	Opium	—
	Heroin	—
	Morphine	—
	Codeine	—
	Hydromorphone	Dilaudid
	Oxycodone	Percodan
	Methadone	Dolophine
	Propoxyphene	Darvon
	Meperidine	Demerol
	Diphenoxylate	Lomotil
	Pentazocine	Talwin
Antagonists	Naloxone	Narcan
	Nalorphine	Nalline
	Levallorphan	Lorfan
	Cyclazocine	—
	Naltrexone	Trexan

(Demerol) (Table 6.1). The relative potency of these drugs has been described in other texts and can be roughly gauged by the usual dosage, with a standard of 10 mg of morphine producing analgesia for the average individual.[7] In this context, 3–4 mg of morphine is roughly equivalent to 1–2 mg of heroin, 0.5 mg of dilaudid, 20 mg of meperidine, and 30 mg of codeine.[8]

These drugs undergo similar metabolism in the body, but differ in their degree of oral absorption (ranging from a low for heroin to a high for propoxyphene). Heroin is rapidly converted by the body into morphine.[9] Detoxification occurs primarily in the liver, and the resulting metabolites are excreted through the urine and the bile. Over 90% of the excretion of doses of these drugs (with the exception of a very long-acting substance such as methadone) occurs within the first 24 hours, although metabolites can be seen for 48 hours or more.[7]

6.1.1.2. Predominant Effects

These substances all produce analgesia, drowsiness, changes in mood, and at high doses, a clouding of mental functioning through the depression of central nervous system (CNS) and cardiac activity.[7] Although there are some major differences in the way these drugs affect particular systems, the actions are homogeneous enough to allow for some generalizations.

The acute intake of an opiate, especially when administered intravenously (IV), is highly reinforcing.[7] The first minute or two after IV injection of heroin is characterized as a kick or rush of feelings in the lower abdomen (resembling an orgasm) accompanied by a warm flushing of the skin. This is followed by a floating, intoxicated feeling accompanied by euphoria, decreases in the respiratory rate, and slowing of peristaltic movement in the colon with resulting constipation. Autonomic nervous system changes for most opiates include a decrease in pupillary size, with the exception of meperidine, for which atropinelike effects result in dilated pupils along with twitching muscles, a tremor, and possibly signs of confusion.[7]

6.1.1.3. Tolerance and Dependence

6.1.1.3.1. Tolerance

Tolerance develops rapidly to most opiates, particularly the more potent analgesics, but the changes in organ sensitivity develop unevenly.[10] For example, high levels of tolerance can be expected for the opiate effects on respiratory depression, analgesia, sedation, and vomiting, as well as for the euphoric properties. However, the same pattern of chronic use is likely to yield little tolerance for pupillary constriction (miosis) or for constipation.[7] The final level of tolerance can be marked, and some addicts can administer over 2 g of heroin without signs of severe toxicity. As is true of most drugs within a class, cross-tolerance is common among the opiates, with a somewhat predictable level of variability among drugs that depends at least in part on the opiate receptor type most prominently affected.

6.1.1.3.2. Dependence

These substances are very addicting (i.e., they have attractive effects and quickly produce tolerance and dependence), and physical dependence develops after relatively short-term use. The degree of dependence varies directly with the potency of the particular drug, the doses taken, and the length of exposure. Therapeutic doses of morphine given twice a day [BID (Latin *bis in die*)] for 2 weeks or four times a day (QID) for 3 days can result in a mild withdrawal syndrome, especially if precipitated by a narcotic antagonist.[11]

6.1.1.4. Recent Findings on Brain Mechanisms

Recent discoveries concerning the pharmacology of opiates have been very exciting and are worthy of mention here. The work began with the hypothesis that there might be opiate receptors in specific areas of the brain. Logically, if there are endogenous opiate receptors, there might be endogenous opiates to occupy those receptors. This line of reasoning has resulted in the discovery of a series of substances (the endorphins and enkephalins) that are present in various parts of the body, especially the CNS, and that appear to function in regulating the perception of pain. These substances have also been hypothesized to have some importance in the regulation of normal mood states, the development of psychoses, and the mediation of action of other misused substances. This series of investigations is leading to important breakthroughs in our understanding of the mechanism of action of these drugs, which might, in turn, lead to important information on the causes and treatment of substance misuse.[12,13]

Since the publication of the second edition of this text, additional information has appeared regarding subtypes among opiate receptors.[14–16] While the specific characteristics of such receptors are relatively complex, some generalizations can be presented. *Mu* opiate receptors have prominent actions affecting respiratory depression, analgesia, euphoria, and the development of dependence. It is thus not surprising that the activity of *Mu* receptors is felt to have a major impact on the reinforcing properties of opiates and that morphine and heroin both have prominent *Mu* effects.[7,15] *Kappa* receptors have marked effects on levels of sedation and sleep as well as on diuresis, while *Sigma*-receptor stimulation can result in feelings of emotional unease or dysphoria and can be responsible for hallucinations.[15] Finally, *Delta* receptors have prominent cardiovascular activity and also contribute to analgesia. It can be seen from this description that it is possible that the major rewarding or reinforcing properties of an opiate could be the result of changes in one type of receptor, while the prominent symptoms of withdrawal might relate most closely to another type.[15,17,18] These discoveries contribute to the hope that safer and more effective analgesics with more selective receptor activities might be developed in the near future.[16]

A third clinically relevant aspect of opiate pharmacology and receptor activity is the recent increase in our knowledge about opiate antagonists. These drugs can displace opiates from receptors and thus antagnoize or block their actions. As discussed in the treatment of opiate overdose in Section 6.2.3.2 as well as in the discussion of the use of antagonists in opiate rehabilitation in Section 15.3.2, the evolution of our knowledge about opiate antagonists has important clinical relevance.

A final note on the pharmacology of opiates relates to the development of the so-called "designer drugs."[19,20] Attempts to produce close analogues of meperidine or synthetic heroin in "kitchen laboratories" often result in contamination with 1-methyl-4-phenyl-1,2,3,6-tetrahydropyridine (MPTP). This chemical irreversibly destroys neurons rich in the neurotransmitter dopamine in areas of the brain important in initiation and coordination of movements (e.g., the substantia nigra). This irreversible process results in the rapid onset of a severe but nonprogressive parkinsonian syndrome characterized by a paucity of spontaneous movements, muscular rigidity, a coarse resting tremor of the hand, loss of numerous reflexes, drooling, and muteness.

6.1.2. Epidemiology and Patterns of Abuse

Simplistically, users divide into the small percentage who misuse analgesics in a medical setting (*medical* abusers), those who take opiates obtained from nonmedical sources (*street* abusers), and abusers who get the drug methadone legally.[7] The medical abusers tend to be older, middle-class, and well established in comparison to the street abusers, but there is much overlap between the two groups.

Nevertheless, for clarity, the characteristics of street and medical abusers are (somewhat artificially) separated in this section while methadone maintenance is discussed in Section 15.3.1.

6.1.2.1. Street Abuse

6.1.2.1.1. Patterns of Use

The sale of illicit opiates is a highly profitable business. Most of these drugs enter the United States illegally as part of an intricate economic–manufacturing–marketing complex that begins in the Orient, the Middle East, Mexico, or South and Central America. The socioeconomics of heroin misuse have been outlined by Stimmel,[21] demonstrating that 10 kg of opium grown from poppy plants at a cost of $250 results in street heroin worth $400,000 in the United States after a series of steps of manufacture and dilution with adulterants. The resulting opiates are abused through all routes of administration, including oral (primarily the synthetic and semisynthetic opiates), IN (snorting), smoking (usually opium), and IV (especially heroin).[6]

The usual street abuser begins using opiates occasionally, but may progress to daily use, with tolerance and physical dependence rapidly following. This pattern is certainly the one most likely to come to the attention of medical and mental health personnel as well as the police.

However, there are a number of individuals who continue to take the drug only occasionally over an extended period of time, even when they use it IV. The exact number of people "chipping" these drugs is not known, but it is probable that they show a much higher level of life stability, having family, friends, and job, than is true of the general user.[22]

A related phenomenon is seen in a number of physically addicted individuals who manage to hold jobs and to function fairly well socially.[23] Another important observation grew out of Vietnam, where large numbers of soldiers with little or no prior experience with opiates found themselves in a situation of high stress and with drugs readily available.[24] Under such circumstances, as many as half those given the chance tried opiates. Although many became physically addicted, those who had not used drugs before Vietnam tended to return to a drug-free status when back in their home communities.[25]

In the 1970s, there was evidence that the prevalence of opiate misuse had stabilized in middle-class populations.[26,27] Analyses of both direct and indirect indices of "street" use in New York showed what appears to be a decrease since 1970 in new "intensive" users, that is, those requiring treatment.[28] These data showed a decrease in the number of felony-related opiate arrests from 22,000 in 1970 to 4000 in 1978, a parallel decrease in opiate misdemeanor arrests per year from 16,000 to 2000, decreases in both infectious hepatitis (from 3000 to 500) and serum hepatitis (from 1500 to 500), and a decrease in overall drug mortality (from 800 to 250) during the same time period. The number of new admissions to methadone maintenance treatment programs decreased from a high of 19,000 in 1972 to

2,000 in 1978, and readmissions to methadone maintenance decreased from 6000 in 1976 to 3500 in 1978.[28] According to one report, it is felt that the most likely explanation for the decrease is a change in attitude toward heroin, as the indices began to shrink *before* street drug supplies became less plentiful. Whatever the cause, the downward trend seems to have continued into the 1980s in North America for the number of opiate-related deaths in some locales.[29] However, it is possible that the number of addicts actually increased in Great Britain over the same time frame.[30]

The data generated in the 1980s in the United States and Canada document the extent of street use of opiates in more recent years. Somewhere between 1 and 3% of 18- to 25-year-olds in the general United States population have used opiates "recreationally" at least once.[7,31,32] Among younger groups, between 0.6 and 1.6% of students in grades 7 to 13 have taken opiates at least once, including 0.5% of high school seniors who have used these drugs in the preceding 30 days.[33−36] Consistent with the figures cited above regarding mortality and treatment data, the prevalence of opiate use among younger populations appears to have stabilized and then decreased between 1980 and 1985.

6.1.2.1.2. Natural History

It is difficult to formulate an accurate average picture that applies to the vast majority of opiate abusers. This difficulty reflects the individual variation likely to be expected in the manifestations of any clinical syndrome as well as the fact that most data have been generated through studies of opiate abusers who enter treatment. Thus, the information might not apply equally to those drug abusers who are living in the community and who do not become identified by the treatment or criminal justice systems.[37]

Despite these caveats, some generalizations can be set forth. The average street user tends to be young, a member of a minority group, and male.[38] He usually demonstrates a prior history of delinquent behavior (the more severe the antisocial problems, the greater the chance of continued drug use).[25,39] One study of a group of black addicts demonstrated that the average age of first use of any drug (usually marijuana) was 14; the first arrest for *any* problem occurred at 16.5; the first use of heroin at age 18; the first evidence of physical dependence at age 20, with the first heroin-related arrest following within about 6 months; and the first treatment at approximately age 26.[38] Initiation of opiate use tends to relate to peer pressure and experience,[39] and the "epidemic" of increased use in the late 1960s may have followed a contagionlike epidemiological model.[27] Almost 80% of opiate addicts in treatment had early school problems, and 90% reported truancy, two thirds had been suspended from school, and 80% had dropped out before graduating from high school.[38] As the discussion of alcoholism notes to be true of alcoholics, opiate abusers who qualify for the careful diagnosis of the antisocial personality (on the basis of their antisocial behavior before age 16 and before the onset of serious drug misuse[40]) carry a much worse prognosis for violent behavior and continued drug and antisocial problems than the "average" street abuser.

The short-term prognosis for opiate abusers is relatively poor, with almost 90% returning to drugs within the first 6 months after treatment, but this return is followed by a trend toward an increasing percentage achieving abstinence over time.[41] Although the majority of addicts tend to show repeated exacerbations and remissions like those shown by alcoholics, long-term follow-ups (up to 20 years) have demonstrated that a third or more of opiate abusers, even those impaired severely enough to be treated in a jail–hospital setting like the Federal facility in Lexington, Kentucky, are finally able to achieve abstinence.[42]

The course for the remainder is far from benign, with one quarter of the original total dead at follow-up and one quarter still addicted.[43,44] The mortality rate for opiate abusers is about 5–10 per thousand, with especially high levels of death due to suicide, homicide, accidents, diseases such as tuberculosis, and peripheral infections.[6,45] In one 2.5-year follow-up, 10 of 361 addicts had died, a remarkable statistic in light of their relative youth.[45] The morbidity and mortality appear to reflect complications from "dirty" needles and impure drugs more than the effects of the opiates themselves.[42,46] If remission is going to occur, it can be seen at any age, with a probable peak after the age of 40, but there is no absolute fixed age.[27,32,43,47] When an addict remains abstinent for 3 years or longer, there is a very good chance that he will not go back to drugs.[43] Good prognostic signs for opiate addicts include a history of relatively stable employment, being married, a history of few delinquent acts, and few criminal activities unrelated to drugs.[25,42,43] For those who do relapse to misuse of substances, it is possible that increasing life crises and feelings of depression may play a role, especially for addicts who have never participated in long-term treatment.[45]

One additional aspect of the natural history of opiate abuse, the rate of associated alcohol problems, requires emphasis. Most opiate abusers began their substance problems with tobacco and alcohol and then progressed to marijuana and other drugs of abuse as described in other publications[47,48] and elsewhere in this text. These "stages" of abuse are not mutually distinct, and most periods involve a combination of other drugs with alcohol. Thus, because ethanol is legal, is readily available, and rarely leads to dismissal from drug treatment programs, it makes sense that many opiate abusers will turn to alcohol abuse when their primary drug is not available, as alcohol can be used to boost the effects of other drugs. Although many opiate addicts demonstrate periods of time both "on the street" and during outpatient treatment when their alcohol use is relatively moderate (e.g., in one survey approximately 50% of methadone-maintenance patients reported three to four drinks per day on the average),[49] perhaps as many as 50% of male and 25% of female addicts meet the criteria for alcohol dependence within the first 5 years after active drug treatment.[50] The prevalence of alcohol abuse is higher in drug treatment dropouts than it is in those who stay with therapy, and abuse is more likely in individuals who have a history of alcohol abuse before being identified as drug addicts.[49–51] Although active education regarding alcohol and attempts to prevent alcohol abuse should be included in treatment programs for drug abusers, successful drug therapy without specific efforts aimed at alcohol can also result in a decreased use of alcohol over time.[49]

6.1.2.2. Medical Abuse

The medical-setting abusers have not been well studied, probably because their use of opiates is not associated with a very high rate of unexpected death, serious crimes, or violence. What data there are indicate a preponderance of middle-class individuals, women, and those with pain syndromes.[52] The abuse is frequently one of multiple drugs, including depressants and stimulants as well as analgesics.

Two groups of individuals stand out as being at high risk for this syndrome. First, it has been suggested that a majority of people with pain syndromes abuse their prescribed drugs.[52] The second important subgroup, health-care professionals (especially physicians and nurses), may have the highest rate of analgesic drug abuse of any middle-class population.[43,53,54] Possible explanations include the stresses of caring for other people's problems, the manner in which their job interferes with their ability to relate to their families, the long hours of their jobs, and the ready availability of drugs.[55]

6.1.3. Establishing the Diagnosis

Diagnosis in either the "street" or the "medical" group requires an awareness of the possibility of misuse with all patients,[5,6] and a good medical history. In addition, there are a number of physical symptoms, signs, and behavioral patterns to watch for, including:

1. *Increased pigmentation* over veins.
2. Evidence of clotted or *thrombosed veins*.
3. Other *skin lesions* and *abscesses*.
4. *Clubbing* of the fingers, possibly secondary to phlebitis.[56]
5. *Constricted* or small *pupils* (except with dilaudid).
6. *Swollen nasal mucosa* (if the drug is "snorted").
7. *Swollen lymph glands*.
8. An *enlarged liver*.
9. Abnormal laboratory tests, including *decreased globulins*, evidence of acquired immune deficiency syndrome (AIDS), a positive *latex fixation test* [Venereal Disease Research Laboratory (VDRL), test], *liver-function test* abnormalities, and a relatively high *white blood count*.
10. Evidence of visiting *many physicians* (perhaps to get a supply of drugs), a *complex medical history* that is hard to follow, or a *de novo* visit with complaints of *severe pain* (e.g., kidney pain, back pain, headache, or abdominal pain), even with physical signs, as these signs are easy to produce at will (e.g., by placing a drop or two of blood in a urine sample).

11. Any *health professional* being seen for a syndrome for which analgesics might be prescribed.
12. *Evidence of opiates* on a blood or urine toxocological screen.[32]

6.2. EMERGENCY PROBLEMS

The emergency difficulties most frequently seen with the opiates are toxic reactions and medical problems.

6.2.1. Panic Reactions (see Section 1.6.1)

As is true with all the sedating drugs of abuse, individuals tend to be slowed down rather than panicked. Thus, panic reactions rarely, if ever, occur.

6.2.2. Flashbacks

The relatively short half-life of most of these drugs and their rapid disappearance and active metabolites make flashbacks rare phenomena.

6.2.3. Toxic Reactions (see Sections 2.2.3 and 14.4)

6.2.3.1. Clinical Picture

6.2.3.1.1. History

The opiate overdose is usually an acute, life-threatening event that is most often accidental but that could, at times, represent a deliberate suicide attempt.[7] The patient is likely to be found in a semicomatose condition with evidence of a recent IV injection (e.g., a needle in the arm or nearby) or empty bottles. The picture includes both pharmacological effects of the drug and a response to behavioral factors.[7,57] In support of the contribution of behavioral forces is the observation of increased toxic-reaction mortality in animals given the drug in an environment unassociated with prior drug use, whereas those challenged in surroundings associated with sublethal drug doses in the past have a greater chance of survival.

Whatever the mechanism, toxic reactions or overdoses are a significant cause of mortality in opiate abusers. Rates of such deaths appear to vary with a variety of factors, among which are increasing risk with higher-quality heroin (probably related to an overriding of any existing levels of tolerance); a negative association with price, so that the less the drug costs, the greater is the risk for death; and a positive association between morbidity and the amount of quinine per drug package.[29] The quinine itself can create a major problem, as it can decrease the activity of the cardiac pacemaker, decrease cardiac electrical conductivity, and thereby induce a prolonged refractory period that increases the risk for ventricular fibrillation.[29]

6.2.3.1.2. Physical Signs and Symptoms

The physical condition dominates the clinical picture. Specific symptoms depend on the drug, how long ago it was taken, and the patient's general condition. The range of symptomatology can include:

1. Decreased respirations.
2. Blue lips and pale or blue body.
3. Pinpoint pupils (unless there is brain damage, in which case the pupils may be dilated).
4. Nasal mucosa hyperemia (for a patient snorting a drug).
5. Recent needle marks or perhaps a needle still in the arm.[58]
6. Pulmonary edema characterized by gasping, rattling respirations of unknown etiology (not related to heart failure), and a state of shock.[48]
7. Cardiac arrhythmias and/or convulsions, especially seen with codeine, propoxyphene (Darvon), or meperidine (Demerol).[7,58]
8. Death appears to occur from a combination of respiratory depression and pulmonary and/or cerebral edema.[7] The pulmonary edema may be related to an idiosyncratic reaction to the opiate or may be an allergic response to either the drug or one of the adulterants (such as quinine) in the injected substance. There is no evidence that it is related to either a fluid overload or heart failure.[59] An alternate hypothesized mechanism is the possible development of cardiac arrhythmias, perhaps related to histamine release.

6.2.3.1.3. Psychological State

The patient is usually markedly lethargic or comatose.

6.2.3.1.4. Relevant Laboratory Tests (see Section 2.2.3.1.4)

It is necessary to rule out all other cuases of coma, such as head trauma (with a physical exam, a neurological exam, skull X rays, and so on) and glucose or electrolyte abnormalities (as shown in Table 1.5). The level of cardiac functioning must be established with an electrocardiogram (EKG) and the level of brain impairment with an electroencephalogram (EEG), if appropriate. A toxicologic blood or urine screen may be helpful.

6.2.3.2. Treatment (see Section 2.2.3.2)

It has been suggested that the medical needs of the overdosed opiate abuser can be divided into emergency, acute, and subacute stages.[59,60] As outlined in Table 6.2, the general support given first addresses problems expected in any medical emergency. The order in which the levels of care are listed here is not necessarily to be rigidly followed.

1. Establish an adequate *airway; intubate* and place on a *repirator* if necessary, using compressed air at a rate of 10–12 breaths per minute unless pulmonary edema is present.
2. Be sure the *heart* is beating; carry out external cardiac massage, defibril-

late, or administer intracardiac adrenaline if needed; also, give 50 ml of sodium bicarbonate by IV drip for serious cardiac depression.

3. Prevent *aspiration* either by positioning the patient on his side or by using a tracheal tube with an inflatable cuff.
4. Begin an IV (large-gauge needle), being prepared to replace all fluids lost to urine plus 20 ml per hour for insensible loss if the coma persists.
5. Deal with *blood loss* or hypotension with plasma expanders or pressor drugs as needed.
6. Treat *pulmonary edema* with positive-pressure oxygen, but beware of giving too much oxygen and thus decreasing the respiratory drive.
7. Treat *cardiac arrhythmias* with the appropriate drug.
8. Administer a *narcotic antagonist:*
   a. *Naloxone* (Narcan) is the preferred drug, given in doses of 0.4 mg (1 ml) or 0.01 mg/kg IV and repeated in 3–10 minutes if no reaction occurs. Because this drug wears off in 2–3 hours, it is important to monitor the patient for at least 24 hours for heroin and 72 hours for methadone. Be prepared to deal with a narcotic abstinence syndrome, should you precipitate one with the narcotic antagonist (see Section 6.2.6.2).
   b. If naloxone is not available, use *nalorphine* (Nalline), 3–5 mg IV (1 cc = 5 mg), repeated as necessary.
   c. If neither of these drugs is available, use *levallorphan* (Lorfan), giving 1 mg (1 cc) IV,[60] repeating the dose in 10–20 minutes, if needed.
9. Draw arterial *blood gases* if there are respiratory problems.

Table 6.2
Opiate Overdose: Symptoms and Treatment

Symptoms
  Unconscious and difficult to arouse
  Blue lips and body
  Small pupils
  Needle marks
  Pulmonary and/or cerebral edema
  Hypothermia
  Decreased respiration
Treatment
  Clear airway
  Artificial respiration
  Treat hypotension with expanders or pressors
  Treat arrhythmias
  Positive-pressure oxygen
  Naloxone 0.4 mg (1 ml) IV; repeat Q 2–3 hr as needed
  Monitor 24+ hr

10. Draw bloods for baseline *laboratory tests,* including complete blood count (CBC) and the usual blood panel series, as well as a toxicological screen (10 cc). If *hypoglycemia* is involved, administer 50 cc of 50% glucose IV.

11. Establish *vital signs* every 5 minutes for 4 hours, with continued careful monitoring for 24–72 hours.

12. The more *subacute* and *chronic care* involves careful patient monitoring, dealing with *withdrawal signs,* treating *infections* (over one half of individuals with pulmonary edema go on to develop pneumonia, but prophylactic antibiotics are not justified). You should continue to monitor vital signs and laboratory tests, and it is suggested that *tetanus* immunization be given.

13. It is very important in treating the overdose to beware of the possibility of *mixed drug ingestion.* This may require special measures, including the possible need for dialysis (see Section 14.4.3.2).

6.2.4. Psychosis and Depression (Possibly 292.11 or 292.84 in DSM-III-R) (see Section 1.6.4)

Unlike most other drugs, the opiates are not likely to produce any type of temporary psychosis.[61,62] The major psychiatric symptom likely to be noted in opiate abusers is sadness, similar to that reported for alcohol.[63] Thus, at the time of entrance into treatment, between one third and two thirds of opiate addicts are likely to demonstrate significant elevations on cross-sectional depression measures, such as the D scale of the Minnesota Multiphasic Personality Inventory (MMPI), the Zung, or the Beck.[50,63,64] Perhaps as many as 20% may meet the criteria for major depressive disorders at intake, but these figures decrease to 10% showing major depressions and 33% minor depressions at 3- to 6-month follow-ups, with only 2% of the sample demonstrating significant depression at both points.[63,64] Thus, it appears that the depression associated with opiate misuse may be pharmacologically and/or situationally induced and that it tends to disappear within a relatively short time without active antidepressant treatment.[65] Such pictures are perhaps twice as likely to be seen in female as in male addicts at treatment intake, but follow-ups show no differences between the sexes.[50] It should be remembered, however, that if depressions persist more than 2–4 weeks and still meet the criteria for major affective episodes, a judicious use of antidepressants should be considered (see Section 3.1.2.3 on alcohol-related depressions).[64]

6.2.5. Organic Brain Syndrome (Possibly 305.50, 292.81, or 292.90 in DSM-III-R) (see Section 1.6.5)

This is unusual with opiates except as part of an obvious toxic overdose. A possible exception is the rate of agitated confusion seen with meperidine, perhaps related to its effects on acetylcholine.[66]

6.2.6. Opiate Withdrawal in the Adult (292.00 in DSM-III-R) (see Sections 2.2.6 and 4.2.6)

The opiate withdrawal syndrome, seen for all the analgesics discussed in this chapter including propoxyphene (Darvon), was, along with alcohol withdrawal, among the first well-described abstinence pictures. A somewhat arbitrary distinction between phases of withdrawal is outlined in Table 6.3. However, it is important to note that these phases overlap greatly.

6.2.6.1. Clinical Picture

6.2.6.1.1. Acute Withdrawal

1. *History:* The onset of withdrawal usually begins at the time of the next habitual drug dose, ranging from 4 to 6 hours for heroin to a day or more for methadone. The prevalence and intensity of this picture increase directly with the dose, the duration of use, and the time the dose is postponed and inversely with the healthiness of the abuser.[7] The accurate diagnosis may be fairly obvious when the patient demonstrates the physical signs and symptoms as well as the psychological

Table 6.3
Acute Opiate (Heroin) Withdrawal[7,10]

Begins in hours, peaks in 36–72 hours
   Marked drive for the drug
Begins in 8–12 hours, peaks in 48–72 hours
   Tearing
   Running nose
   Yawning
   Sweating
Begins in 12–14 hours, peaks in 48–72 hours
   Restless sleep
Begins in 12 hours, peaks in 48–72 hours
   Dilated pupils
   Anorexia
   Gooseflesh
   Irritability
   Tremor
At peak
   Insomnia
   Violent yawning
   Weakness
   Gastrointestinal (GI) upset
   Chills
   Flushing
   Muscle spasm
   Ejaculation
   Abdominal pain

state described below and requests opiatés, but frequently the clinician must have an index of suspicion and probe for potential "street" or medical abuse. The most usual withdrawal syndrome of the "street" abuser is a relatively benign mixture of emotional, behavioral, and physical symptoms.[7,67] This is due to the variability in the potency of heroin obtained on the street, ranging from 0 to 77% (with most around 3%). Adulterants, such as lidocaine, procaine, quinine, and lactose, make up most of the substances sold as street opiates.[7,10]

   2. *Physical signs and symptoms:* Although much variability can be expected, it is possible to make some generalizations for heroin and morphine.[7] Variations from the usual "heroinlike" picture outlined below include methadone (slower development of symptoms, a less intense clinical picture, persistence of acute problems for 3 weeks or more once they have developed), dilaudid [small rather than large pupils during withdrawal, along with muscle twitching and only mild gastrointestinal (GI) complaints], and codeine (tendency of symptoms to be relatively mild).[7,68] With these examples aside, the usual heroin or morphine withdrawal can be said to have the following characteristics:

   a. Within 12 hours of the last dose, there is usually the beginning of *physical discomfort,* characterized by tearing of the eyes, a runny nose, sweating, and yawning.

   b. Within 12–14 hours, and peaking on the second or third day, the patient moves into a *restless sleep* (a "yen").

   c. Over the same time period, other symptoms begin to appear, including *dilated pupils, loss of appetite, gooseflesh* (hence the term "cold turkey"), *back pain,* and a *tremor.*

   d. This picture gives way to *insomnia;* incessant *yawning;* a *flulike* syndrome consisting of weakness, GI upset, chills, and flushing; *muscle spasm; ejaculation;* and *abdominal pain.*

   e. In the acute phases of withdrawal, the syndrome *decreases* in intensity and is usually greatly reduced by the fifth day, disappearing in 1 week to 10 days.

   3. *Psychological state:* This is as important as the physical problems and includes a strong *"craving"* along with emotional *irritability.*

   4. *Relevant laboratory tests:* As the patient's degree of physical impairment tends to be less severe than that noted for the CNS depressants, it is usually enough to carry out a good physical exam and to establish the baseline laboratory functions described in Table 1.5. Specific test results can include a decrease in carbon dioxide values secondary to increased respiratory rates, a possible increase in the WBC (e.g., 14,000/cubic mm), and occasionally, evidence of ketosis.[7] A toxicological screen may be helpful in establishing the recent use of opiates and analgesics.

6.2.6.1.2. Protracted Abstinence

   The acute abstinence phase is followed by a more protracted abstinence, with two probable subphases.[6,10,32]

1. The early phase of protracted abstinence lasts from approximately *Week 4 to Week 10* or longer and consists of a mild increase in blood pressure, temperature, respirations, and pupillary diameter.

2. This is followed by a later phase lasting *30 weeks or more,* consisting of a mild decrease in all the aforementioned measures and a decrease in the respiratory center response to carbon dioxide. It is possible to see differences in autonomic nervous system responses to opiates as long as 1 year after acute withdrawal is complete.[7]

Thus, what we recognize most clearly as withdrawal is only the acute phase. The protracted abstinence, consisting of physiological as well as behaviorally mediated aspects, goes on for many months. It is possible that this long-term syndrome produces a vague discomfort that may play an important role in driving the addict back to drug use.

6.2.6.2. Treatment (also review Section 2.2.6.2)

Treatment of the opiate withdrawal syndrome in adults is briefly outlined in Table 6.4 and in references 7 and 10. Helping the patient achieve relative comfort during this period may be associated with a higher rate of retention of patients in rehabilitation.[68,69]

1. The first phase of therapy involves a good medical examination, as these patients have high rates of medical disorders as discussed below.
2. The physician must do all he can to develop physician–patient rapport to maximize patient comfort and cooperation. It is important that one physician be in charge.
3. After estimating the probable degree of dependence and thereby deciding whether active treatment of withdrawal is needed, it is important to explain carefully to the patient the symptoms he can expect and that they cannot be

Table 6.4
Treatment of Opiate Withdrawal

General support:
  Physical and laboratory exam
  Rest
  Nutrition
  Reassurance
  Honest appraisal of what is to be expected
  Keep one doctor in charge
One type of specific treatment:
  Example: Give methadone 15–20 mg orally as a test
  Determine dose on Day 1 or 2
  Give dose BID
  Decrease by 20%/day or over 2 weeks

totally eliminated. However, you should reassure him that you will do everything you can to minimize his discomfort.

4. You should establish a flow sheet of symptom severity and the treatments.[70]

5. One treatment approach for physical withdrawal symptoms begins with the readministration of an opiate to the point at which symptoms are greatly reduced, after which the drug dose is slowly decreased over a period of 5–14 days. Any of a variety of specific drugs can be used.[71] Most states have rather severe restrictions on the prescription of opiates to addicts. Unless the physician or clinic possesses a special license for opiate prescription, treatment is usually limited to 72 hours, and then only in case of a medical emergency.[72] Even if a permit is granted, detoxification is usually limited to a month or less. Therefore, although I will first outline detoxification using opiates (the most "physiological" way to treat the syndrome), I will then discuss alternate approaches.

a. Any opiate can be used, but most authors recommend oral methadone.

   i. Give a test dose of about 20 mg of methadone orally and repeat the dose if the symptoms are not alleviated, thus determining the minimum dose needed to control symptoms during the first 24–36 hours. Note that 1 mg of methadone roughly equals 2 mg of heroin or 20 mg of meperidine (Demerol).

   ii. Most addicts achieve some comfort at doses of 20 mg of methadone the first day. The necessary drug is then divided into twice-daily doses, with daily decreases of 10–20% of the first day's dose, depending on the development of symptomatology.

b. An alternate approach is to administer 10 mg of methadone intramuscularly (IM) and observe the effects, reexamining the patient in 8 hours and monitoring the amount of drug necessary to abolish the symptoms.[70] This procedure makes it possible to determine the amount of drug needed to control the symptoms in the first 24 hours, after which the doses can be given orally two to three times a day and can be decreased as described above.

c. It is possible to administer any opiate, establishing the necessary first-day dose and decreasing the drug by 10–20% per day. One example is propoxyphene (Darvon) treatment, in which an initial detoxification dose of 600–800 mg/day has been used in a 21-day withdrawal program.[73] Propoxyphene hydrochloride can be administered in doses of 110–220 mg by mouth given three or even four times a day, whereas the napsylate may need to be given in slightly higher doses of 165–330 mg by mouth three times a day; 600 mg of the hydrochloride a day is roughly equivalent to 20–25 mg per day or morphine subcutaneously [SQ (Latin *sub cuti*)] or 10 mg per day of oral methadone.[74] Another example is the treatment of withdrawal through use of the relatively weak opiatelike drug diphenoxylate (Lomotil), using 2 or 3 tablets three times per day for the first several days, followed by 2 tablets three times per day on Day 3 or 4, after which the drug can be decreased and stopped.[75]

d. A special case occurs when an individual has been taking part in a methadone maintenance program. Under these circumstances, it is advisable to decrease the drug slowly to minimize the chance of the development of symptoms. This usually means a diminution of approximately 3 mg from the daily dose each week, but even at this rate, some symptoms will be seen.

6. Recognizing the need to develop nonopiate approaches to both outpatient and inpatient detoxification, Tennant and Uelmen[72] described a "cocktail" of medications, giving the usual dose administered on Day 1 in an attempt to decrease the symptoms (but not to abolish them) and then decreasing the dose to zero over the next 10–14 days. This regimen includes carisoprodol (Soma), 300 mg QID for muscle pain and tension as needed; prochlorperazine (Compazine), 10 mg QID by mouth for nausea as needed; and a relatively mild opiate that is legal for such use in many states, pentazocine (Talwin), 50–100 mg every 4–6 hours by mouth for pain.

7. Another symptom-oriented nonopiate approach to withdrawal utilizes clonidine (Catapres). This drug decreases sympathetic nervous system overactivity during withdrawal by blocking alpha-2 receptors, especially in the locus coeruleus area of the brain and perhaps in spinal sympathetic neurons.[76–78] When the drug is given in doses of approximately 5 μg/kg (the average adult patient receiving approximately 0.3 mg QID), most patients undergoing opiate withdrawal report a decrease in autonomic nervous system dysfunction.[79–81]

A variant of the clonidine approach to opiate withdrawal following heroin use or methadone maintenance has recently been proposed by Kleber et al.[82] For methadone, after doses have been decreased to 20 mg or less per day, therapy is begun with a naloxone challenge (0.8 mg IM) at 9:00 A.M. to establish the grade and severity of the future withdrawal symptoms. Patients who are more uncomfortable 10–30 minutes after the challenge are then treated with 0.1 mg of clonidine, a dose that is repeated 1 hour later if needed. If the naloxone challenge results in few or no symptoms, the narcotic antagonist is repeated within approximately 30 minutes; a resulting relatively benign clinical picture then indicates that no active medications are needed. If withdrawal symptoms are observed, the active treatment regimen is begun at approximately 10:00 A.M. with 0.2–0.3 mg of clonidine three times a day (10:00 P.M., 2:00 P.M., and 8:00 P.M.). On the second day of treatment, naltrexone (Trexan), 1 mg, as a challenge is used with the institution of additional clonidine as needed. This is then a prelude to the institution of naltrexone every 4 hours (up to 8 mg) as described in Section 15.3.2.2.

A third variant of withdrawal treatment with clonidine uses a transdermal skin patch.[83] Treatment of withdrawal begins with a total of approximately 1 mg/day of clonidine orally in divided doses on Day 1. This reflects the fact that it takes approximately 24 hours for the transdermal patch to produce adequate blood levels. After the first oral dose (usually 0.2 mg), a Catapres TTS (clonidine) transdermal patch is placed on the upper arm, where it is to remain for approximately 7 days for heroin abusers and approximately 10 days for methadone maintenance patients. Adjunctive therapy with diflunisal (Dolobid), 100 mg twice a day for pain, can be used. Finally, other alpha agonists have been proposed to be used in an approach similar to oral clonidine.[84]

However, no matter how it is applied, clonidine appears to be inferior to opiates in the relief of subjective discomfort and pain, and it produces high levels of sedation and hypotension and thus is often not well tolerated by patients.[79,85] In the final analysis, this mode of treatment may be inferior to the use of opiates in relieving most withdrawal symptoms.

8. Additional treatments of potential interest are the use of acupuncture, hypnosis, or any other mechanism for possibly increasing the body's own opiates, the endorphins and enkephalins.[86,87] However, few if any controlled data on the use of these approaches to treating opiate withdrawal are available.

9. During detoxification, it is very important that some thought be given to plans for rehabilitation. It should be recognized that many patients enter detoxification solely to decrease their high drug levels or in response to immediate life problems. Under such circumstances, the individual may not want to participate in a rehabilitation program—only 10% of those who complete a detoxification program seek long-term care.[88] However, for those who might consider rehabilitation, the detoxification period is an excellent time to introduce the need for permanent abstinence, and counseling should be offered to *everyone*.

6.2.7. Opiate Withdrawal in the Neonate (292.00 in DSM-III-R)

A special case of opiate withdrawal is seen in the newborn, passively addicted by the mother's drug abuse during the latter part of pregnancy.[6,7,10,89,90] However, addiction of the infant is only one part of the wide span of severe problems likely to accompany abuse of opiates by pregnant women.[90] Difficulties also include elevated rates of intrauterine death, low-birth-weight infants, premature delivery, and a 2–5% risk for neonatal mortality. In one series, only 31% of children delivered to opiate-abusing women were free of potentially serious complications.

Up to one half to two thirds or more of live births to opiate addicts produce children who demonstrate a withdrawal syndrome that is likely to increase the length of hospital stay and itself carry a mortality of 3–30%. However, when more accurate instruments are used to measure the level of symptomatology, it *may be* that as few as 25% of the infants of *methadone*-maintenance mothers may require active treatment, and this for usually less than 2 weeks. Therefore, the reader is advised to carefully evaluate the levels of symptoms before actively beginning treatment.[91]

6.2.7.1. Clinical Picture

The syndrome consists of *irritability, crying,* a *tremor* (seen in 80%), increased *reflexes,* increased *respiratory* rate, *diarrhea, hyperactivity* (seen in 60%), *vomiting* (seen in 40%), and *sneezing/yawning/hiccuping* (seen in 30%).[92] The child usually has a *low birth weight* but may be otherwise unremarkable until the first or second day, when the symptoms usually begin. For children of methadone addicts, symptoms might not appear until Day 3 or 4 or even later.[7]

6.2.7.2. Treatment

1. A first step should be prevention. For pregnant addicts on methadone maintenance, it is important that the drug be reduced to 20 mg a day or less during the last 6 weeks of pregnancy.[93]
2. Of course, symptoms may indicate other disorders as well, and the clinician must carefully rule out hypoglycemia, hypocalcemia, infections including those of the CNS, CNS trauma, or anoxia and must aggressively treat any such syndromes uncovered.[91]
3. Treatment of neonatal withdrawal consists of general support and observation, including keeping the child in a warm, quiet environment and observing electrolytes, glucose, and other physiological parameters.
4. In addition, the child with *moderate to severe* symptoms can be treated with paregoric, a total of 4 drops/kg per day, which translates to about 0.2 ml orally every 3–4 hours as needed to control symptoms.[7] Doses can be increased up to a total of about 2 ml/kg per day in divided doses if needed.[89] The interested reader is referred to a more detailed discussion by Finnegan.[89] Other approaches include a daily total of *methadone,* 0.3–1.5 mg/kg; or *phenobarbital,* 8 mg/kg; or *diazepan,* 2–5 mg, with any of these drugs being given in divided doses three or four times a day.[7] Medications should be given for 10–20 days, the amounts being decreased toward the end of that period.
5. Following all the caveats mentioned above, the clinician may also consider attempting to control the symptoms with clonidine. In this approach, the infant may be given a test dose of 0.5–1.0 µg/kg, which, if it is tolerated well and produces a reduction in symptoms, can be followed 24 hours later with 3 µg/kg per day by mouth divided into six hourly doses and continued over 10–16 days in decreasing amounts.[92]
6. It is also possible to treat, at least primarily, the addicted infants of mothers on methadone maintenance by having them breast-feed while they continue to take their methadone. Additional drugs can be given to the child as needed.

6.2.8. Medical Problems

When opiates are taken in their pure form in appropriate doses, even their long-term use is not necessarily associated with severe medical problems.[7,46] However, opiate abusers, especially those taking street drugs, frequently present for care in some sort of medical crisis. This may be an overdose or other serious medical problem as a consequence of the adulterants in opiate mixtures or the poor hygienic practices involved in the use of needles. The medical problems and their treatment have been covered in detail in a variety of texts[70] and will be mentioned only briefly here. My goal is to increase your level of awareness of the problems so that you can then use the proper medical procedures.

Some of the more common problems include:

1. AIDS as spread through "dirty" needles[94,95]
2. Abscesses and other infections of the skin and muscle
3. Tetanus or malaria
4. Hepatitis and other liver abnormalities[96]
5. Gastric ulcers
6. Heart arrhythmias
7. Endocarditis
8. Anemias
9. Electrolyte abnormalities, especially hyperkalemia
10. Bone and joint infections
11. Eye-ground abnormalities, as they reflect emboli from the adulterant added to the street drug
12. Kidney failure secondary to infections or adulterants
13. Muscle destruction
14. Pneumonia
15. Lung abscesses
16. Tuberculosis
17. Bronchospasm and wheezing, especially likely after inhalation of opiate fumes ("chasing the dragon")[97]

In addition, addicts may present with a series of emotional and social problems, including:

18. Depression, frequently seen during methadone maintenance as described above[98,99]
19. Sexual functioning abnormalities, which may partially reflect the transiently low testosterone level seen during chronic administration and lasting at least a month after the opiate is stopped[100]
20. Police problems
21. Social and interpersonal problems

These problems point out the absolute necessity for a careful evaluation of medical and emotional problems in *any* opiate abuser undergoing treatment.

6.3. REHABILITATION

After identification and acute treatment of the opiate abuser, all such individuals should be advised of the need for rehabilitation to try to help them achieve abstinence. Such rehabilitation is usually done through methadone-maintenance clinics, drug-free residential programs, or a variety of outpatient approaches. In keeping with my emphasis on acute drug problems, rehabilitation is discussed separately in Section 15.3.

REFERENCES

1. Vandam, L. D. Butorphanol. *New England Journal of Medicine 302*:381–384, 1980.
2. Hayes, J. R. Gentanyl. *Newsletter: California Society for the Treatment of Alcoholism and Other Drug Dependencies 8*:3–5, 1981.
3. Inturrisi, C. E., Max, M. B., Foley, K. M., *et al.* The pharmacokinetics of heroin in patients with chronic pain. *New England Journal of Medicine 310*:1213–1217, 1984.
4. Berridge, V. Opium and the historical perspective. *Lancet 2*:78–80, 1977.
5. Musto, D. F. *The American Disease: Origins of Narcotic Control.* New Haven, Connecticut: Yale University Press, 1973.
6. Stimmel, B. *Heroin Dependency: Medical, Economic, and Social Aspects.* New York: Stratton Intercontinental Medical Book Corp., 1975.
7. Jaffe, J. H. Drug addiction and drug abuse. In A. G. Gilman, L. S. Goodman, T. W. Rall, & F. Murad (Eds.), *The Pharmacological Basis of Therapeutics* (7th ed.). New York: Macmillan, 1985, pp. 532–581.
8. Woods, J. H., & Winger, G. Opioids, receptors, and abuse liability. In H. Y. Meltzer (Ed.), *Psychopharmacology: The Third Generation of Progress.* New York: Raven Press, 1987, pp. 1555–1564.
9. Jaffe, J. H., & Martin, W. R. Opioid analgesics and antagonists. In A. G. Gilman, L. S. Goodman, T. W. Rall, & F. Murad (Eds.), *The Pharmacological Basis of Therapeutics* (7th ed.), New York: Macmillan, 1985, pp. 491–531.
10. Marshall, B. E., & Wollman, H. General anesthetics. In A. G. Gilman, L. S. Goodman, T. W. Rall, & F. Murad (Eds.), *The Pharmacological Basis of Therapeutics* (7th ed.). New York: Macmillan, 1985, pp. 276–301.
11. Koob, G. F., & Bloom, F. E. Behavioral effects of opioid peptides. *British Medical Bulletin 39*:89–94, 1983.
12. Cohen, M. R., Cohen, R. M., Pickar, D., *et al.* Behavioural effects after high dose naloxone administration to normal volunteers. *Lancet 2*:1110, 1981.
13. Bloom, F., Segal, D., Ling, N., *et al.* Endorphins: Profound behavioral effects in rats suggest new etiological factors in mental illness. *Science 194*:630–632, 1976.
14. Mathiasen, J. R., Raffa, R. B., & Vaught, J. L. Mice: Differential sensitivity in the tail flick test to centrally administered Mu- and Delta-opioid receptor agonists. *Life Sciences 40*:1989–1994, 1987.
15. Woods, J. H., & Winger, G. Behavioral characterization of opioid mixed agonist–antagonists. Paper presented at the Committee on Problems in Drug Dependence Annual Meeting, Philadelphia, June 16, 1987.
16. Pfeiffer, A., Brantl, V., Herz, A., & Emrich, H. M. Psychotomimesis mediated by κ opiate receptors. *Science 233*:774–776, 1986.
17. Kleber, H. D. *Trexan: A Pharmacologic Adjunct for the Detoxified Opioid Addict.* Wilmington, Delaware: E. I. du Pont de Nemours, 1984.
18. Bozarth, M. A., & Wise, R. A. Anatomically distinct opiate receptor fields mediate reward and physical dependence. *Science 224*:514–517, 1984.
19. Burns, R. S., LeWitt, P. A., Ebert, M. H., *et al.* The clinical syndrome of striatal dopamine deficiency. *New England Journal of Medicine 312*:1418–1421, 1985.

20. Langston, J., Ballard, P., Tatrud, J., & Irwin, I. Chronic parkinsonism in humans due to a product of meperidine-analog synthesis. *Science 219*:9789–9790, 1983.
21. Stimmel, B. The socioeconomics of heroin dependency. *New England Journal of Medicine 287*:1275–1280, 1972.
22. Zinberg, N. E., & Jacobson, R. C. The natural history of "chipping." *American Journal of Psychiatry 133*:37–40, 1976.
23. Caplovitz, D. *The Working Addict*. New York: The Graduate School and the University Center of the City University of New York, 1976.
24. Dess, W. J., & Cole, F. C. The medically evacuated Viet-Nam narcotic abuser: A follow-up rehabilitative study. *Bulletin on Narcotics 24*:55–65, 1977.
25. Robins, L. N., Helzer, J. E., & Davis, D. H. Narcotic use in Southeast Asia and afterward. *Archives of General Psychiatry 32*:955–961, 1975.
26. Wechsler, H., & Rohman, M. E. Patterns of drug use among New England college students. *American Journal of Drug and Alcohol Abuse 8*:27–37, 1981.
27. Messeri, P. A., & Brunswick, A. F. Heroin availability and aggregate levels of use: Secular trends in an urban black cohort. *American Journal of Drug and Alcohol Abuse 13*:109–133, 1987.
28. Des Jarlais, D. C., & Uppal, G. S. Heroin activity in New York City, 1970–1978. *American Journal of Drug and Alcohol Abuse 7*:335–346, 1980.
29. Ruttenbar, A. J., & Luke, J. L. Heroin-related deaths: New epidemiologic insights. *Science 226*:14–20, 1984.
30. Hartnoll, R., Lewis, R., Mitcheson, M., & Bryer, S. Estimating the prevalence of opioid dependence. *Lancet 1*:203–205, 1985.
31. Kandel, D. B., & Logan, J. A. Patterns of drug use from adolescence to young adulthood: Periods of risk for initiation, continued use, and discontinuation. *American Journal of Public Health 74*:660–666, 1984.
32. Editorial: Alcohol and politics. *Lancet 1*:1358–1359, 1987.
33. Smart, R. G., & Adlaf, E. M. Patterns of drug use among adolescents: The past decade. *Social Science Medicine 23*:717–719, 1986.
34. Editorial: National survey finds continuing decline in use of illicit drugs by high school seniors. *Hospital and Community Psychiatry 36*:1011, 1985.
35. Smart, R. G., Goodstadt, M. S., Adlaf, E. M., et al. Trends in the prevalence of alcohol and other drug use among Ontario students: 1977–1983. *Canadian Journal of Public Health 76*:157–161, 1985.
36. Nicholi, A. M. The nontherapeutic use of psychoactive drugs. *New England Journal of Medicine 308*:925–933, 1983.
37. Rounsaville, B. J., & Kleber, H. D. Untreated opiate addicts. *Archives of General Psychiatry 42*:1072–1077, 1985.
38. Halikas, J. A., Darvish, H. S., & Rimmer, J. D. The black addict. 1. Methodology, chronology of addiction, and overview of the population. *American Journal of Drug and Alcohol Abuse 3*:529–543, 1976.
39. Maddux, J., & Desmond, D. P. Heroin addicts and nonaddicted brothers. *American Journal of Drug and Alcohol Abuse 1*:237–248, 1984.
40. Croughan, J. L., Miller, J. P., Waggelin, D., et al. Psychiatric illness in male and female narcotic addicts. *Journal of Psychiatry 43*:225–228, 1982.
41. Langenauer, B. J., & Bowden, C. L. A follow-up study of narcotic addicts in the NARA program. *American Journal of Psychiatry 128*:73–78, 1971.
42. O'Brien, C. P., Woody, G. E., & McLellan, A. T. Long-term consequences of opiate dependence. *New England Journal of Medicine 304*:1098–1099, 1981.
43. Vaillant, G. E. A 20-year follow-up of New York narcotic addicts. *Archives of General Psychiatry 29*:237–241, 1973.
44. Snow, M. Maturing out of narcotic addiction in New York City. *International Journal of the Addictions 8*:921–938, 1973.
45. Kosten, T. R., Rounsaville, B. J., & Kleber, H. D. A 2.5-year follow-up of depression, life crises,

and treatment effects on abstinence among opioid addicts. *Archives of General Psychiatry 43:*733–738, 1986.

46. Kreek, M. J. Health consequences associated with methadone. In J. Cooper, & F. Altman (Eds.), *NIDA Research Monograph Series,* Department of Health and Human Services Publication (ADM) 83-1281. Washington, D.C.: U.S. Government Printing Office, 1983, pp. 456–482.

47. Winick, C. The life cycle of the narcotic addict and of addiction. *Bulletin on Narcotics 26:*1–11, 1964.

48. Kandel, D. B. *Longitudinal Research on Drug Use.* New York: Halstead Press, 1978.

49. Simpson, D. D., & Lloyd, M. R. Alcohol use following treatment for drug addiction. *Journal of Studies on Alcohol 42:*323–335, 1981.

50. Croughan, J. L., Miller, J. P., Whitman, B. Y., & Schober, J. G. Alcoholism and alcohol dependence in narcotic addicts: A prospective study with a five-year follow-up. *American Journal of Drug and Alcohol Abuse 8:*85–94, 1981.

51. McGlothlin, W. H., & Anglin, M. D. Shutting off methadone: Costs and benefits. *Archives of General Psychiatry 38:*885–892, 1981.

52. Lass, H. Most chronic pain patients misuse drugs, study shows. *Hospital Tribune World Service 6:*2, 1976.

53. McAuliffe, W. E., Rohman, M., Santangelo, S., et al. Psychoactive drug use among practicing physicians and medical students. *New England Journal of Medicine 315:*805–810, 1986.

54. Maddux, J. F., Hoppe, S. K., & Costello, R. M. Psychoactive substance use among medical students. *American Journal of Psychiatry 143:*187–191, 1986.

55. Jones, R. E. A study of 100 physician psychiatric inpatients. *American Journal of Psychiatry 134:*1119–1122, 1977.

56. Chotkowski, L. A. Clubbing of the fingers in heroin addiction. *New England Journal of Medicine 311:*262, 1984.

57. Siegel, S., Hinson, R. E., Krank, M. D., & McCully, J. Heroin "overdose" death: Contribution of drug-associated environmental cues. *Science 216:*436–437, 1982.

58. Greene, M. H., & DuPont, R. L. The treatment of acute heroin toxicity. In P. G. Bourne (Ed.). *A Treatment Manual for Acute Drug Abuse Emergencies.* Washington, D.C.: U.S. Government Printing Office, 1974, pp. 11–16.

59. Dimijian, G. G. Differential diagnosis of emergency drug reactions. In P. G. Bourne (Ed.). *A Treatment Manual for Acute Drug Abuse Emergencies.* Washington, D.C.: U.S. Government Printing Office, 1974, pp. 1–7.

60. Kleber, H. D. The treatment of acute heroin toxicity. In P. G. Bourne (Ed.), *A Treatment Manual for Acute Drug Abuse Emergencies.* Washington, D.C.: U.S. Government Printing Office, 1974, pp. 17–21.

61. Oppenheimer, E., Stimson, G. V., & Thorley, A. Seven-year follow-up of heroin addicts: Abstinence and continued use compared. *British Medical Journal 2:*627–630, 1979.

62. McLellan, A. T., Woody, G. E., & O'Brien, C. P. Development of psychiatric illness in drug abusers. *New England Journal of Medicine 301:*1310–1314, 1979.

63. Kosten, T. R., & Rounsaville, B. J. Suicidality among opioid addicts. *American Journal of Drug and Alcohol Abuse 14:*357–369, 1988.

64. Rousaville, B. J., Weissman, M. M., Crits-Christoph, K., et al. Diagnosis and symptoms of depression in opiate addicts. *Archives of General Psychiatry 39:*151–156, 1982.

65. Dorus, W., & Senay, E. C. Depression, demographics, and drug abuse. *American Journal of Psychiatry 137:*699–704, 1980.

66. Eisendrath, S. J., Goldman, B., Dougland, J., et al. Meperidine-induced delirium. *American Journal of Psychiatry 144:*1062–1065, 1987.

67. Siegel, S. Evidence from rats that morphine tolerance is a learned response. *Journal of Comparative Physiology and Psychology 89:*498–506, 1975.

68. Gossop, M., Green, L., Phillips, G., & Bradley, B. What happens to opiate addicts immediately after treatment: A prospective follow-up study. *British Medical Journal 294:*1377–1380. 1987.

69. Sorenson, J. L., Hargreaves, W. A., & Weinberg, J. A. Withdrawal from heroin in three or six weeks. *Archives of General Psychiatry 39:*167–171, 1982.

70. Shapira, J. *Drug Abuse: A Guide for the Clinician.* New York: American Elsevier, 1975.
71. Wen, H. L., Ho, W. K. K., & Wen, P. Y. C. Comparison of the effectiveness of different opioid peptides in suppressing heroin withdrawal. *European Journal of Pharmacology 100:*155–162, 1984.
72. Tennant, F. S., & Uelman, G. F. Prescribing narcotics to habitual and addicted narcotic users: Medical and legal guidelines in California and some other Western states (medicine and the law). *Western Journal of Medicine 133:*539–545, 1980.
73. Tennant, F. S., Russell, B. A., Casas, S. K., et al. Heroin detoxification: A comparison of propoxyphene and methadone. *Journal of the American Medical Association 232:*1019–1022, 1975.
74. Jasinski, D. R., Pevnick, J. S., Clark, S. C., & Griffith, J. D. Therapeutic usefulness of propoxyphene napsylate in narcotic addiction. *Archives of General Psychiatry 34:*227–233, 1977.
75. Ives, T. J., & Stults, C. C. Short-course diphenoxylate hydrochloride for treatment of methadone withdrawal symptoms. *British Journal of Psychiatry 143:*513–514, 1983.
76. Franz, D. N., Hare, B. D., & McCloskey, K. L. Spinal sympathetic neurons: Possible sites of opiate-withdrawal suppression by clonidine. *Science 215:*1643–1645, 1982.
77. Charney, D. S., Riordan, C. E., Kleber, H. D., et al. A safe, effective, and rapid treatment of abrupt withdrawal from methadone therapy. *Archives of General Psychiatry 39:*1327–1332, 1982.
78. Charney, D. S., Heninger, G. R., & Kleber, H. D. The combined use of clonidine and naltrexone as a rapid, safe, and effective treatment of abrupt withdrawal from methadone. *American Journal of Psychiatry 143:*831–837, 1986.
79. Jasinski, D. R., Johnson, R. E., & Kocher, T. R. Clonidine in morphine withdrawal. *Archives of General Psychiatry 42:*1063–1066, 1985.
80. Schuckit, M. Clonidine and the treatment of withdrawal. *Drug Abuse and Alcoholism Newsletter 17*(3):1–4, 1988.
81. Charney, D. S., Sternberg, D. E., Kleber, H. D., et al. The clinical use of clonidine in abrupt withdrawal from methadone. *Archives of General Psychiatry 38:*1273–1277, 1981.
82. Kleber, H. D., Topazian, M., Gaspari, J., et al. Clonidine and naltrexone in the outpatient treatment of heroin withdrawal. *American Journal of Drug and Alcohol Abuse 13:*1–17, 1987.
83. Clark, H. W., & Longmuir, N. Clonidine transdermal patches: A recovery oriented treatment of opiate withdrawal. *Newsletter: California Society for the Treatment of Alcoholism and Other Drug Dependencies 13,* 1986.
84. Schubert, H., Fleischhacker, W. W., Meise, U., & Theohar, C. Preliminary results of guanfacine treatment of acute opiate withdrawal. *American Journal of Psychiatry 141:*1271–1273, 1984.
85. Jasinski, D. R., Johnson, R. E., & Makhxoumi, H. Efficiency of clonidine in morphine withdrawal. Paper presented at the 20th Annual American College of Neuropsychopharmacology meeting in San Diego, December 16–18, 1981.
86. Wen, G., & Keith, L. Drug addiction in pregnancy. In J. J. Sciarra (Ed.), *Gynecology and Obstetrics.* Philadelphia: Harper and Row, 1983, pp. 119–127.
87. Clement-Jones, V., Tomlin, S., Rees, L. H., et al. Increased β-endorphin but not metenkephalin levels in human cerebrospinal fluid after acupuncture for recurrent pain. *Lancet 2:*946–948, 1980.
88. Sheffet, A., Quinones, M., Levenhar, M. A., et al. An evaluation of detoxification as an initial step in the treatment of heroin addiction. *American Journal of Psychiatry 133:*337–340, 1976.
89. Finnegan, L. P. Neonatal abstinence syndrome: Assessment and pharamcotherapy. In F. F. Rubaltelli & B. Granati (Eds.), *Neonatal Therapy: An Update.* New York: Elsevier, 1986, pp. 122–146.
90. Fitzsimmons, J., Tunis, S., Webster, D., et al. Pregnancy in a drug-abusing population. *American Journal of Drug and Alcohol Abuse 12:*247–255, 1986.
91. Green, M., & Suffet, F. The neonatal narcotic withdrawal index: A device for the improvement of care in the abstinence syndrome. *American Journal of Drug and Alcohol Abuse 8:*203–213, 1981.
92. Hoder, E. L., Leckman, J. F., Ehrenkranz, R., et al. Clonidine in neonatal narcotic-abstinence syndrome. *New England Journal of Medicine 305:*1284, 1981.
93. Strass, M. E., Andresko, M., Stryker, J. C., et al. Relationship of neonatal withdrawal to maternal methadone dose. *American Journal of Drug and Alcohol Abuse 3:*339–345, 1976.

94. Friedland, G. H., & Klein, R. S.: Transmission of the human immunodeficiency virus. *New England Journal of Medicine 317:*1125–1135, 1987.
95. Ancelle-Park, R., Brunet, J. B., & Downs, A. M. AIDS and drug addicts in Europe. *Lancet 2:*626–627, 1987.
96. Lettau, L. A., McCarthy, J. G., & Smith, M. J. Outbreak of severe hepatitis due to delta and hepatitis B viruses in parental drug abusers and their contacts. *New England Journal of Medicine 317:*1256–1262, 1987.
97. Oliver, R. M. Bronchospasm and heroin inhalation. *Lancet 1:*915, 1986.
98. Rounsaville, B., Kosten, T., Weissman, M., & Kleber, H. Prognostic significance of psychopathology in treated opiate addicts. *Archives of General Psychiatry 43:*739–745, 1986.
99. Wolters, E., Stam, F. C., Lousberg, R. J., *et al.* Leucoencephalopathy after inhaling "heroin" pyrolysate. *Lancet 2:*1233–1238, 1982.
100. Mendelson, J. H., Mendelson, J. E., & Patch, V. D. Plasma testosterone levels in heroin addiction and during methadone maintenance. *Journal of Pharmacology and Experimental Therapeutics 192:*211–217, 1975.

Cannabinols

7.1. INTRODUCTION

Marijuana is among the most widely used of the drugs described in this text. The health-care problems involved with delta-9-tetrahydrocannabinol (THC) (the most active ingredient in marijuana and hashish), include panic reactions, toxic reactions, and a great deal of anxiety in the general population about possible mental and physiological damage to young users. Because you will be called on, as a health-care deliverer, to give information about this drug to worried parents and to teenagers attempting to make decisions about future use, this chapter presents information on the history, the physiology, and the medical effects of the cannabinols.

THC is an ancient drug; its use dates back to at least 2700 B.C.[1,2] It has been used in many cultures, including the Middle East, the Orient, and Western countries. As a result it has had a variety of names, including hashish and charas (the dried resin from the flowering tops of marijuana plants), bhang (the less potent dried leaves and flowering shoots), ganja (the resins from the small leaves), and so on.[2] In North America, THC is obtained as marijuana or hashish. [Pure THC is not available "on the streets," and samples so labeled are usually phencyclidine (PCP) or other substances that are relatively inexpensive or easy to produce (see Chapters 8 and 9).] At low to moderate doses, THC produces fewer physiological and psychological alterations than do most other classes of drugs, including alcohol. However, the fact that this drug does affect the nervous system, and that the peak age of use occurs in late adolescence when the brain and sexual systems are still developing, makes the substance a legitimate concern.

Diagnosing the misuse or abuse of marijuana poses many of the same problems seen with alcohol. Although, in contrast to alcohol, marijuana is illegal, its acceptance by the general population and the high prevalence of users make it important to differentiate among use, misuse (implying temporary problems that may disappear), and abuse or dependence (implying a high potential for future problems).

Using this approach, no one has developed objectively stated criteria for cannabinol abuse that have been tested through follow-ups to demonstrate that they predict pervasive and persistent future difficulties. One exception may be a 5-year follow-up of a moderate-size sample reported by Weller and Halikas[1] using criteria for cannabinol abuse based on the presence of problems in at least three of four areas of potential difficulties: (1) adverse physical and psychological reactions to the drug (e.g., health problems and signs of physical addiction), (2) problems with control of use (e.g., using the drug in the morning and going on binges of heavy use for days), (3) social or interpersonal problems (e.g., arrests, traffic accidents, and fights), and (4) the opinion of the patient or significant others that use has been too high. The authors found a correlation between the daignosis of abuse and the frequency of use, the level of initial intake, early age of onset, and future drug problems.

7.1.1. Pharmacology

THC comes from the marijuana plant, *Cannabis sativa*, which grows readily in warm climates. The percentage of active THC produced parallels the amount of sunlight received by the plant. Marijuana, the less potent source of THC, is the dried plant leaves, and hashish and other more potent sources of the drug are the resins of the plant flowers.

7.1.1.1. General Characteristics

Although this drug is sometimes called a hallucinogen, at the doses most frequently taken the predominant effects are euphoria and a change in the level of consciousness without frank hallucinations. The drug can be ingested through smoking, eating, and (rarely) intravenous (IV) injection. The average cigarette contains 2.5–5.0 mg of the most active THC, delta-9-THC; however, only one half of the drug is absorbed through this route of administration.[2] The potency of a cigarette depends on the quality of the marijuana used (whether from the stems, leaves, or flowering tops, in increasing order of potency) and the amount of time elapsed since the plant was harvested (there is a decrease in potency over time[3]).

When the drug is smoked, its peak plasma level is reached in approximately 10 minutes, but the most prominent physiological and subjective effects may not develop for 20–30 minutes.[2] Intoxication usually lasts between 2 and 3 hours, depending on the dose.[4,5] When the plant is eaten, a greater percentage of the drug is absorbed, and the result is a longer (but less predictable) "high." In this case, the onset is seen in 0.5–1 hour, a peak blood level is reached in 2–3 hours, and the effects last up to 8 hours.

Other forms of cannabinols and related substances have been manufactured and tested for their psychopharmacological properties. Each has been developed for oral administration. The drugs include nabilone, a synthetic analogue with modest antiemetic properties and sedative side effects, but few euphorogenic attributes, except at high doses.[2,6,7]

The relationship between THC blood levels and clinical effects is complex, and few readily available measures for THC in the blood have yet been developed.[5] Once ingested, the drug tends to disappear from the plasma rapidly, becoming absorbed in tissues, especially those with high levels of fat, such as the brain and testes.[2] The half-life is believed to be 7 days,[8] primarily a result of THC in tissues, and active ingredients are found for as long as 8 or more days.[9] The drug is first metabolized to an 11-hydroxylated derivative with some psychoactivity; however, the remaining metabolites do not change levels of consciousness. THC is excreted primarily as metabolites, mostly in the feces, but also in the urine.[9]

Although the mechanisms of action of THC are not completely understood, there is some evidence of disruption of cellular metabolism and prevention of the proper formation of proteins, including DNA and RNA.[8] More recent studies have raised the possibility that THC has important effects on the dopamine system, as well as some possible interactions between this drug and benzodiazepine receptor binding sites.[10]

7.1.1.2. Predominant Effects

The greatest effects of THC are on the brain, the heart or cardiovascular system, and the lungs. Most changes, if not all, occur acutely and appear to be reversible.

The changes in mood seen with THC depend not only on the amount of drug but also on the setting in which the substance is taken and, as with any more "mild" drugs, what one expects to happen.[11] It is also important to consider the form in which the drug was taken (e.g., hashish vs. marijuana tobacco), the route of administration (e.g., smoking vs. eating), and the purity of the drug (ranging from 0.5 to greater than 10%).[2]

In addition to euphoria, the individual usually experiences a feeling of relaxation, sleepiness, and heightened sexual arousal; is unable to keep accurate track of time; experiences hunger; and exhibits decreased social interaction. The user develops problems with short-term memory and may demonstrate an impairment of the ability to carry out multistep tasks.[2,12] Intoxication may be associated with mild levels of suspiciousness or paranoia along with some loss of insight.[13] If intoxication occurs during a state of high stress, a heightened level of aggressiveness may occur; however, most frequently one sees a decrease in this attribute.[12] At higher doses, frank hallucinations may occur, usually visual, sometimes accompanied by paranoid delusions. Like any toxic reaction, this can be associated with confusion, disorientation, and panic, as described in Section 7.2.[2]

A variety of physiological problems can accompany moderate intoxication. These include fine shakes or tremors, a slight decrease in body temperature, a decrease in muscle strength and balance, a decreased level of motor coordination, dry mouth, and bloodshot eyes (injected conjunctivae).[2,12,14] Some individuals experience nausea, headache, nystagmus, and mildly lowered blood pressure.[12,15] THC may also precipitate seizures in epileptics.[16]

Along with an increased breathing rate, the respiratory effects of an acute administration of THC include an increase in the diameter of the bronchial tubes, of potential significance in treating asthma.[12,16,17] However, chronic use results in a decrease rather than an increase in the diameter and a worsening of breathing problems.[8,18]

Marijuana affects the heart by increasing the heart rate, resulting in an increased cardiac work load. Thus, this drug can be dangerous for individuals with preexisting cardiac disease.[19]

7.1.1.3. Tolerance and Dependence

7.1.1.3.1. Tolerance

Neither tolerance nor physical dependence is a major clinical problem with marijuana. Toleration of increasing doses of the drug does develop through both metabolic and pharmacodynamic mechanisms, but the most important aspect is the mild level of cross-tolerance to alcohol that has been demonstrated.[2,20,21]

7.1.1.3.2. Dependence

There is some debate about whether there is an actual withdrawal syndrome from marijuana. If it does occur, the strength probably parallels the amount of and length of exposure to the drug and consists of nausea, lowered appetite, mild anxiety, a rebound in rapid-eye-movement (REM) sleep and dreaming, and insomnia, as well as a mild tremor and increased body temperature.[2,20,22] It is possible, however, that with higher doses a syndrome resembling mild opiate withdrawal may be noted.[22]

7.1.2. Epidemiology and Patterns of Abuse

The usual distinction made in this text between medical use and "street" use is not as relevant to marijuana as it is to many other drugs. Although some medical use of this drug is being evaluated, all but an infinitesimal amount of use of THC-containing substances takes place illegally.

Marijuana is used as a "recreational" drug by all strata of society, reaching into all job levels and ages, although the predominant use is among younger people. It has been tried on at least one occasion by 50–60 million Americans, an increase of nearly 100% since 1971.[2,20,23] At the time of the second edition of this book, there was a hint (but little convincing evidence) that the percentage of users of marijuana had begun to decrease.[23-25] New evidence continues to support this conclusion. For example, while approximately 56% of high school seniors admitted to having used marijuana at least once in 1977 and 59% in 1982, the figure had decreased to 56% by 1985.[26] When grades 7 through 13 were considered together, a similar moderate decrease for lifetime use was apparent in Canada, from approximately 24% in 1983 to 21% in 1985.[27] Other surveys have also focused on histories of use of marijuana in the preceding 12 months, demonstrating moderate decreases between 1979 and 1983 for high school seniors (from 44 to 36%),[28] with similar data noted for high school students who had used marijuana within the last 30 days, with figures falling from 37% in 1979 to 27% in 1983.[2,29] At the same time, over the last decade, approximately 5.5–7% of young adults and late adolescents admit to having used marijuana daily, without any marked change over the years.[2,29] In summary, while in recent years 72% of people in the United States have used marijuana by age 25, including about 55% who have taken this drug by the end of high school, frequent or daily use is more uncommon, and there appears to be a trend for a moderate decrease in the prevalence of use of this drug over the last several years.[30,31]

The average marijuana user is in the 18–25 age range, and, reflecting the aging of young people who were first introduced to marijuana in the 1960s and 1970s, the age of the using population is now increasing.[32] As is true with almost all drugs, there appears to be a correlation between the frequency and intensity of use of marijuana and experience with other drugs or heavier intake of alcohol.[32] There is also a probable association between heavier intake of the cannabinols and experience with other life problems, including delinquency, as well as between heavier intake and an increased risk for drug-related health difficulties.[33]

7.1.3. Medical Uses

The purported medicinal properties of THC resulted in wide general use until legislation limiting its availability was introduced shortly after the turn of the century.[2] The drug was listed in the *Pharmacopoeia* until the 1930s as having antibacterial activity, decreasing intraocular pressure, decreasing the perception of pain, helping in the treatment of asthma, having anticonvulsant properties (although recent evidence disputes this[16]), increasing appetite, and helping with general morale.[2,18] Currently, THC is being used for glaucoma which has been otherwise resistant to therapy, and for terminal cancer.

Recent interest in the medicinal properties of these drugs has resulted in their being tested as antianxiety agents, antidepressants, analgesics, and antitumor substances; the results have been basically negative.[18,25] However, their ability to lower intraocular pressure in glaucoma has been substantiated by controlled research, and they may be of at least temporary help in treating acute asthma attacks.[6,18,25,34] Their greatest therapeutic usefulness has been in controlling the severe nausea often associated with cancer chemotherapy. The doses change with the specific substance administered, but in one paradigm, delta-9-THC was given at 10 mg/m^2 of body surface every 3 hours for a total of five doses, to help with nausea.[34] Although the long-term use of some of the synthetic cannabinols, such as nabilone, may have some toxic effects,[6] most (although not all) researchers do report that this drug is of benefit during chemotherapy and for decreasing intraocular pressure.[6,34] Nabilone is available in some countries, but has not been marketed in the United States.

7.1.4. Establishing the Diagnosis

Recognizing whether psychiatric and medical problems are associated with marijuana and hashish use requires knowledge of the drug and an adequate history.

Although THC is thought to exacerbate depression and to intensify any preexisting psychosis,[35,36] there are no known pathognomonic physical signs and no available laboratory tests to help. Again, the key is to have a high index of suspicion.

7.2. EMERGENCY PROBLEMS

The vast majority of individuals who present with marijuana-related problems show either panic or toxic reactions. These involve high levels of anxiety and/or confusion.

7.2.1. Panic Reactions (e.g., 305.20 or 292.89 in DSM-III-R) (see Sections 1.6.1, 5.2.1, 8.2.1, and 14.2)

7.2.1.1. Clinical Picture

This is a classic drug-induced panic, lasting at most 5–8 hours.[4] The clinical picture includes an exaggeration of the usual marijuana effects, which commonly are perceived as threatening by the naive or inexperienced user. The feeling of anxiety, the fear of losing control or going crazy, and the fear of physical illness can be seen in individuals with no preexisting psychopathology as well as in those who have a history of erratic or maladaptive behavior.

7.2.1.2. Treatment

Treatment is predicated on careful diagnosis, ruling out the involvement of other drugs and preexisting psychopathology,[36] and gentle reassurance.

1. A physical examination is necessary to rule out signs of other drugs of intoxication and preexisting medical disorders. It is advisable to draw blood (10 cc) or collect urine (50 ml) for a toxicological screen for cannabinols and other drugs.
2. A quick history should establish the does taken and the individual's prior experience with the drug.
3. The individual should be reassured that his problems will clear within the next 4–8 hours.
4. It helps to place the patient in a quiet room, constantly reassure him, and allow friends to help "talk him down."
5. The level of intoxication may fluctuate over the next 5 hours or so, as the active drug is released from the tissues.
6. No specific type of drug should be used to treat every panic reaction. If, however, the anxiety cannot be controlled in any other manner, the drugs of choice would be antianxiety medications, such as chlordiazepoxide (Librium), 10–50 mg orally, which may be repeated in an hour, if needed.
7. Because of the persistence of THC metabolites in the body, patients should

be warned that they may experience some mild feelings of drug intoxication over the next 2–4 days.

8. If the reaction is unusually intense, the patient, as well as the family, should be advised to seek evaluation for the possibility of preexisting psychopathology. Referral to a physician or a health-care practitioner experienced with drug problems is best.

7.2.2. Flashbacks (Possibly 292.90 in DSM-III-R) (see Sections 1.6.2 and 8.2.2)

7.2.2.1. Clinical Picture

Flashbacks involve the spontaneous recurrence of feelings and perceptions experienced in the intoxicated state. They are classically seen for marijuana and the hallucinogens,[4] in both frequent and infrequent users.

The clinical picture involves a change in time sense or a feeling of slowed thinking, generally at a lower level of intensity than that experienced when the user is high. Because flashbacks tend to be time-limited (usually lasting only minutes), the major difficulty comes if the individual panics, fearing brain damage. It has also been reported that marijuana may "induce" flashbacks in individuals who have taken hallucinogens in the past.[15] In rare instances, the symptoms may be "chronic" or persistent, but this is so unusual that the presence of additional neurological or psychiatric disorders should be evaluated.

7.2.2.2. Treatment

The treatment for a flashback is simple reassurance, following all the steps outlined for the treatment of the panic reaction in Section 7.2.1.2.

7.2.3. Toxic Reactions (see Section 1.6.3)

7.2.3.1. Clinical Picture

When an individual takes a high level of marijuana, toxic reactions can occur, but are usually characterized by an organic brain syndrome (OBS) and/or paranoia as discussed in Sections 7.2.4 and 7.2.5. The relatively low potency of marijuana and the lack of availability in the United States of more toxic forms, such as ganja, combine to make this an infrequent problem. Life-threatening overdose is very rare for the cannabinols, even hashish.[22]

7.2.3.2. Treatment

The treatment is identical to that outlined for panic reactions in Section 7.2.1.2. The approach involves offering good general support and reassurance and allowing the passage of time in a room with no excessive external stimuli. It is best to treat this disorder symptomatically, avoiding the administration of other drugs.

7.2.4. Psychiatric Symptoms (e.g., 292.11 in DSM-III-R) (see Sections 5.2.4, 1.6.4, and 8.2.4)

A *temporary* psychotic state, characterized by paranoia and hallucinations without confusion, can be seen with marijuana, but there is no evidence that it results in permanent mental impairment.

7.2.4.1. Clinical Picture

The temporary paranoid state accompanied by visual hallucinations is probably a reaction to excessive doses of the drug.[13,37,38] Retrospective studies indicate bizarre behavior, violence, and panic in some heavy users in India, but this reaction appears to be temporary, lasting for up to a few days or at most several weeks.[10,24,37,39]

If a frankly pyschotic state does not clear within that time, the patient generally has a prior psychiatric disorder, as marijuana probably worsens prior psychotic problems.[39–42] In addition, I have seen a number of people who had clear evidence of prior depressions or demonstrated a prior psychotic picture, but complained that their present symptoms were caused by marijuana. In taking a history from the individual and relatives, the preexisting illness became obvious, and in some instances the history of drug ingestion was a delusion.

Anecdotal reports indicate the development of apathy, decreased self-awareness, impaired social judgment, slow thinking, and a decrease in goal-directed drives in chronic THC users.[2,4,42,43] However, these reports do not address the question of whether any changes in personality occurred *before* marijuana use, perhaps predisposing users to heavy doses of the drug. An equally acceptable explanation is that individuals who are becoming apathetic and withdrawing from competition and from society in general also find the chronic use of marijuana attractive.[20,25] However, although no cognitive deficits have been objectively demonstrated in chronic users,[12,44] it is possible (although unlikely) that an *amotivational syndrome* exists, in which the person loses interest in tasks and accomplishments.

Several follow-up studies of marijuana users have been carried out in an effort to establish the actual rate of psychiatric disorders subsequent to marijuana use. For example, one 6- to 7-year follow-up of 97 regular marijuana smokers and 50 controls showed no significant increases in rates of depression or other major psychiatric disorders among the smokers.[40] This information in combination with the data described above makes it unlikely that marijuana use alone often precipitates major, long-lasting psychiatric disorders.

7.2.4.2. Treatment

It is imperative that a history of prior psychiatric problems be obtained for all individuals who present with what appears to be a marijuana-related psychiatric problem. Any underlying prior psychiatric diagnosis (e.g., affective disorder or schizophrenia, as described by Goodwin and Guze[45]) is an important factor to be addressed in treatment.

1. If the individual is out of contact with reality, a short-term hospitalization can keep him out of trouble until the psychosis clears.
2. Understanding and reassurance are the cornerstone of treatment of these disorders. The individual should be told that his problem is temporary, and attempts should be made to help him with reality testing by, for example, giving him insight into his hallucinations and delusions.
3. Antipsychotic medication can be initiated for a psychosis on a short-term basis if behavior control is absolutely necessary. You might use haloperidol (Haldol) at approximately 5 mg/day in divided doses (rarely up to 20 mg daily) or chlorpromazine (Thorazine) at 25–50 mg intramuscularly (IM) or 50–150 mg by mouth.
4. Anyone demonstrating a grossly psychotic reaction that lasts more than a day should be carefully evaluated for other major psychiatric disorders. The most frequent will probably be schizophrenia or affective disorder, as described in Goodwin and Guze.[45]

7.2.5. Organic Brain Syndrome (Possibly 305.20 or 292.81 in DSM-III-R) (see Section 1.6.5 and 14.6)

7.2.5.1. Clinical Picture

1. Temporary clouding of mental processes, consisting of impaired and dull thinking, impaired tracking ability, decreased short-term memory, decreased concentration, and impaired learning can occur with marijuana and hashish. This is really a toxic reaction and clears fairly rapidly.[20,25,46–48] It is possible that this clinical picture might be produced at least in part by adulterants in the marijuana, including formaldehyde or paraquat.[47]

2. More startling is a report of cerebral ventricular dilation (which may indicate cerebral hemisphere shrinkage) in 10 heavy drug users whose major drug was marijuana[48]—but attempts to replicate these findings have failed.[3,20,25] To date, no convincing evidence of permanent decreased brain functioning in heavy users of THC substances has been shown.[49,50]

7.2.5.2. Treatment

The temporary type of clinical picture and the relatively mild level of impairment make the focus of treatment careful observation and reassurance. Treatment involves the same steps outlined for the treatment of panic reactions (Section 7.2.1.2).

7.2.6. Withdrawal

It is not certain whether any form of withdrawal of clinical significance occurs with marijuana and hashish. If symptoms develop, the picture can be expected to be limited and to clear with time alone.

7.2.7. Medical Problems

No drug can be taken into the body with complete safety. The medical disorders associated with the frequent use of marijuana tend to be relatively mild and transient. However, because of the purely recreational nature of this drug, it is hard to justify its use even if the possibility of serious medical complications is remote. Despite the long history of use of marijuana, only in recent years has serious research into the possible medical consequences been carried out.

The risk of adverse consequences, of course, increases with increasing amount, frequency of intake, and length of exposure to these drugs.[51] Some of the more important areas of possible damage are presented below, primarily to help you in answering questions from patients and their relatives.

7.2.7.1. Lungs[2,8,12,18,51]

1. Marijuana and other inhaled compounds are irritating and produce a bronchitis that usually disappears with the discontinuation of drug use.

2. Although the acute administration of marijuana causes dilatation of the bronchial tree, chronic administration is thought to cause constriction, with a resulting asthmalike syndrome.

3. The chronic use of any substance that irritates the lungs can cause temporary or permanent destruction of lung architecture, and there is evidence of a decreased vital capacity in chronic smokers—even healthy young men.[12]

4. Although it is extremely difficult to document accurately, there is some evidence that heavy marijuana smokers have increased rates of precancerous lung lesions. Marijuana has 50% higher levels of carcinogenic hydrocarbons than tobacco, and animal experiments have corroborated a possible increased rate of cancer after many years of heavy marijuana intake.[2,18,25]

7.2.7.2. Nose and Throat

A chronic inflammation of the sinuses (sinusitis), as well as pharyngitis, has been reported in heavy smokers of marijuana.[18,25] There is also the possibility (without any good direct evidence) that heavy marijuana smokers have the same increased risk of cancers of the head and neck as heavy tobacco smokers.

7.2.7.3. Cardiovascular System

Marijuana produces an increased heart rate and a decreased strength of heart contractions.[2,17,20,25] This reaction is dangerous for heart patients, as there is an associated decrease in oxygen delivery to heart muscle and a decrease in the amount of exercise an individual can tolerate before the onset of heart pain or angina.[19]

7.2.7.4. Immune System

Some research indicates that lymphocytes are sensitive to THC, which decreases their ability to carry out the usual immune responses.[2,18,25] It has not yet been determined whether this impairment results in a clinically significant increase in infections in marijuana users. A related problem is possible contamination of the drug with pathogens such as salmonella.[52]

7.2.7.5. Reproductive System

THC has been demonstrated to impair sperm production in heavy users[7] and has been associated with an increased rate of chromosomal breakage. Chronic marijuana use in humans has also been shown to be associated with a decrease in the size of the prostate and testes in males and to block ovulation in females, although these changes are reversible.[18,25] In mice, chronic exposure to marijuana in the perinatal period decreases the reproductive functioning of adult males.[53]

It is also likely that THC can have an effect on the developing fetus. Smoking by pregnant mothers is likely to produce problems with oxygenation of the baby and can be associated with altered behavior and learning by the neonate.[2,54] The clinical importance of the findings discussed above has not yet been demonstrated, and the purported teratogenic action of the cannabinols has also been questioned.[55]

7.2.7.6. Endocrine System

Decreased levels of various hormones, including testosterone, have been demonstrated in heavy marijuana smokers,[18,25,38] but these abnormalities appear to be temporary and are usually seen only after 3 weeks of regular use. It is also possible that growth-hormone production is decreased in heavy marijuana smokers, but the clinical significance to humans of this and other hormonal findings has not been established.[56] Marijuana intake has also been reported to affect prolactin levels in animals, but it has not yet been demonstrated whether these changes are relevant to humans.[56]

7.2.7.7. Brain

CNS problems were briefly discussed in Sections 7.2.3, 7.2.4, and 7.2.5. Heavy marijuana smokers may show changes in electroencephalographic (EEG) tracings that may last for 3 months or more after chronic use, and in animals some ultrastructural brain changes have been reported.[8,57] THC has also been noted to act on the septal area of the limbic system—an area important in the control of emotions. These findings may have some importance for CNS disease, especially in adolescents, with their rapidly growing brains. In any event, THC does produce acute memory impairment.[51]

7.2.7.8. Diabetes

The use of marijuana by diabetics can result in a potentially life-threatening alteration in the body's acid–base metabolism, ketoacidosis.[58]

7.2.8. Other Emergency Problems

7.2.8.1. Accidents

One of the greatest known dangers of marijuana is accidents as a consenquence of the decreased judgment, the impaired ability to estimate time and distance, and the impaired motor performance that follow use.[2,18,25] These effects are similar to those of alcohol, and it appears that the two substances may potentiate each other.[2,12] Thus, there is impressive evidence that marijuana smoking significantly decreases automobile-driving ability for up to 8 hours after smoking, and a recent report shows that up to 17% of drivers in fatal auto accidents tested positive for cannabinols.[59] This drug also significantly decreases the ability of even experienced pilots to properly fly airplanes 24 hours after their last "recreational use."[60] One can expect that there is great loss of property and lives from driving under the influence of marijuana and related substances.[61]

7.2.8.2. Precipitation of Use of Other Drugs

A brief notation is necessary to deal with public fears that the use of marijuana is the first step on the road to more dangerous drugs, such as heroin. Such exaggerated reports have been prevalent since the 1920s and have done little to establish the credibility of individuals teaching that THC-containing substances have some real dangers.

The data in this area are very complex, as marijuana (as well as tobacco and alcohol) *is* frequently one of the first drugs taken by those who go on to the use of stimulants, depressants, or heroin.[31,33] There is, however, no convincing evidence that marijuana plays a role in "causing" the use of more potent substances. There is probably an association between an earlier age of first use of cannabinols and later development of delinquency, unemployment, and health problems.[31,33,51] It is also likely that individuals with characteristics that lead them to use drugs like heroin also tend to use marijuana (and alcohol, caffeine, and other drugs).

7.2.9. Conclusion and Caveat

Thus, THC is not a benign drug, and individuals who choose to use this substance should recognize the potential dangers. On the other hand, in educating people about THC, it is important to portray the dangers accurately and to avoid scare tactics that might lead the young user, especially, to mistrust *all* information about the drug.

REFERENCES

1. Weller, R. A., & Halikas, J. A. Objective criteria for the diagnosis of marijuana abuse. *Journal of Nervous and Mental Disease 168*:98–103, 1980.
2. Jaffe, J. H. Drug addiction and drug abuse. In A. G. Gilman, L. S. Goodman, & A. Gilman (Eds.), *The Pharmacological Basis of Therapeutics* (7th ed.). New York: Macmillan, 1985, pp. 558–561.
3. Liskow, B. Marijuana deterioration. *Journal of the American Medical Association 214*:1709, 1970.

4. Talbott, J. A. The emergency management of marijuana psychosis. In P. G. Bourne (Ed.), *A Treatment Manual for Acute Drug Abuse Emergencies.* Washington, D.C.: U.S. Government Printing Office, 1974, pp. 83–87.

5. Domino, L. E., Domino, S. E., & Domino, E. F. Do plasma levels of delta-9-tetrahydrocannabinol reflect a marijuana high? *Psychopharmacology Bulletin 19:*760–765, 1983.

6. Sallan, S. E. Antiemetics in patients receiving chemotherapy for cancer. *New England Journal of Medicine 302:*135–138, 1980.

7. Harris, L. S. Cannabinoids as analgesics. In R. F. Beers & T. Basset (Eds.), *Pain and Analgesic Compounds.* New York: Raven Press, 1979, pp. 467–473.

8. Nahas, G. Biomedical aspects of cannabis usage. *Bulletin on Narcotics 24:*13–27, 1977.

9. Dackis, C. A., Pottash, A. L. C., Annito, W., *et al.* Persistence of urinary marijuana levels after supervised abstinence. *American Journal of Psychiatry 139:*1196–1198, 1982.

10. Sethi, B. G. B., Trivedi, J. K., Kumar, P., *et al.* Antianxiety effect of cannabis: Involvement of central benzodiazepine receptors. *Biological Psychiatry 21:*3–10, 1986.

11. Stillman, R., Galanter, M., & Lemberger, L. Tetrahydrocannabinol (THC): Metabolism and subjective effects. *Life Sciences 19:*569–576, 1976.

12. Mendelson, J. H., Rossi, A. M., & Meyer, R. E. *The Use of Marihuana: A Psychological and Physiological Inquiry.* New York: Plenum Press, 1974.

13. Galanter, M., Stillman, R., Wyatt, R. J., *et al.* Marihuana and social behavior: A controlled study. *Archives of General Psychiatry 30:*518–521, 1974.

14. Weil, A. T., Zinberg, N. E., & Nelsen, J. M. Clinical and psychological effects of marihuana in man. *Science 162:*1234–1242, 1968.

15. Weil, A. T. Adverse reactions to marihuana: Classification and suggested treatment. *New England Journal of Medicine 282:*997–1000, 1970.

16. Feeney, D. M. Marihuana and epilepsy. *Science 197:*1301–1302, 1977.

17. Nicholi, A. M. The nontherapeutic use of psychoactive drugs. *New England Journal of Medicine 308:*925–933, 1983.

18. Cohen, S., & Stillman, R. C. *The Therapeutic Potential of Marihuana.* New York: Plenum Press, 1976.

19. Gottschalk, L. A. Aronow, W. S., & Prakash, R. Effect of marijuana and placebo-marijuana smoking on psychological state and on psychophysiological cardiovascular functioning in anginal patients. *Biological Psychiatry 12:*255–266, 1977.

20. Jones, R. T. Clinical relevance of cannabis tolerance and dependence. *Journal of Clinical Pharmacology 211:*1435–1475, 1981.

21. Perez-Reyes, M., Hicks, R., Bumberry, J., Jeffcoat, A. R., & Coak, C. E. Interaction between marijuana and alcohol. *Alcoholism: Clinical and Experimental Research 12:*268–272, 1988.

22. Kaymakcalan, S. Potential dangers of cannabis. *International Journal of the Addictions 10:*721–735, 1975.

23. Smart, R. G., & Murray, G. F. A review of trends in alcohol and cannabis use among young people. *Bulletin on Narcotics 33:*77–90, 1981.

24. Wechsler, H., & Rohman, M. E. Patterns of drug use among New England college students. *American Journal of Drug and Alcohol Abuse 8:*27–37, 1981.

25. Relman, A. S. Marijuana "justifies serious concern." In *Marijuana and Health.* Washington, D.C.: National Academy Press, 1982.

26. Kozel, N. J., & Adams, E. H. Epidemiology of drug abuse: An overview. *Science 234:*970–974, 1986.

27. Smart, R. G., Adlaf, E. M., & Goodstadt, M. S. Alcohol and other drug use among Ontario students: An update. *Canadian Journal of Public Health 77:*57–58, 1986.

28. Smart, R. G., Goodstadt, M. S., Adlaf, E. M., *et al.* Trends in the prevalence of alcohol and other drug use among Ontario students: 1977–1983. *Canadian Journal of Public Health 76:*157–161, 1985.

29. Editorial: National survey finds continuing decline in use of illicit drugs by high school seniors. *Hospital and Community Psychiatry 36:*1011–1012, 1985.

30. Editorial: Epidemiology of drug usage. *Lancet 1:*147, 1985.

31. Kandel, D. B. Marijuana users in young adulthood. *Archives of General Psychiatry 41:*200–209, 1984.

32. Lex, B. W., Griffin, M. L., Mello, N. K., & Mendelson, J. H. Concordant alcohol and marihuana use in women. *Alcohol 3:*193–200, 1986.

33. Kandel, D. B., Davies, M., Karus, D., & Yamaguchi, K. The consequences in young adulthood of adolescent drug involvement. *Archives of General Psychiatry 43:*746–754, 1986.

34. Rose, M. Cannabis: A medical question? *Lancet 1:*703, 1980.

35. Halikas, J. A., Goodwin, D. W., & Guze, S. B. Marihuana use and psychiatric illness. *Archives of General Psychiatry 27:*162–165, 1972.

36. Treffert, D. A. Marihuana use in schizophrenia: A clear hazard. Paper presented at the 130th Annual Meeting of the American Psychiatric Association, Toronto, Ontario, Canada, May 5, 1977.

37. Edwards, G. Psychopathology of a drug experience. *British Journal of Psychiatry 143:*509–512, 1983.

38. Smart, R. G., & Adlaf, E. M. Adverse reactions and seeking medical treatment among student cannabis users. *Drug and Alcohol Dependence 9:*201–211, 1982.

39. Miszzek, K. A. Behavioral effects of chronic marijuana. *Psychopharmacology 67:*195–201, 1980.

40. Weller, R. A., & Halikas, J. A. Marijuana use and psychiatric illness: A follow-up study. *American Journal of Psychiatry 142:*848–850, 1985.

41. Andreasson, S., Allebeck, P., Engstrom, A., & Rydberg, U. Cannabis and schizophrenia: A longitudinal study of Swedish conscripts. *Lancet 2:*1483–1484, 1987.

42. Szmanzki, H. V. Prolonged depersonalization after marijuana use. *American Journal of Psychiatry 138:*231–233, 1981.

43. Schaeffer, J. Cognition and long-term use of ganja. *Science 13:*465, 1981.

44. Brill, N. Q., & Christie, R. L. Marihuana use and psychosocial adaptation. Follow-up study of a collegiate population. *Archives of General Psychiatry 31:*713–719, 1974.

45. Goodwin, D. W., & Guze, S. B. *Psychiatric Diagnosis* (4th ed.). New York: Oxford University Press, 1988.

46. Meyer, R. E. Psychiatric consequences of marijuana use. In J. R. Tinklenberg (Ed.), *Marijuana and Health Hazards.* New York: Academic Press, 1975, pp. 133–152.

47. Spector, I. AMP: A new form of marijuana. *Journal of Clinical Psychiatry 46:*498–499, 1985.

48. Campbell, A. M. G., Evans, M., Thomason, J. L. G., *et al.* Cerebral atrophy in young cannabis smokers. *Lancet 2:*1219–1224, 1974.

49. Grant, I., & Mohns, L. Chronic cerebral effects of alcohol and drug abuse. *International Journal of the Addictions 10:*883–920, 1975.

50. Stefanis, C., Laikos, A., Boulougouris, J., *et al.* Chronic hashish use and mental disorder. *American Journal of Psychiatry 13:*225–227, 1976.

51. Wu, T. C., Tashkin, D. P., Djahed, B., & Rose, J. E. Pulmonary hazards of smoking marijuana as compared with tobacco. *New England Journal of Medicine 318:*347–351, 1988.

52. Taylor, D. N., Washsmuth, I. K., Shangkuan, Y. H., *et al.* Salmonellosis associated with marijuana: A multistate outbreak traced by pasmid fingerprinting. *New England Journal of Medicine 306:*1249–1253, 1982.

53. Dalterio, S., Badr, F., Bartke, A., *et al.* Cannabinoids in male mice: Effects on fertility and spermatogenesis. *Science 216:*315–316, 1982.

54. Clapp, J. F., Wesley, M., Cooke, R., *et al.* The effects of marijuana smoke on gas exchange in ovine pregnancy. *Alcohol and Drug Research 7:*85–92, 1986.

55. Smith, C. G., & Asch, R. H. Drug abuse and reproduction. *Fertility and Sterility 48:*355–373, 1987.

56. Mendelson, J. H., Ellingboe, J., & Mello, N. K. Acute effects of natural and synthetic cannabis

compounds on prolactin levels in human males. *Pharmacology, Biochemistry and Behavior 20:*103–106, 1984.

57. Heath, R. G. Cannabis: Effects on brain function and ultrastructure. *Biological Psychiatry 15:*657–690, 1980.

58. Bier, M. M., & Steahly, L. P. Emergency treatment of marihuana complicating diabetes. In P. G. Bourne (Ed.), *A Treatment Manual for Acute Drug Abuse Emergencies.* Washington, D.C.: U.S. Government Printing Office, 1974, pp. 88–94.

59. Fortenberry, J. C., Brown, D. B., & Shevlin, L. T. Analysis of drug involvement in traffic fatalities in Alabama. *American Journal of Drug and Alcohol Abuse 12:*257–267, 1986.

60. Yesavage, J. A., Leirer, V. O., Denari, M., & Hollister, L. E. Carryover effects of marijuana intoxication on aircraft pilot performance: A preliminary report. *American Journal of Psychiatry 142:*1325–1329, 1985.

61. Sutton, L. The effects of alcohol, marihuana and their combination on driving ability. *Journal of Studies on Alcohol 44:*438–445, 1983.

Hallucinogens and Related Drugs

8.1. INTRODUCTION

Both marijuana and the hallucinogens produce a change in the level of consciousness, and both are capable of inducing hallucinations. However, in the usual doses taken, the predominant effect of cannabis is to alter the "feeling state" with less intensity and without frank hallucinations. The drugs discussed in this chapter produce more intense changes and often yield abnormal sensory inputs of a predominantly visual nature (illusions or hallucinations), even at low doses.

This chapter covers a variety of substances, as exemplified Table 8.1. These related drugs are amenable to a number of different types of categorizations, each with its own assets and liabilities.[1] No matter how they are broken down, the hallucinogens are structurally similar; many resemble amphetamine, some (e.g., LSD) are synthetic, and others are plant products of cacti (e.g., peyote or mescaline) and fungi (e.g., psilocybin). Despite unsubstantiated and potentially dangerous claims to the contrary regarding LSD and MDMA (ecstasy), hallucinogens have no proven medical uses in which their assets are known to outweigh their liabilities.[2,3]

The hallucinogens are by no means new substances. They have been used as part of religious ceremonies and at social gatherings by native Americans for over 2000 years and are still utilized by some native groups.[4-6]

8.1.1. Pharmacology

All drugs of this class, except DMT, are well absorbed orally, exert effects at relatively low doses, and have adrenergic (e.g., adrenalinelike) properties.[1] Despite many clinical similarities, there are, of course, differences in the doses that are required for the most prominent clinical effects. For example, on a milligram basis, LSD has 100 times the potency of the "magic mushroom" constitutents of psilocybin and psilocin, and is 4000 times more potent that mescaline, but is weaker than STP or DOM.[1] These relative potencies are of limited clinical importance because users adjust the self-administered dose of each so that all yield similar effects. The

Table 8.1

Some Hallucinogenic Drugs[1,3,13,34,62]

Indolealkylamines
  Lysergic acid diethylamide (LSD[a])
  Psilocybin
  Psilocyn
  Dimethyltryptamine (DMT)
  Diethyltryptamine (DET)
Phenylethylamines
  Mescaline (peyote)
Phenylisopropylamines
  2,5-Dimethoxy-4-methylamphetamine (DOM or STP)
  Methylene dioxyamphetamine (MDA)
  Methylene dioxymethamphetamine (MDMA)
  4-Bromo homolog of STP (DOB)
Related drugs
  Phencyclidine (PCP) (see Chapter 9)
  Nutmeg
  Morning glory seeds
  Catnip
  Nitrous oxide
  Amyl or butyl nitrite

[a]As a point of interest, the abbreviation LSD (like EKG) comes from the original German: *Lyserg Säure Diethylamid.*

drugs also demonstrate different side-effect profiles (e.g., there is a greater likelihood of vomiting with mescaline at even low doses) and different ratios between feelings of euphoria and self-awareness vs. actual hallucinations (e.g., DOM and DET tend to show more euphoria at lower doses and may require higher levels of intake before hallucinations are observed). Overall, however, about 200 µg of LSD produces a fairly typical hallucinogenic reaction. Thus, the generalizations given for LSD at this dose can be assumed to hold for the other drugs as well, unless specifically noted.

The exact mechanism of action of these substances is not known, but much study has centered on their structural similarities to the brain transmitters, especially serotonin, with prominent effects on both major subtypes of serotonin brain receptors.[1,7-10] The effects of hallucinogens have been documented in most areas of the brain, ranging from the cortex to the brain stem.

The term *psychotomimetic* has also been used, implying a possible relationship between the hallucinogen psychoses and schizophrenia.[11] The visual hallucinations and the strong emotional state seen with these substances, however, do not resemble the auditory hallucinations accompanied by the flat (or unchanging) affect seen in schizophrenics.[9,12]

The hallucinogens differ in length of action, with the "high" from LSD having an onset after 40–60 minutes, peaking at 90 minutes, and lasting as long as

6–12 hours; most other hallucinogens have clinically relevant actions for between 2 and 8 hours.[1,3] The rate of metabolism tends, of course, to parallel the length of action.

8.1.1.1. Predominant Effects

The state induced by these substances includes an increased awareness of sensory input with vivid colors and a sharpened sense of hearing, a subjective feeling of enhanced mental activity, a perception of usual environmental stimuli as novel events, altered body images, a turning of thoughts inward, and a decreased ability to tell the difference between oneself and one's surroundings.[1] Some clinicians have felt that these experiences, especially as they relate to LSD or MDMA (ecstasy), might serve to increase actual mental insights and feelings of empathy. Because of this, it was hoped that use of these agents might enhance treatment efforts, but there is *no evidence* that the potential dangers of these substances are justified as part of psychotherapy or that any improvement is likely to occur.[3] In addition to the possibility that the drugs will increase feelings of anxiety and sadness, hallucinogens are also said to produce a "knight's move" pattern of jumping in logical sequences and nonlinear thinking—making it harder to reason one's way through problems.[3,13]

LSD and the group of related drugs tend to produce adrenalinelike or adrenergic effects in addition to hallucinations. Thus, the intoxicated individual usually exhibits dilated pupils, a flushed face, a fine tremor, increased blood pressure, elevations in blood sugar, and an increase in body temperature.[1,14,15]

8.1.1.2. Tolerance and Dependence

8.1.1.2.1. Tolerance

Toleration of larger and larger doses, reflecting both behavioral and pharmacological mechanisms, develops rapidly after as little as 3 or 4 days at one dose per day and disappears within 4 days to a week after stopping use.[13,16,17] Cross-tolerance exists among most of the hallucinogens, including LSD, mescaline, and psilocybin, but this cross-tolerance does not appear to extend to marijuana.[1,6,18]

8.1.1.2.2. Dependence

There is no known clinically significant withdrawal syndrome with the hallucinogens.

8.1.1.3. Specific Drugs

Thus far in this text, most of the drugs described are readily available on the street and are usually the drugs that the seller advertises them to be [a notable exception being the virtual nonexistence of pure tetrahydrocannabinol (THC)]. This, however, is *not* the case for the hallucinogens. Studies have demonstrated that although 87% of LSD samples are pure, as many as 95% of mescaline or peyote units contain either no drug or phencyclidine (PCP) (see Chapter 9), or LSD, and the figures are probably similar for the other hallucinogens.[19] In addition, even those samples that actually contain the alleged substance usually also contain an adulterant, such as amphetamines.[18-20] Thus, it is *not* safe to assume that one can predict the reaction just by knowing what substance the individual *thinks* he has taken.

Briefly, the more common drugs include those discussed below.

8.1.1.3.1. Lysergic Acid Diethylamide (LSD)

This is a very potent drug that produces frank hallucinations at doses as low as 20–35 μg, with the usual street dose ranging from 50 to 300 μg.[1,6] At doses as low as 0.5–2.0 μg/kg, the individual experiences dizziness, weakness, and a series of physiological changes that are replaced by euphoria and hallucinations lasting from 4 to 12 hours. The actual "high" depends on the dose, the individual's emotional set, the environment, prior drug experiences, and psychiatric history.

LSD can be purchased as a powder, a solution, a capsule, or a pill. The colorless, tasteless substance is also sold dissolved on sugar cubes or pieces of blotter. Although the drug is usually taken orally, it has been known to be administered subcutaneously or intravenously. LSD can be placed on tobacco and smoked, but the intoxication obtained by this method is usually quite mild.[6]

8.1.1.3.2. Mescaline or Peyote

The hard, dried brown buttons of the peyote cactus contain mescaline, the second most widely used hallucinogen.[6] Mescaline effects have a slower onset than those of LSD and are frequently accompanied by unpleasant side effects, such as nausea and vomiting. The hallucinations commonly last 1–2 hours after a usual dose.

8.1.1.3.3. Psilocybin

Psilocybin is obtained from mushrooms, many of which grow wild in the United States, and the resulting hallucinations are similar to those noted for LSD and mescaline. It is usually taken by mouth and has a rapid onset: Effects are demonstrated within 15 minutes after a dose of 4–8 mg. Reactions peak at about 90 minutes and begin to wane at 2–3 hours, but they do not disappear for 5–6 hours. Larger doses tend to produce longer periods of intoxication.[6]

8.1.1.3.4. 2,5-Dimethoxy-4-methylamphetamine (DOM or STP)

This is a synthetic hallucinogen, bearing a structural resemblance to both amphetamine and mescaline and resembling LSD in its effects. The usual dose is 5 mg or more; thus, the drug is between 50 and 100 times less potent than LSD. The onset of effects is usually within 1 hour of ingestion, and peak effects occur at 3–5 hours, disappearing by 7 or 8 hours.[6] The physiological changes are adrenalinelike, paralleling those of LSD. It may be that the effects of this substance are intensified following the administration of chlorpromazine (Thorazine).[6]

8.1.2. Epidemiology and Patterns of Abuse

The hallucinogens were, along with marijuana, the first of the "middle-class" street drugs to cause public concern in the 1960s.[1] Although it is impossible to be certain of the extent of abuse, studies of the street culture, as well as emergency room admissions, indicate a peak prevalence in 1966–1967, with a subsequent leveling off and decline.[6,15] Hallucinogens remain in general use, but have been somewhat replaced in popularity by the stimulants, especially cocaine, as well as by PCP.

In 1982, approximately 25% of people aged 18–25 in the United States had used a hallucinogen at some time during their lives, including 1–2% who had used the substance in the preceding 30 days.[1,21] This translates to approximately 9% of high school students who admitted to using hallucinogens in a 1983 survey, a figure that decreased closer to 7% in a similar survey in 1985.[22–24] With the exception of native Americans' use of peyote as part of religious ceremonies, the use of hallucinogens by various subcultural groups has diminished.

8.2. EMERGENCY PROBLEMS ASSOCIATED WITH ABUSE OF LSD-TYPE DRUGS

The most common hallucinogen-related difficulties seen in emergency rooms are panic reactions, flashbacks, and toxic reactions. In addition, temporary psychoses (which are probably toxic reactions) and a limited number of medical problems have been noted and need to be discussed.

8.2.1. Panic Reactions (Possibly 305.30 or 292.89 in DSM-III-R) (See Sections 1.6.1, 5.2.1, 7.2.1, and 14.2)

8.2.1.1. Clinical Picture

Because these drugs cause both stimulation and altered feeling states at relatively low doses, it is not surprising that the most common problem connected with hallucinogens seen in emergency room settings is the high level of anxiety and fear that characterize the panic reaction.[1,3] In the panic state, the individual is highly stimulated, frightened, may be hallucinating, and is usually fearful of losing his mind. This is one example of a "bad trip," the other being the toxic reaction seen in individuals who have taken higher doses (see Section 8.2.3).[1]

Panic reactions are most likely to be found in people with limited prior exposure to hallucinogens. The emotional discomfort tends to last for the length of action of the drug, for example, up to 8–12 hours for LSD and closer to 2–4 hours for mescaline and peyote.[13]

8.2.1.2. Treatment

1. Therapy is based on reassurance by explaining the process of a panic reaction to the individual and reassuring him that he will totally recover.[1,13]
2. For added comfort, care should be given in the presence of friends or family members if possible.[25]
3. It is important to establish a supportive, nonthreatening environment in which constant verbal contact can be maintained.[26]
4. Hospitalization is not usually needed if a temporary quiet, safe atmosphere can be arranged.[27]
5. Medications are usually *not* needed. However, if it is impossible to control the patient otherwise, most authors suggest the use of an antianxiety drug such as:
   a. Diazepam (Valium), 10–30 mg orally, repeated in 1–2 hours as needed.[15] or
   b. Chlordiazepoxide (Librium) in doses of 10–50 mg orally, which may be repeated in 1–2 hours.[28]
   c. Be careful regarding the use of chlorpromazine (Thorazine) or any other antipsychotic drug because of the possibility that the hallucinogen might be STP (see Section 8.1.1.3.4) or that the antipsychotics might increase any anticholinergic effects of adulterants in the ingested drug.[26]
6. It is important to obtain a clear history of drug abuse and prior psychiatric disorders and to establish a differential diagnosis, particularly ruling out mania and schizophrenia.[26,29]
7. It is suggested that a follow-up visit be arranged to help the individual deal with his drug-taking problems and to rule out any major coexisting psychiatric disorder.[26]

8.2.2. Flashbacks (e.g., 292.89 in DSM-III-R) (see Sections 1.6.2, 7.2.2, and 14.3)

8.2.2.1. Clinical Picture

This relatively *benign* condition usually comes to the attention of the health-care practitioner because an individual becomes concerned that the recurrence of drug effects represents permanent brain damage.[1,30] Experiences that have been termed *flashbacks* include simple visual images, lines or tracing of objects, and complex emotional experiences similar but not identical to the prior drug experience.[31] In the midst of such a state, the patient may demonstrate sadness, anxiety, or even paranoia, which may recur periodically for days to weeks after taking the drug.[30] It is thought that this recurrence of hallucinogen effects may be set off by taking a milder drug such as marijuana or by an acute crisis.

The actual incidence of flashback experiences depends on the specific definition used and the study methods invoked. The prevalence of such problems probably increases with the number of times an individual has taken the hallucinogen, but it is probable that somewhere between 15 and 30% of users have at some time had a discrete flashback of some sort.[1,31]

The person usually notes a feeling of euphoria and detachment, which is frequently associated with visual illusions (actual sensory inputs that are misinterpreted by the individual) lasting several minutes to hours.[15] The hallucinations are usually lights or geometric figures seen out of the corner of the eye, often when entering darkness or just before falling asleep, or a trail of light following a moving object. Only rarely do they interfere with an individual's ability to function. Other types of flashbacks, including isolated feelings of depersonalization or a recurrence of distressing emotional reactions experienced while under the drug effects, can also occur.[15]

8.2.2.2. Treatment

Therapy for the self-limited picture is relatively simple[15]:

1. Care is based on reassurance that the syndrome will gradually decrease in intensity and disappear.
2. The subject should be educated about the course and the probable causes (e.g., residual drug) of the flashback.
3. It is important that all other medications, especially marijuana, antihistamines, and stimulants, be avoided.[14]
4. If medication is needed to relax the individual during the experience (I usually choose to use no medication), use diazepam (Valium) in doses of 10–20 mg orally, repeated at 5-mg doses if the flashback recurs,[15] or comparable oral doses of chlordiazepoxide (e.g., 10–30 mg).
5. As is true in any drug-related disorder, in an emergency situation it is important to consider the possibility that the problem is a reflection of a preexisting psychiatric disorder and not really a flashback. Therefore, a careful *history of prior psychiatric problems* and a *family history of psychiatric illness* (which may indicate a propensity toward illness for this individual) must be taken.

8.2.3. Toxic Reactions (see Sections 1.6.3, 2.2.3, 5.2.3, 6.2.3, and 14.4)

8.2.3.1. Clinical Picture

8.2.3.1.1. History

The usual toxic reaction consists of the rapid onset (over minutes to hours) of a loss of contact with reality and the physical symptoms described below for an individual taking a hallucinogen. The markedly disturbed behavior usually leads friends or relatives to bring the patient in for care. While death following LSD appears quite rare, ingestion of high levels of methylene dioxyamphetamine (MDA) and probably of methylene dioxymethamphetamine (MDMA) might carry significantly higher risk.[3]

8.2.3.1.2. Physical Signs and Symptoms

Although the psychological state dominates the picture for the average patient after LSD or psilocybin, vital sign abnormalities that are consistent with the state of anxiety and panic are also seen. These include palpitations, increases in blood pressure and temperature, perspiration, and possibly blurred vision. Very high levels of overdose, especially with MDA, MDMA, and bromo-MDA, may include exceedingly high body temperatures (greater than 103°F orally), cardiovascular collapse, and convulsions.[3,32–34]

8.2.3.1.3. Psychological State

This is an exaggeration of the effects of a panic reaction. The individual, frequently an experienced user, has taken a higher than usual dose of the drug, with a resulting high anxiety state along with frank hallucinations and loss of contact with reality.[35] Depersonalization, paranoia, and confusion are often demonstrated.[15] The clinical picture diminishes as the drug is metabolized, but the symptoms tend to wax and wane over the subsequent 8–24 hours.[34]

8.2.3.1.4. Relevant Laboratory Tests

There are no specific laboratory tests to be noted except for the possible use of a toxicological screen (10 cc of blood or 50 ml of urine). It is important to monitor the vital signs, especially the blood pressure and the body temperature. If signs of organicity are present, it is necessary to rule out ancillary causes, including head trauma and infection.

8.2.3.2. Treatment (see Sections 2.2.3.2, 5.2.3.2, and 6.2.3.2)

1. Although quite rare with LSD, the overdose may involve markedly elevated drug levels, and the patient may present with convulsions or hyperthermia. The treatment steps for any life-threatening drug emergency must be carried out.[36] These include:
    a. Careful observation of vital signs.
    b. Establishing an airway.
    c. Treatment of convulsions with anticonvulsants and a slow injection of diazepam (5–20 mg IV), if needed (see Section 5.2.3.2).
    d. The use of ice baths or a hypothermic blanket.
    e. Cardiac monitoring, support of blood pressure by medications, if needed (see Sections 6.2.3.2 and 14.4.3), and so on.
2. For the usual patient with relatively stable vital signs, a rapid physical

examination, including a neurological evaluation, should be carried out. The vital signs should be monitored for at least 24 hours.[34]

3. It is important to gain the patient's confidence with an understanding but firm approach. Consistent verbal contact and reality-orienting cues must be given, generally for up to 24 hours.

4. The rapid absorption of most of these drugs would indicate that gastric lavage is of little use and may only serve to frighten the patient.[30]

5. Once again, I prefer to avoid all medications but when necessary, I usually fall back on:

   a. Diazepam (Valium), 15–30 mg orally, repeating 5–20 mg every 4 hours as needed.

   or

   b. Chlordiazepoxide (Librium), at 10–50 mg orally, followed by up to 25–50 mg every 4 hours as needed.

   c. It may be best to *avoid* chlorpromazine (Thorazine) or any other antipsychotic drug.

6. If the clinical problem does not clear within 24 hours, suspect that the drug ingested was STP (which might last for several days to 2 weeks) or PCP, as discussed in Chapter 9. Treatment in this situation is very similar to that outlined above; however, the vital signs must be carefully monitored.

8.2.4. Psychosis (e.g., 292.11 in DSM-III-R) (see Sections 1.6.4, 4.2.4, 5.2.4, 7.2.4, and 14.5)

8.2.4.1. Clinical Picture

In my experience, hallucinogen-induced psychoses (most often marked by visual hallucinations) clear within hours to days and for bromo-MDA and STP, certainly within a matter of weeks. The clinical symptoms can range from paranoid delusions to hallucinations and may even encompass maniclike pictures.[37] As the patient often realizes that the drug caused the symptoms (i.e., he has insight), this picture rarely meets the criteria for a drug-induced psychosis given in Section 1.6.4. The literature substantiates that those rare individuals for whom the psychosis does not clear usually have a preexisting psychiatric problem, often mania, schizophrenia, or a psychotic depression.

If a state of psychopathology persists for a month or more, it probably relates to a preexisting psychiatric disorder. The prognosis is not always benign, and perhaps as many as 50% of these individuals for whom problems persist have long-term psychiatric difficulties.[20]

The causes of hallucinogen psychoses are difficult to study and are frequently complicated by multiple drug use.[38] As would be expected, the psychotic syndrome has a wide variety of presentations, including depression, panic, uncontrolled hallucinations, and/or intensification of a preexisting paranoid picture.[1,39]

One special area for consideration is a crime committed under the apparent influence of LSD or other hallucinogens. If the criminal act is a well-thought-out, goal-oriented one, and especially if criminal behavior is consistent with the individual's prior experiences and activities, I would tend to discount the role played by LSD in the commission of the crime.[40]

8.2.4.2. Treatment

The actual treatment must depend on the clinical picture.

1. If on reevaluation one finds an intense panic or toxic reaction, the treatment is as described in Sections 8.2.1.2 and 8.2.3.2.
2. In an individual with a preexisting affective disorder, obvious preexisting schizophrenia, and so on, emergency treatment for a psychotic reaction resembles that outlined in Section 8.2.3.2, but the most important therapy is aimed at the specific psychiatric disorder.[29]
3. A drug-induced psychosis occurring in an individual without a preexisting psychiatric disorder is treated with reassurance, education, and comfort in a manner similar to that outlined in Sections 8.2.1.2 and 8.2.3.2.[14] Hospitalization may be required if the loss of contact with reality is severe.
4. There is one report that 200 mg of niacin, or enough of this vitamin to cause cutaneous vasodilatation, might improve the clinical condition.[41] However, this finding will require corroboration before it can be implemented in clinical settings.
5. If the psychosis does not clear within 1 or 2 days and no prior psychiatric disorder is apparent, it is imperative that the individual be carefully evaluated for any neurological damage, that a thorough physical examination and laboratory tests be carried out, and that the practitioner recognize the unusual nature of the syndrome. As with any atypical picture, treatment is symptomatic, requiring careful observation, good history-taking, and constant reevaluation for possible underlying pathological diagnoses. There is no set procedure in this instance, and antipsychotic drugs, if used, should be carefully monitored.

8.2.5. Organic Brain Syndrome (Possibly 292.81 or 292.90 in DSM-III-R) (see Section 1.6.5, 2.2.5, 4.2.5, and 14.6)

8.2.5.1. Clinical Picture

An organic picture can develop in the midst of a toxic reaction or a severe overdose, or it can be part of a drug-induced psychosis. The treatment of these syndromes was outlined in Sections 8.2.3.2 and 8.2.4.2.

A second major concern is that prolonged exposure to these drugs may cause decreased intellectual functioning and even an organic brain syndrome (OBS). People chronically taking hallucinogens have been noted to demonstrate a syndrome similar to the purported "amotivational syndrome" discussed in relation to marijuana in Section 7.2.4. It is extremely difficult to establish a "cause-and-effect" relationship, as persons likely to use these drugs regularly may have tended toward social withdrawal, lack of motivation, and even brain impairment before the drug use was begun. The problem of establishing cause and effect is even more acute when multiple substances are taken.

There is some evidence, however, of a decrease in abstract reasoning in heavy users,[1] but this has not been corroborated in all groups studied.[42] Brain damage should be considered in the evaluation of any chronic abuser of hallucinogens, but the probability of clinically significant impairment is remote.

8.2.5.2. Treatment

The individual suffering possible organic brain damage from continued hallucinogen use should be dealt with symptomatically. The treatment should include a recommendation of abstinence from drugs and all other medications (including alcohol), a reevaluation of the degree of impairment over time, and vocational or educational rehabilitation, if appropriate.

8.2.6. Withdrawal

No clinically significant withdrawal picture is known for the hallucinogens.[1]

8.2.7. Medical Problems

Evaluation of chronic users of hallucinogens has rarely demonstrated unique physiological impairment directly related to the drugs.[43,44] One area of great concern has been the possibility of *chromosomal damage*.[45] Although broken chromosomes have certainly been demonstrated with LSD-type drugs, and birth abnormalities have been seen in the offspring of mothers using hallucinogens (especially LSD in the first trimester), the nature of the relationship has not been established. Many substances (including aspirin) cause chromosomal breakage but have not been demonstrated to have definitely affected the fetus. Nonetheless, these substances are very potent; they may pose a danger of fetal abnormality when they are used by pregnant women, and they may be associated with a significant increase in spontaneous absorptions.[1,45-47] Additional potential medical problems include the reported high levels of toxicity of MDA to serotonin-rich nerve cells and the possibility of a progressive and widespread spasm of arteries in the arms and legs after ingestion of the 4-bromo homolog of DOM (DOB).[48,49]

8.3. RELATED DRUGS AND EMERGENCY PROBLEMS ASSOCIATED WITH THEIR ABUSE

It is necessary to discuss separately a series of drugs that produce effects similar to the more common substances but the structures of which do not allow for generalizations. The more exotic (and usually less potent) substances that require mention include *nutmeg, morning glory seeds, catnip, nitrous oxide,* and *amyl* or *butyl nitrite.* The active ingredients of most "hallucinogenlike" plants and mushrooms are usually LSD-like or atropinelike substances. The reader is advised to review Section 8.2 as well as the anticholinergic syndrome and its treatment as presented in Section 11.9.

8.3.1. Nutmeg

The nutmeg plant can be ground up and either inhaled or ingested in large amounts to produce a change in consciousness.[1] The unpleasant side effects of these substances (including vomiting) limit their use to places where other drugs are not available, such as prisons.[1,50] The oral ingestion of two grated nutmeg pods will produce, after a latency of several hours, a feeling of heaviness in the arms and legs, depersonalization (a feeling of not being oneself), derealization (a feeling of unreality), and apprehension. Along with this reaction come physiological changes such as dry mouth, thirst, increased heart rate, and flushing.[1,50–52]

The specific mechanism of the action of nutmeg is not known, but it is felt that it might inhibit prostaglandin.[50] One of the side effects of chronic use may be constipation.[51]

The usual recovery from signs of intoxication occur within 24–48 hours. No specific treatment for the toxic reaction is needed. None of the other categories of drug abuse problems is known to occur with nutmeg.

8.3.2. Morning Glory Seeds

The seeds of the more common varieties of morning glory flowers contain an LSD-related substance[53,54] that, if ingested in high enough amounts, can produce a mild hallucinatory state. The usual effect of this substance, known as *heavenly blue* or *pearly gates,* is a change in self-awareness and visual hallucinations, which may be very dangerous and has been shown to produce a lethal, shocklike state.[54]

The treatment of any panic, toxic, or potential psychotic reactions would follow that outlined for the hallucinogens in Sections 8.2.1.2, 8.2.3.2, and 8.2.4.2.

8.3.3. Catnip and Locoweed

Catnip is derived from the plant *Nepeta cataria* (a member of the mint family) and has a long history as a folk-medicine prescription for abdominal irregularities.[1] The plant contains a variety of substances, including tannin and atropinelike drugs. It can be obtained in pet stores and has been given to cats to make them appear happy, contented, and somewhat intoxicated. When catnip is used by humans, usually smoked, the intoxication can be quite similar to that from marijuana. Visual hallucinations, euphoria, and fairly rapid changes in mood are frequently associated with headaches, but these tend to clear rather quickly. There is no known treatment needed for the panic or toxic state that can be noted with the substance.

An interesting and somewhat related substance is locoweed (*Astragalus* and *Oxytropis*), which is widely distributed in the western United States.[55] This plant is usually associated with accidental ingestion in animals, the result of which is a clinical picture of incoordination, depression, and difficulty in eating, as well as an exaggerated reaction to stress. The active ingredients involved are indolizidine alkaloids that have some characteristics in common with the hallucinogens described in this section.

8.3.4. Nitrous Oxide (N_2O)

This is a relatively weak general anesthetic that is either used as an adjunct to other agents or given on its own by dentists and/or obstetricians.[1,56] This drug is reinforcing, and animals will self-administer it.[1] Abuse of this inhalant tends to occur among professionals, but one recent case study indicated the abuse of N_2O used as a propellant for canned whipped cream.[57] Use of the drug for a number of months on a daily basis can result in a paranoid psychotic state accompanied by confusion. As would be expected, this clears fairly rapidly when the drug use is stopped.[58]

8.3.5. Amyl or Butyl Nitrite

These potent vasodilators appear to be widely used in homosexual groups in an attempt to postpone and enhance orgasm during sexual intercourse.[1,59−61] The substance is marketed under a variety of names, including Vaporole, and is sold in "adult" bookstores as Rush, Kick, Belt, and so on. Although medically the drug dilates the blood vessels and has been used in the treatment of angina, it now has limited medical usefulness.[61] It is reported in the street culture that the nitrites cause a slight euphoria and flushing and may slow down time perception, in addition to having subjective effects during intercourse.

In recent surveys, approximately 17% of 18- to 25-year-olds and 60% of a series of 150 homosexuals admitted using amyl nitrite, including almost 20% of the latter who took the substance once or twice a week or more often.[1] Heavier use was associated with urban residents and, either directly or indirectly, with greater evidence of promiscuity, group sexual practices, and heavy intake of alcohol.[59] Regarding the latter, approximately 48% of the heavier amyl nitrite users vs. 23% of light users or nonusers reported being drunk at least weekly over the prior year.

The most common clinical problems of intoxication are a toxic reaction and a panic reaction, which are expected to clear spontaneously with simple reassurance. In addition, the drug can cause nausea, dizziness, and faintness, associated with a drop in blood pressure. Theoretically, it can also change the red-blood-cell pigment hemoglobin to methemoglobin and thereby impair the oxygen-carrying capacity of the blood. Butyl nitrite might aggravate the immune deficiency seen with AIDS and contribute to the development of Kaposi's sarcoma.[62]

REFERENCES

1. Jaffe, J. H. Drug addiction and drug abuse. In A. G. Gilman, L. S. Goodman, T. W. Rall, & F. Murad (Eds.), *The Pharmacological Basis of Therapeutics* (7th ed.). New York, Macmillan, 1985, pp. 532–581.

2. Leonard, H. L., & Rapoport, J. L. Treatment of anorexia nervosa patient with fluoxetine. *American Journal of Psychiatry 144:*1239–1240, 1987.
3. Hollister, L. E. Clinical aspects of use of phenylalkylamine and indolealkylamine hallucinogens. *Psychopharmacology 22:*977–979, 1986.
4. Dorrance, D. L., Janiger, O., & Teplitz, R. L. Effect of peyote on human chromosomes: Cytogenetic study of the Huichol Indians of Northern Mexico. *Journal of the American Medical Association 234:*299–302, 1975.
5. Dobkin de Rios, M. Man, culture and hallucinogens: An overview. In V. Rubin (Ed.), *Cannabis and Culture.* The Hague: Mouton, 1975, pp. 76–92.
6. Hofmann, F. G., & Hofmann, A. D. *A Handbook on Drug and Alcohol Abuse.* New York: Oxford University Press, 1975.
7. White, F. J., & Appel, J. B. Lysergic acid diethylamide (LSD) and lisuride: Differentiation of their neuropharmacological actions. *Science 216:*535–537, 1982.
8. Jacobs, B. L., & Trulson, M. E. Mechanisms of action of LSD. *American Scientist 67:*396–404, 1979.
9. Weaver, K. E. C. LSD and schizophrenia. *Archives of General Psychiatry 41:*631, 1984.
10. Jacobs, B. L. Effects of classical hallucinogenic drugs are mediated by an action at postsynaptic serotonergic sites. Paper presented at the American College of Neuropsychopharmacology Annual Meeting, Maui, Hawaii, December 10, 1985.
11. Vardy, M. M., & Kay, S. R. LSD psychosis or LSD-induced schizophrenia? *Archives of General Psychiatry 40:*877–883, 1983.
12. Segal, D. S., & Schuckit, M. A. Animal models of stimulant-induced psychosis. In I. Creese (Ed.), *Stimulants: Neurochemical, Behavioral and Clinical Perspectives.* New York: Raven Press, 1982, pp. 131–168.
13. Cohen, S. The hallucinogens. *Drug Abuse and Alcoholism Newsletter 13,* July 1984.
14. Diagnosis and management of reactions to drug abuse. *Medical Letter 19:*13–16, 1977.
15. Ungerleider, J. T., & Frank, I. M. Emergency treatment of adverse reactions to hallucinogenic drugs. In P. G. Bourne (Ed.). *A Treatment Manual for Acute Drug Abuse Emergencies.* Washington, D.C.: U.S. Government Printing Office, 1974, pp. 73–76.
16. Davis, M., Kehne, J. H., Commissaris, R. L., & Geyer, M. A. Effects of hallucinogens on unconditioned behaviors in animals. In B. L. Jacobs (Ed.), *Hallucinogens: Neurochemical, Behavioral and Clinical Perspectives.* New York, Raven Press, 1984, pp. 35–75.
17. Schlemmer, R. F., Nawara, C., Heinze, W. J., *et al.* Influence of environmental context on tolerance to LSD-induced behavior in primates. *Biological Psychiatry 21:*314–317, 1986.
18. Cohen, S. (Ed.). Pharmacology of drugs of abuse. *Drug Abuse and Alcoholism Newsletter 5:*1–4, 1976.
19. Brown, J. K., & Malone, M. H. Some U.S. street drug identification programs. *Journal of the American Pharmaceutical Association 13:*670–675, 1973.
20. Bowers, M. B., Jr. Psychoses precipitated by psychotomimetic drugs: A follow-up study. *Archives of General Psychiatry 34:*832–835, 1977.
21. Editorial: Epidemiology of drug usage. *Lancet 1:*147–148, 1985.
22. Smart, R. G., Adlaf, E. M., & Goodstadt, M. S. Alcohol and other drug use among Ontario students: An update. *Canadian Journal of Public Health 77:*57–58, 1986.
23. Editorial: National survey finds continuing decline in use of illicit drugs by high school seniors. *Hospital and Community Psychiatry 36:*1011, 1985.
24. Blackford, L. *Student Drug Surveys—San Mateo County, California, 1968–1975.* San Mateo, California: San Mateo County Department of Public Health and Welfare, 1975.
25. Shapira, J., & Cherubin, C. E. *Drug Abuse: A Guide for the Clinician.* New York: American Elsevier, 1975.
26. Taylor, R. L., Maurer, J. I., & Tinklenberg, J. R. Management of "bad trips" in an evolving drug scene. *Journal of the American Medical Association 213:*422–425, 1970.
27. Frosch, W. A., Robbins, E. S., & Stern, M. Untoward reactions to lysergic acid diethylamide (LSD) resulting in hospitalization. *New England Journal of Medicine 273:*1235–1239, 1965.
28. Levy, R. M. Diazepam for LSD intoxication. *Lancet 1:*1297, 1971.

29. Goodwin, D. W., & Guze, S. B. *Psychiatric Diagnosis* (4th ed.). New York: Oxford University Press, 1988.
30. Cohen, S. (Ed.). Flashbacks. *Drug Abuse and Alcoholism Newsletter 6:*1–3, 1977.
31. Yager, J., Crumpton, E., & Rubenstein, R. Flashbacks among soldiers discharged as unfit who abused more than one drug. *American Journal of Psychiatry 140:*857–861, 1983.
32. Forrest, J. A. H., & Tarala, R. A. 60 hospital admissions due to reactions to lysergide (LSD). *Lancet 2:*1310–1313, 1973.
33. Winek, C. L., Collom, W. D., & Bricker, J. D. A death due to 4-bromo-2,5-dimethoxyamphetamine. *Clinical Toxicology 18:*261–266, 1981.
34. Shoichet, R. Emergency treatment of acute adverse reactions to hallucinogenic drugs. In P. G. Bourne (Ed.). *A Treatment Manual for Acute Drug Abuse Emergencies.* Washington, D.C.: U.S. Government Printing Office, 1974, pp. 80–82.
35. Abruzzi, W. Drug-induced psychosis. *International Journal of the Addictions 12:*183–193, 1977.
36. Friedman, S. A., & Hirsh, S. E. Extreme hyperthermia after LSD ingestion. *Journal of the American Medical Association 217:*1549–1550, 1971.
37. Lake, C. R., Stirba, A. L., Kinneman, R. E. *et al.* Mania associated with LSD ingestion. *American Journal of Psychiatry 138:*1508–1509, 1981.
38. Liskow, B. LSD and prolonged psychotic reactions. *American Journal of Psychiatry 128:*1154, 1972.
39. Glass, G. S., & Bowers, M. B. Chronic psychosis associated with long-term psychotomimetic drug abuse. *Archives of General Psychiatry 23:*97–102, 1970.
40. Ungerleider, J. T. LSD and the courts. *American Journal of Psychiatry 126(8):*1179, 1970.
41. Goldstein, J. A. Niacin and acute psychedelic psychosis. *Biological Psychiatry 19:*272–273, 1984.
42. Grant, I., Mohns, L., Miller, M., & Reitan, R. M. A neuropsychological study of polydrug users. *Archives of General Psychiatry 33:*973–978, 1976.
43. Abraham, H. D. A chronic impairment of colour vision in users of LSD. *British Journal of Psychiatry 140:*518–520, 1982.
44. Culver, C. M., & King, F. W. Neuropsychological assessment of undergraduate marihuana and LSD users. *Archives of General Psychiatry 31:*707–711, 1974.
45. Smith, C. G., & Asch, R. H. Drug abuse and reproduction. *Fertility and Sterility 48:*355–373, 1987.
46. Emanuel, I., & Ansell, J. S. LSD, intrauterine amputations, and amniotic-band syndrome. *Lancet 2:*158–159, 1971.
47. Bloom, A. D. Peyote (mescaline) and human chromosomes. *Journal of the American Medical Association 234:*313, 1975.
48. Ricuarte, G., Bryan, G., & Strauss, L. Hallucinogenic amphetamine selectively destroys brain serotonin nerve terminals. *Science 229:*986–988, 1985.
49. Bowen, J. S., Davis, G. B., Kearney, T. E., & Bardin, J. Diffuse vascular spasm associated with 4-bromo-2,5-dimethoxyamphetamine ingestion. *Journal of the American Medical Association 249:*1477–1479, 1983.
50. Dietz, W. H., Jr., & Stuart, M. J. Nutmeg and prostaglandins. *New England Journal of Medicine 294:*503, 1976.
51. Schulze, R. G. Nutmeg as a hallucinogen. *New England Journal of Medicine 295:*174, 1976.
52. Faguet, R. A., & Rowland, K. F. "Spice cabinet" intoxication. *American Journal of Psychiatry 135:*860–861, 1973.
53. Fink, P. J., Goldman, M. J., & Lyons, I. Morning glory seed psychosis. *Archives of General Psychiatry 15:*209–213, 1966.
54. Domino, E. F. The hallucinogens. In R. W. Richter (Ed.). *Medical Aspects of Drug Abuse.* New York: Harper & Row, 1975, pp. 210–217.
55. Molyneux, R. J. Loco intoxication: Indolizidine alkaloids of spotted locoweed (*Astragalus lentiginosus*). *Science 216:*190–191, 1982.
56. Lane, G. A. Nitrous oxide is fetotoxic. *Science 210:*889–890, 1980.

57. Block, S. H. The grocery store high. *American Journal of Psychiatry 135:*126, 1978.
58. Gillman, M. A. Safety of nitrous oxide. *Lancet 2:*1397, 1982.
59. Goode, E., & Troiden, R. R. Amyl nitrite use among homosexual men. *American Journal of Psychiatry 136:*1067–1069, 1979.
60. McManus, T. F. Amyl nitrite. *Lancet 1:*503, 1982.
61. Lange, W. R., Haertzen, C. A., Hickey, J. E., *et al.* Nitrite inhalants: Patterns of abuse in Baltimore and Washington, D.C. *American Journal of Drug and Alcohol Abuse 14:*29–39, 1988.
62. Mirvish, S. S., & Haverkos, H. W. Butyl nitrite in the induction of Kaposi's sarcoma in AIDS. *New England Journal of Medicine 317:*1603, 1987.

CHAPTER 9

Phencyclidine (PCP)

9.1. INTRODUCTION

In the intervening years between the editions of this text, the misuse of PCP has expanded. Phencyclidine has become one of the more widely misused drugs in the Western cultures (along with alcohol, tobacco, stimulants, and caffeine), being taken both deliberately as a drug of intoxication and inadvertently by individuals who believe that they are buying another substance.

Analogues of this interesting substance were first introduced as general anesthetics for both humans and animals (Sernyl or Sernylan, Ketamine, Ketalar, Ketaject, and Ketavet). PCP-like drugs have the benefit of allowing anesthesia (lack of pain) through a dissociative state in which the subject is not in a deep "coma." Thus, they produce relatively little depression of blood pressure, respiration, and other vital signs.[1] However, their use soon became limited in humans after it was recognized that approximately 20% of individuals developed agitation and even hallucinations during the immediate postoperative period.[1]

PCP has become widely misused as an adulterant of other, more expensive street drugs. One of the major attractions on the illegal market is the relative ease of synthesis in the "kitchen" laboratory, with the result that by the mid-1970s, a majority of the drugs marketed as more esoteric substances [e.g., tetrahydrocannabinol (THC), as well as mescaline] were really PCP.

In its own right, the drug has become widely misused as a "hallucinogen" known on the street by a variety of names (Table 9.1). In addition to its wide use as an adulterant or a substitute for other street substances, PCP can be smoked or ingested orally, or injected intravenously (IV) or sprayed on other drugs, such as marijuana.[2] The most usual routes of administration, however, are smoking (about 50% of ingestions) and eating.[3]

9.1.1. Pharmacology

PCP is readily absorbed by mouth or IV, as well as by smoking or snorting.[1] It is estimated that the average tobacco, marijuana, or parsley cigarette with PCP

Table 9.1
Some "Street" Names for PCP

Angel dust	Hog	Rocket fuel
Aurora	Horse tranquilizers	Shermans
Busy bee	Jet	Sherms
Cheap cocaine	K	Special L.A. coke
Cosmos	Lovely	Superacid
Criptal	Mauve	Supercoke
Dummy mist	Mist	Supergrass
Goon	Mumm dust	Superjoint
Green	Peace pill	Tranq
Guerrilla	Purple	Whack

powder contains 12–25 mg up to 100mg of this substance.[1,4] Metabolism is primarily in the liver. There is no known pharmacological activity for metabolites, and excretion is through hydroxylation and conjugation with glucuronic acid, as only a small amount of the active drug is excreted directly in the urine.[1,2]

This crystalline, water-soluble, and lipophilic substance penetrates easily into fat stores and thus has a long half-life (e.g., half of a fairly large dose may be present 3 days later).[1] PCP, an arylcycloalkylamine, is moderately attractive as a drug of abuse and will be self-administered by animals, whereas other "hallucinogens" will not be.[1,4,5]

The drug has relatively complex interactions with a number of different systems. It has been shown to be *sympathomimetic,* increasing central nervous system (CNS) catecholamines such as dopamine and norepinephrine, with a subsequent rise in blood pressure, heart rate, respiratory rate, and reflexes—the latter probably resulting in muscle rigidity.[6–10] PCP also has *cholinergic* effects, increasing CNS acetylcholine, with resulting sweating, flushing, drooling, and pupillary constriction.[9] CNS serotonin systems might also be affected, and effects on the cerebellum are fairly prominent, with resulting dizziness, incoordination, slurred speech, and nystagmus.[1,11,12] More recent evidence indicates possible additional actions in the gamma-aminobutyric acid system and the likelihood of direct binding sites for PCP in the CNS that might in turn out to be related to some opioid receptors.[1,8] Many investigators hypothesize that the states of psychopathology seen with this drug may relate more to the altered relationship among the various neurotransmitters than to any one specific change.

The behavioral toxicity of PCP is dose-related, and the effects range from mild intoxication to lethal overdoses.[1,13] Doses of 1–5 mg produce incoordination, a floating feeling of euphoria, and heightened emotionality, along with mild increases in heart rate, sweating, and lacrimation, with the usual intoxication lasting 4–6 hours.[1] A dose of 10 mg results in a drunken state, with possible numbness of the extremities and perceptual illusions (misconceptions of sensory inputs).[1,14,15] The toxic effects noted at doses above 10 mg are described in greater detail in Section

9.2.3, but can include signs of psychosis and catatonia, along with moderate to severe physical toxicity.

Tolerance to various aspects of PCP's actions have been noted to develop, but there are marked differences among animal species.[1] In humans, the documentation of the intake of up to 1 g of this substance in 24 hours in some users indicates that this phenomenon occurs in clinical settings. Abrupt cessation of PCP use, however, does not appear to produce a dramatic *abstinence syndrome,* with most patients showing relatively minor symptoms including feelings of fearfulness, tremor, and possibly facial twitching.[1]

9.1.2. Epidemiology and Patterns of Abuse

The patterns of *both* deliberate and inadvertent misuse of this substance make it difficult to determine accurate statistics on its epidemiology. An additional complicating factor is that most PCP users rarely take only one drug, with an estimate that at least 40% have ingested multiple drugs at the time of identification.[16,17]

There is indirect evidence of widespread misuse. The substance appears to be taken by people in all ethnic groups and at all socioeconomic strata, and it may be one of the most commonly used substances available on the "street."[12,18] It is one of the few drugs that had shown little sign of a leveling off or decrease in drug use in the early 1980s, although in the time between the second and third editions of this text a decrease in prevalence does appear to have occurred.[18–20]

The study of patterns of intake has been advanced by the development of detection techniques that can measure 5 pg/ml in the blood.[21,22] Use patterns increase with age, and it has been estimated that approximately 3% of young people in the 12–17 age range had taken PCP in the early 1980s, a figure that decreased slightly to 2% of children in grades 7 to 13 who in both 1983 and 1985 reported having taken PCP at least once, including only 1% of high school seniors reported taking the drug over the preceding 12 months.[23,24] Between 10 and 15% or more of those over 18 have used the substance at least one time, often having taken it with other substances.[1,15] Because of the high rate of both medical and psychiatric pathology, the rates increase when individuals attending urban emergency rooms are studied, as in some settings between one third and one half have detectable blood levels of PCP.[4,21] The importance of the blood determinations is demonstrated by the fact that only half those with positive blood levels admitted use, and only 20% of the population of users had been correctly diagnosed by staff before the blood or urine results were made available.[4,12,21] In one recent study, up to 80% of the acute psychiatric admissions to the central Los Angeles hospital had PCP levels detectable in their blood,[22] although not all investigations have related such dramatic findings.[19]

The average user is probably a male in his mid 20s, and if the drug is detected in an emergency room or psychiatric facility, it is likely that he has had experience with it for 4 years.[3,12] Most ingest the substance as smoke at an average daily cost of at least \$25.[12] The most usual pattern of intake is relatively casual (one ingestion per week), but some individuals report "runs" of continuous intake lasting 2 or 3 days or longer.[1]

9.2. EMERGENCY PROBLEMS

Knowledge of the pharmacology and the behavioral toxicity of this substance can be used to predict its pattern of problems. Clinical pictures in emergency settings are most likely to include confusion, paranoia, violent outbursts, and hallucinations.[3]

9.2.1. Panic and Violence (e.g., 305.90 in DSM-III-R) (see Sections 1.6.1, 5.2.1, and 8.2.1)

9.2.1.1. Clinical Picture

Any drug with sympathomimetic properties can produce a state of panic. However, most PCP patients who present in a hyperstimulated state have some level of associated confusion and a decrease in behavioral controls. Thus, an important aspect of a "panic" can be violence.

A history of physical or verbal aggressiveness, often impulsive, bizarre, and unprovoked, is prevalent among chronic PCP users.[25] Clinical observations have indicated a possible progression from anger and irritability to violence as PCP use is continued, and a history of physical acting out has been reported by up to 75% of chronic abusers.[4,13,25]

9.2.1.2. Treatment

The treatment of violence is symptomatic. As discussed below, physical restraints should be avoided if at all possible, because of fear of muscle damage, but inactivation through holding by personnel may be required. Of course, as is true in all panic-type syndromes, it is best to avoid medication and to attempt to reason with a patient not showing signs of obvious toxicity or psychosis and to use medication only as a last resort. The medications that can be used are discussed in Section 9.2.3.2 (item 10).

9.2.2. Flashbacks (Possibly 292.90 in DSM-III-R)

Although not well documented, anecdotal reports indicate that a recurrence of mild drug effects (e.g., feelings of unreality or mild sympathomimetic symptoms) can occur.[26] Flashbacks are generally not disturbing to the patient and are probably best treated with reassurance, although antianxiety drugs [e.g., chlordiazepoxide, 10–20 mg orally, or diazepam (Valium), 5–10 mg] can be used on a one- or, at most, two-dose schedule.

9.2.3. Toxic Reactions (see Sections 1.6.3, 2.2.3, 6.2.3, and 14.4)

9.2.3.1. Clinical Picture

PCP has marked medical and psychological effects that vary greatly among individuals, social settings, doses, and whether the patient is being observed on the rising or falling PCP blood levels.[1] There is a narrow range between the amount responsible for the usual "mild" intoxication and the dose that causes a life-threatening toxic reaction. Thus, in attempting to understand the clinical picture, it is important that the clinician review all relevant parts of Section 9.2.3.

Medically, the toxic reaction consists of a combination of sympathetic and cholinergic overactivity, and symptoms appear at oral doses as low as 5–10 mg. The intensity of the symptoms varies directly with the clinical dose, although the lipophilic nature of this drug makes total reliance on blood or (even worse) urinary levels hazardous, as the active substance may be repeatedly released from fat stores. Longitudinal monitoring of urinary levels appears to be of little direct help.[27]

Although some level of confusion and prominent psychological changes are often noted even with low doses, each of these symptoms intensifies with higher blood levels. Moderate doses (i.e., 10 mg and above) can result in catalepsy, mutism, and even a "light" level of coma with associated stupor. The vital signs and autonomic changes intensify at the higher doses, and anything in excess of 25–50 mg is capable of producing a coma and/or convulsions.[6] At these levels, the patient is likely to demonstrate sweating and a fever; the blood pressure may be alarmingly high; the increase in deep tendon reflexes (DTRs) can progress to muscle rigidity and thence convulsions; and the changes in heart and respiratory rate can progress to failure in both systems.[1]

Although moderate to severe toxic reactions may develop rather rapidly, the clinical picture is likely to clear less quickly. One can expect a progression of recovery from severe intoxication (e.g., coma) through more moderate intoxication and on to light levels of impairment, with the entire picture taking perhaps 2–6 weeks to clear. Thus, the coma may progress to a severe organic brain syndrome (OBS), with or without psychotic symptoms, which then, in turn, slowly disappears. Therefore, a toxic reaction to PCP not only is life-threatening but also tends to be the longest-lasting of any produced by drugs of abuse.[4,28,29] The combination of a comalike state, open eyes, nystagmus, increased DTRs, decreased brain perception, and temporary periods of excitation should raise suspicion that a PCP toxic state is being observed.[12,26]

9.2.3.2. Treatment

There are no specific antagonists to PCP intoxication.[4] Treatment of the toxic state follows the commonsense rules of offering general support while avoiding the use of other medications unless absolutely necessary.[1] When a second medication is chosen to treat the PCP intoxication, the side effects must be kept in mind, and low doses should be used over as short a time as possible. Thus, the treatment is symptomatic, but the clinical picture may take many weeks to clear.

The most important part of treating this medical emergency is support of the vital signs. In dealing with patients, it is important to have some general understanding of the treatment of toxic conditions, as outlined in Sections 2.2.3.2, 4.2.3.2, 6.2.3.2, and 14.4.3. The necessary steps (with the exception of the first several lifesaving procedures) are not given in any rigid order and are to be executed in as quiet an atmosphere as possible.

1. Support vital signs. Respiratory depression should be treated with a respirator if needed (take care to avoid laryngospasm).[4]
2. Serious hypertension may be treated with hydralazine or phentolamine (Regitine)—the latter as an IV drip of 2–5 mg over 5–10 minutes.
3. Serious hyperthermia should be addressed with a hypothermic blanket or ice.[1]
4. Rule out all other possible causes of the obtunded condition and physical impairment. This procedure will require an accurate neurological evaluation and drawing blood (10 cc) or obtaining a urine sample (50 ml) for a toxicological screen. A test injection with naloxone [0.25 mg IV, subcutaneously (SQ), or intramuscularly (IM)] may be advisable to rule out the possibility that opiates were involved.
5. When PCP has been taken orally, gastric lavage should be considered, including a rinsing with saline until a clear return is seen. Of course, the precaution of using an inflatable cuff for the tracheal tube should be taken to prevent aspiration in patients who are in coma.
6. Copious salivation may need to be treated with oral suction.[1]
7. As is true in any emergency situation, an IV should be begun with a large-gauge needle, as it may be necessary to replace fluid lost in the urine (along with 20 ml/hour of insensible loss).[1]
8. Acidification of the urine can be helpful. Cranberry juice, vitamin C, and/or ammonium chloride can decrease the half-life of PCP from 72 to 24 hours—if the pH of the urine is kept less than 5.0.[1] Ammonium chloride should be given at doses of 500 mg every 3–4 hours, and urine acidification may be required for as long as 1–2 weeks for longerlasting toxic states.[1,2]
9. Although some authors have recommended diuresis either through the use of furosemide (Lasix) at doses of 40–120 mg as often as is necessary to maintain 250 ml or more of urinary output per hour *or* through the use of excessive IV fluids, there is little evidence that this treatment actually increases the excretion of PCP.[1,4,6] Thus, it is probably not advisable to use diuresis.[11,26]
10. Control of behavior may be difficult and poses a number of clinical dilemmas, especially in light of the desire to avoid physical restraints. Chemical restraint using phenothiazines has been advised, but these drugs may result in excessive orthostatic hypotension, may increase the risk of seizures, and may enhance the cholinergic imbalance.[30–32] However, this

type of drug has been used in clinical settings, and there are anecdotal reports that toxic reactions that had not responded to other therapies may improve rapidly with neuroleptics.[27,31] The butyrophenones [e.g., haloperidol (Haldol)] may have less effect on the cholinergic systems than the phenothiazines, but have been reported to be associated with potentially greater muscle damage.[1,4]

Other clinicians have suggested the use of benzodiazepines to decrease the risk of convulsions while helping to keep patients calm, but these run the theoretical risk of slowing down the excretion of PCP (although one study found no evidence of this[1,4]). In the final analysis, no "perfect" chemical restraint is available, and the clinician might be best advised to use benzodiazepines, keeping the doses as low as possible for the shortest time possible (e.g., diazepam at 5–10 mg every 4 hours, as needed) while taking care to avoid accumulation of the drug over time.

11. Other drugs have been recommended in the treatment of PCP toxic reactions, but few data are available to back up clinical claims. For instance, control of the heart rate and other signs of sympathetic nervous system overactivity may be approached with propranolol (Inderal) in doses of 20–40 mg by mouth up to 3 times a day. Anticholinergic problems may also be reversed with physostigmine, 2 mg IM, which may be repeated as needed, as the drug tends to wear off after 2 hours.[4,31] Reserpine has been reported to be of use in some cases,[33] and, related to the possible effects of PCP on the opioid systems, it is possible that opioid receptor agonists [e.g., meperidine (Demerol), 50 mg IM] can help improve the clinical picture.[8] Finally, in the context of severe and persistent clinical impairment, one study reported that electroconvulsive therapy (ECT) may be of help.[10] However, any of the approaches mentioned in this paragraph must be considered experimental, and in keeping with the general bias of this text, these medications should be avoided unless absolutely needed.

9.2.4. Psychosis (e.g., 292.11 in DSM-III-R) (see Sections 1.6.4, 5.2.4, and 14.5)

9.2.4.1. Clinical Picture

The psychotic picture with PCP can occur with moderate intoxication and is rarely seen in the presence of a totally clear sensorium (i.e., *a true PCP psychosis in a clear sensorium is rare*). Also, hallucinations and/or delusions (usually in a clouded sensorium) are to be expected during the process of improvement from a serious toxic reaction. With PCP, the state may fluctuate, so that many individuals who developed the toxic reaction or OBS will "improve" to the point of demonstrating what appears to be a psychosis alone.[26,34]

The psychotic picture may consist of paranoia and/or manic behavior (e.g., grandiosity, hyperactivity, and rapid thoughts and speech).[34,35] The patient may show great emotional changes, including hostility accompanied by violent outbursts as described in Section 9.2.1.1 for the panic reaction.[11,26] The degree and persistence of the psychosis appear to relate to the amount of drug ingested, and it can last from 24 hours to 1 month.[34] In one group of psychiatrically hospitalized PCP abusers, 94% reported histories of feelings of unreality associated with drug use in the past, 75% reported various levels of paranoia, and 62% related a history of hallucinations.[12,21]

9.2.4.2. Treatment

Because the psychosis is part of a continuum with the toxic reaction, the treatment parallels that outlined in Section 9.2.3.2. The best approach is to offer the patient a quiet, sheltered environment where his psychosis is not likely to lead to harm to himself or to those around him (i.e., a closed psychiatric ward). Care should include acidification of the urine as described in Section 9.2.3.2 (item 8); sparing use of physical restraints, the preference being to hold the patient rather than use leather or cloth immobilization; and the judicious use of IM or oral anti-psychotics or benzodiazepines (e.g., diazepam in doses up to 60 mg or chlor-diazepoxide in doses up to 100 mg/day, if needed). Of course, the adequate treatment of any psychotic state requires a careful evaluation to rule out preexisting psychiatric disorders that may require treatment (e.g., manic–depressive disease or schizophrenia).

9.2.5. Organic Brain Syndrome (e.g., 292.81 in DSM-III-R) (see Sections 1.6.5, 2.2.5, 4.2.5, and 14.6)

A state of confusion and/or decreased intellectual functioning is a usual part of the toxic and psychotic reactions. Thus, the reader is referred to Sections 9.2.3 and 9.2.4. The confusion may last for 4 weeks or longer and may be associated with violence.[12,25] Some residual level of impairment of recent memory and ability to carefully think through problems has been reported to last in some individuals for as long as 6–12 months.[1]

9.2.6. Withdrawal

Because of the structure of PCP (which resembles that of the CNS depressants), there could theoretically be a withdrawal syndrome after chronic administration. However, this has not yet been reported in the literature, and there is no evidence of withdrawal in monkeys who have been maintained on the drug for up to 2 months.[1] A "rebound" can be expected after abrupt discontinuation of any medication (even aspirin), and patients may relate some level of discomfort, although there is no evidence that active treatment is required.[36]

A related problem concerns the high rate of relapse observed in chronic PCP users. This could reflect a chronic abstinence phase similar to that seen with alcohol or opiates (see Chapters 4 and 6). Because of this, some authors have recommended aggressive treatment of possible withdrawal symptoms over 2 weeks or more with trycyclic antidepressants (e.g., desipramine, 50–100 mg on the first day, decreasing over the next 2 weeks.[36] Until further evidence is presented, I do not use this approach.

9.2.7. Medical Problems

One important area of medical problems associated with PCP involves the results of physical violence. In the context of confusion and severe agitation, patients can inadvertently harm themselves through accidents, and the emotional lability associated with confusion can result in apparent suicide attempts.[16] It is likely that alcohol can contribute significantly to the risk that these problems will arise.[16]

It is not yet known whether the chronic abuse of this very toxic substance is associated with failure of any specific major organ system. However, the importance of muscle rigidity and other physiological consequences is discussed elsewhere in this chapter. There is also a possibility of impairment in lymphocytes and immune functioning with PCP. Thus, clinicians must carefully evaluate the physical condition of all such patients. Most of the data to date come from studies of the toxic reactions described in Section 9.2.3.

REFERENCES

 1. Jaffe, J. H. Drug addiction and drug abuse. In A. G. Gilman, L. S. Goodman, T. W. Rall, & F. Murad (Eds.), *The Pharmacological Basis of Therapeutics* (7th ed.). New York: Macmillan, 1985, pp. 565–568.
 2. Gelenberg, A. H. Psychopharmacology update. *McLean Hospital Journal 2*:89–96, 1977.
 3. Garey, R. E., Dual, G. C., Samuels, M. S., *et al.* PCP abuse in New Orleans: A six-year study. *American Journal of Drug and Alcohol Abuse 13*:135–144, 1987.
 4. Aniline, O., & Pitts, F. N. Incidental intoxication with PCP. *Journal of Clinical Psychiatry 41*:393–394, 1980.
 5. Woolverton, W. L., & Balster, R. L. Tolerance to the behavioral effects of phencyclidine: The importance of behavioral and pharmacological variables. *Psychopharmacology 64*:19–24, 1979.
 6. Domino, E. F. Neurobiology of PCP: An update. In R. C. Petersen & R. C. Stillman (Eds.), *PCP Abuse*. Rockville, Maryland: *NIDA Research Monograph 21*:210–217, 1978.
 7. Montgomery, P. T., & Mueller, M. E. Treatment of PCP intoxication with verapamil. *American Journal of Psychiatry 142*:882, 1985.
 8. Giannini, A. J., Loiselle, R. J., Price, W. A., & Giannini, M. C. Chlorpromazine vs. meperidine in the treatment of phencyclidine psychosis. *Journal of Clinical Psychiatry 46*:52–54, 1985.
 9. Castellani, S., & Adams, P. M. Effects of dopaminergic and cholinergic agents on phencyclidine behaviors in rats. *Neuropharmacology 20*:371–374, 1981.
10. Grover, D., Yeragani, V. K., & Keshavan, M. S. Improvement of phencyclidine-associated psychosis with ECT. *Journal of Clinical Psychiatry 47*:477–478, 1986.
11. Marwaha, J. Candidate mechanisms underlying phencyclidine-induced psychosis: An electrophysiological, behavioral, and biochemical study. *Biological Psychiatry 17*:155–162, 1982.
12. Khajawall, A. M. Characteristics of chronic phencyclidine abusers. *American Journal of Drug and Alcohol Abuse 8*:301–310, 1981.
13. Fauman, M. A., & Fauman, B. J. The psychiatric aspects of chronic PCP use. In R. C. Petersen & R. C. Stillman (Eds.), *PCP Abuse*. Rockville, Maryland: *NIDA Research Monograph 21*:183–200, 1978.
14. Cohen, S. (Ed.). Flashbacks. *Drug Abuse and Alcoholism Newsletter 6*:1–3, 1977.

15. McCarron, M. M., Schulze, B. W., Thompson, G. A., *et al.* Acute phencyclidine intoxication: Clinical patterns, complications, and treatment. *Annals of Emergency Medicine 10:*290–297, 1981.

16. Brunet, B. L., Reiffenstein, R. J., Williams, T., & Wong, L. Toxicity of phencyclidine and ethanol combination. *Alcohol and Drug Research 6:*341–349, 1986.

17. McCarron, M. M., Schlze, V. W., Thompson, D. M., & Winsauer, P. J. Effects of opioids and phencyclidine intoxication: Incidence of clinical findings in 1000 cases. *Annals of Emergency Medicine 10:*347–242, 1981.

18. Fauman, M. A., & Fauman, B. J. Violence associated with PCP abuse. *American Journal of Psychiatry 136:*1584–1586, 1979.

19. Ragheb, M. Drug abuse among state hospital psychiatric inpatients with particular reference to PCP. *Journal of Clinical Psychiatry 46:*339–340, 1985.

20. Davis, B. L. The PCP epidemic: A critical review. *International Journal of the Addictions 17:*1137–1155, 1982.

21. Yago, K. B., Pitts, F. N., Burgoyne, R. W., *et al.* The urban epidemic of phencyclidine (PCP) use: Clinical and laboratory evidence from a public psychiatric hospital emergency service. *Journal of Clinical Psychiatry 42:*193–196, 1981.

22. Aniline, O., Allen, R. E., Pitts, F. N., *et al.* The urban epidemic of phencyclidine use: Laboratory evidence from a public psychiatric hospital inpatient service. *Biological Psychiatry 15:*813–817, 1980.

23. Smart, R. G., Goodstadt, M. S., Adlaf, E. M., *et al.* Trends in the prevalence of alcohol and other drug use among Ontario students: 1977–1983. *Canadian Journal of Public Health 76:*157–161, 1985.

24. Smart, R. G., Adlaf, E. M., & Goodstadt, M. S. Alcohol and other drug use among Ontario students: An update. *Canadian Journal of Public Health 77:*57–58, 2986.

25. Fauman, M. A., & Fauman, B. J. Violence associated with phencyclidine abuse. *American Journal of Psychiatry 136:*1584–1586, 1979.

26. Cohen, S. (Ed.), PCP: New trends in treatment. *Drug Abuse and Alcoholism Newsletter 5:*1–4, 1978.

27. Walker, S., Yesavage, J. A., & Tinklenberg, J. R. Acute phencyclidine (PCP) intoxication: Quantitative urine levels and clinical management. *American Journal of Psychiatry 138:*674–675, 1981.

28. Crosby, C. J., & Binet, E. F. Cerebrovascular complications in PCP intoxication. *Journal of Pediatrics 94:*316–318, 1979.

29. Johnson, K. M. Neurochemical pharmacology of PCP. In R. C. Petersen & R. C. Stillman (Eds.), *PCP Abuse.* Rockville, Maryland: *NIDA Research Monograph 21:*44–52, 1978.

30. Giannini, A. J., Loiselle, R. H., DiMarzio, L. R., & Giannini, M. C. Augmentation of haloperidol by ascorbic acid in phencyclidine intoxication. *American Journal of Psychiatry 144:*1207–1209, 1987.

31. Castellani, S., Giannini, J., & Adams, P. M. Physostigmine and haloperidol treatment of acute phencyclidine intoxication. *American Journal of Psychiatry 139:*508–510, 1982.

32. Done, A. K., Aranow, R., & Miceli, J. N. Pharmacokinetics of PCP in overdosage and its treatment. In R. C. Petersen & R. C. Stillman (Eds.), *PCP Abuse.* Rockville, Maryland: *NIDA Research Monograph 21:*210–217, 1978.

33. Berglant, J. L. Reserpine and phencyclidine-associated psychosis: Three case reports. *Journal of Clinical Psychiatry 46:*542–544, 1985.

34. Yesavage, J. A., & Freman, A. M. Acute PCP intoxication. *Journal of Clinical Psychiatry 39:*664–666, 1978.

35. Slavney, P. R., Rich, G. B., Pearlson, G. D., *et al.* Phencyclidine abuse and symptomatic mania. *Biological Psychiatry 12:*697–700, 1977.

36. Tennant, F. S., Rawson, R. A., & McCann, M. Withdrawal from chronic phencyclidine (PCP) dependence with desipramine. *American Journal of Psychiatry 138:*845–847, 1981.

Glues, Solvents, and Aerosols

10.1. INTRODUCTION

10.1.1. General Comments

This short chapter deals with a heterogeneous group of industrial substances that share the ability to produce generalized central nervous system (CNS) depression and signs of confusion through disturbances in physiological functioning within neurons.[1-4] Although the intermittent use of solvents was noted in the last century,[4] more widespread misuse began with the inhalation of model airplane glue in the early 1960s.[4,5] Despite the efforts of the hobby industry to modify its products by removing some of the more toxic substances and adding an irritating smell, the abuses have continued, and intoxication through inhalation has spread to aerosol propellants and industrial solvents.[4]

The more frequently abused agents and their contents (Table 10.1) include cleaning solvents such as carbon tetrachloride, toluene, gasoline, lighter fluids, typewriter correction fluid, nail polish remover, and the fluorinated hydrocarbons used in aerosols. These products are popular because they induce euphoria and are readily available, cheap, legal, and easy to conceal.[8] The onset of mental change

Table 10.1
Some Commonly Used Agents[1,2,4,6,7]

Glues	Toluene, naphtha, acetates, hexane, benzene, xylene, chloroform, and others
Aerosols	Fluorinated hydrocarbons, Freon, bromochlorodifluoromethane (fire extinguishers), and others
Cleaning solutions	Trichloroethylene, petroleum products, carbon tetrachloride
Nail polish removers	Acetone and others
Lighter fluids	Naphtha, aliphatic hydrocarbons, and others
Paints and paint thinners	Toluene, butylacetate, acetone, naphtha, methanol, and others
Other petroleum products	Gasoline, tetraethyl lead, benzene, toluene, petroleum ether

occurs rapidly and disappears fairly quickly, and with the exception of headache, serious hangovers are usually not seen.[9-12]

10.1.2. Pharmacology

10.1.2.1. General Characteristics

The solvents are all fat-soluble organic substances that easily pass through the blood–brain barrier to produce a change in the state of consciousness similar to the more mild Stage I or II level of anesthesia.[2] It is difficult to make detailed generalizations, as the substances themselves are diverse in structure and most commercial products contain a combination of solvents along with other chemicals. However, much of their action probably centers on alterations in the lipid–rich neuroglial membranes in the central nervous system (CNS), with associated changes in turnover and production of brain neurotransmitters.[3,13-16] Whatever the mechanisms, some of these substances are reinforcing, as animals will self-administer solvents such as toluene.[8] The metabolism of most solvents occurs in both the kidneys and the liver.

10.1.2.2. Predominant Effects

The usual "high" begins within minutes and lasts a quarter to three quarters of an hour, during which the individual feels giddy and light-headed.[4,10] Most users report a decrease in inhibitions along with a floating sensation, misperceptions or illusions, clouding of thoughts and drowsiness, and occasionally amnesia during the height of the inhalation episode.[2,4,5]

Acute intoxication is accompanied by a variety of potentially disturbing physi-

Table 10.2
Common Signs and Symptoms of Acute
Solvent Intoxication[2,5,17]

Sensory	Light sensitivity
	Eye irritation
	Double vision
	Ringing ears
Respiratory	Sneezing
	Runny nose
	Cough
Gastrointestinal	Nausea
	Vomiting
	Diarrhea
	Loss of appetite
Other	Chest pain
	Abnormal heart rhythm
	Muscle and joint aches

ological symptoms (Table 10.2), including irritation of the eyes, sensitivity to light, double vision, ringing in the ears, irritation of the lining or mucous membranes of the nose and mouth, and a cough.[18,19] The abuser may also complain of nausea, vomiting, and diarrhea and may become faint or (especially with a fluorinated hydrocarbon aerosol) may demonstrate heartbeat irregularities or arrhythmias.[1,4,8] Intoxication is usually associated with a slowing of the brain waves on the electroencephalogram (EEG) to an 8–10/sec pattern.[2]

10.1.2.3. Tolerance and Dependence

Toleration of higher doses of solvents appears to develop fairly quickly, but there is little evidence of cross-tolerance among substances.[4] Clinically relevant withdrawal symptoms do not appear to develop, even with protracted use.[2,4]

10.1.3. Epidemiology and Patterns of Abuse

Solvents are usually taken intermittently, and often as part of a "fad" among adolescents in their early teens or among groups with limited access to drugs.[2,4,10,18−22] Teenagers tend to abandon the use of solvents after a year or two as they mature and move on to other substances, but a small percentage continue with solvents as their drug of choice for periods of 15 years or more.[7,21,23] Although the actual scope of the use of solvents is unknown, recent surveys indicate that as many as 20% of adolescent girls and 33% of adolescent boys in an urban setting had used solvents at least once, with the percentage of continuing users *decreasing* from junior high school to high school and into college.[8,24,25] These rates appear to be higher in some minority groups, including native Americans and Mexican–Americans. Regarding the latter, in one recent survey almost 50% of Spanish Americans coming for counseling had in the past taken some form of solvents "recreationally."[26,27] No matter what the population group, the probability of having used solvents increases among those with histories of poor school performance, difficulties with jobs, and arrests.[28−30]

Solvents are usually taken by groups of young people, using any one of a variety of modes of administration. With the glues, it is common to inhale from a paper or plastic bag, perhaps increasing the intensity of the fumes by gentle warming. Unfortunately, this procedure also markedly increases the chances of suffocation, especially when plastic bags are used.[2,4] Liquids, such as the industrial solvents and paint thinners, can be inhaled directly from a container or by sniffing a cloth or placing the cloth in the mouth. Gasoline is sometimes inhaled directly from gas tanks.[2,4,11] Propellants may be inhaled directly, but most users attempt to remove the particulate contents by straining the gases through a cloth.[4,11] In the survey cited above, 75% of users reported inhaling a substance from a plastic bag, and over 50% used paint, 40% glue, 37% gasoline, 27% nail polish, and 25% lacquer.[24]

10.2. EMERGENCY PROBLEMS

The most common emergency situations seen with the solvents are toxic reactions, organic brain syndromes (OBSs), and medical complications.

10.2.1. Panic Reactions (e.g., 305.90 or 292.89 in DSM-III-R) (see Sections 1.6.1, 5.2.1, 7.2.1, and 14.2)

Because the period of intoxication is short (15–45 minutes), panic states usually abate by the time an individual would seek professional care.[31] Panic attacks and enhanced feelings of general anxiety can be seen with deliberate intoxication as well as with inadvertent exposure to these substances at home or in the workplace.[32] As is true of all panic episodes, education, reassurance, and supplying a comfortable and nonthreatening atmosphere form the basis of treatment.

10.2.2. Flashbacks (see Sections 1.6.2, 8.2.2, and 14.3)

With the exception of possible residual OBSs, flashbacks are not known to occur with these drugs.

10.2.3. Toxic Reactions (see Sections 1.6.3, 2.2.3, 4.2.3, 6.2.3, and 14.4)

10.2.3.1. Clinical Picture

10.2.3.1.1. History

The patient usually experiences a very abrupt onset (within minutes) of severe physical distress while inhaling a solvent.[1,6,33] This is usually done as part of a group activity involving young teenagers.

10.2.3.1.2. Physical Signs and Symptoms

A life-threatening toxic picture characterized by respiratory depression and cardiac arrhythmias can follow the administration of solvents, especially fluorinated hydrocarbons. The result may be a rapid loss of consciousness and sudden death.[1,6,9,10,17,30] There is also a chance of death from suffocation in those individuals who inhale deeply from a plastic bag which then collapses.[4,8]

10.2.3.1.3. Psychological State

The physically ill individual may present with anxiety and some level of mental impairment, ranging from OBS to coma.

10.2.3.1.4. Relevant Laboratory Tests

These are rarely helpful in establishing the diagnosis. It is important, however, to carry out a thorough physical examination and to establish baseline vital signs. It is also necessary to monitor cardiac functioning through an electrocardiogram (EKG) and to establish the RBC and WBC counts (see Table 1.5), as well as the level of liver function and kidney function (see Section 10.2.7).

10.2.3.2. Treatment

There are no specific antidotes for the solvent overdose. The treatment consists of offering good supportive care, symptomatically controlling arrhythmias, and aiding the respirations. Thus, the therapy would be similar to the general life supports outlined for opiates in Section 6.2.3.2, except that naloxone (Narcan) has no use here.

10.2.4. Psychosis and Depression (e.g., 292.11 and 292.84 in DSM-III-R) (see Section 5.2.4)

Any change in mentation occurring with the solvents is likely to involve an OBS, not the delusions and/or hallucinations that might be seen with stimulants or depressants. In the course of this confusion, hallucinations can occur.[10,34] Another clinical state associated with solvents involves emotional lability and depression, which can be associated with occasional violent outbursts during intoxication.[3,11,12] Of course, as is true of all drugs of abuse, these agents can exacerbate any preexisting state of psychopathology and might precipitate longer–term depressions or states of confusion in people who are so predisposed.[10,30,35]

The treatment of any of these states of psychopathology is aimed at controlling behavior for the short period of intoxication. Efforts include reassurance and physical or pharmacological controls such as diazepam (Valium) (15–30 mg or more by mouth, or chlordiazepoxide, 25–50 mg or more, which can be repeated in 1 hour, if needed). If symptoms do not clear within days, the possibility of a concomitant or preexisting organic or psychiatric disorder must be considered. This means that the clinical picture must be reviewed again and any possible ancillary information should be obtained from resource persons. There are data to indicate that patients with more persistent abuse of solvents are more likely to have prominent symptoms of psychopathology.[36]

10.2.5. Organic Brain Syndrome (e.g., 305.90, 292.81, or 292.82 in DSM-III-R)

10.2.5.1. Clinical Picture (see Sections 1.6.5, 2.2.5, and 14.6)

Frequently, individuals abusing solvents present with a rapid onset of confusion and disorientation.[37] The patient may have a rash around the nose or mouth from inhaling, may have the odor of a solvent on his breath, and may have been found in a semiconscious state with solvents near him. Or he may be brought in by somebody who knows that he has been taking solvents.

The most frequent neurological positive finding is an EEG pattern of diffuse encephalopathy with an otherwise basically normal clinical neurological examination.[21] There is evidence that protracted long-term abuse can result in brain damage as demonstrated by a course tremor, a staggering gait, and scanning speech, perhaps reflecting cerebellar impairment.[21,38,39] This brain damage may be accompanied by disorders of thought, such as tangentiality, but is usually without evidence of gross delusions or hallucinations. At this stage, nystagmus may be observed. Although long-term follow-ups have not been carried out, this type of brain–damage picture has been observed for 5 months or longer after abstinence and may be permanent.[8,40]

10.2.5.2. Treatment

This is usually a short-lived OBS that clears within a matter of hours. As with any delirium state, treatment centers on reassurance; the elimination of any ambiguous or misleading stimuli, such as shadows or whispers; protection of the patient from the consequences of hostile outbursts; and the provision of a generally supportive environment. Few data are available on the optimal care for longer–term cognitive impairment, and most clinicians offer supportive therapy.

10.2.6. Withdrawal

No clinically relevant withdrawal syndrome from solvents has been described.

10.2.7. Medical Problems

10.2.7.1. Clinical Picture

These substances interfere with the normal functioning of most body systems. However, because abuse is generally intermittent and relatively short-lived and the typical user is young and healthy, permanent sequelae are relatively rare. Nonetheless, the range of problems must be noted, as deaths do occur. The medical disorders associated with the solvents include the following:

1. Cardiac irregularities or arrhythmias can be seen with inhalation, especially with aerosol use.[8,30]
2. Hepatitis with possible liver failure has been noted following chronic exposure to solvents.[3,4,17,41,42]
3. Kidney failure may be seen with chronic abuse of toluene and benzene.[4,18,24,43]
4. Transient impairment of lung functioning may be noted in tests immediately after inhalation.[37,44,45]
5. Decreased production of all types of blood cells may occur and may result in a life-threatening aplastic anemia.[18,42]
6. Skeletal muscle weakness may develop as a result of muscle destruction, especially with toluene abuse.[18]
7. Transient mild stomach or gastrointestinal upsets can be seen with any of these substances.[18]
8. Peripheral neuropathies have been reported, especially for naphtha- and

lead-induced nerve damage to the innervation of the hands and feet associated with the chronic inhalation of gasoline.[46]

9. There is *anecdotal* evidence that these substances produce permanent CNS damage, but reports in the literature are not consistent.[2,4,11]

10. Because of the probability that the solvents easily cross to the developing fetus, there is evidence that the chronic inhalation of solvents during pregnancy can be associated, either directly or indirectly, with infant abnormalities.[47,48]

10.2.7.2. Treatment

Most of these disorders are transient and disappear with general supportive care. In the case of severe liver or kidney damage, the treatment is the same as that used for insults to these organs from any source. Any patient presenting with an encephalopathy should be carefully evaluated for other causes of the OBS, including intracranial bleeding.

REFERENCES

1. Garriott, J., & Petty, C. S. Death from inhalant abuse: Toxicological and pathological evaluation of 34 cases. *Clinical Toxicology 16:*305–315, 1980.

2. Glaser, F. B. Inhalation psychosis and related states. In P. G. Bourne (Ed.), *A Treatment Manual for Acute Drug Abuse Emergencies.* Washington, D.C.: U.S. Government Printing Office, 1974, pp. 95–104.

3. Struve, G., Knave, B., & Mindus, P. Neuropsychiatric symptoms in workers occupationally exposed to jet fuels: A combined epidemiological and causal study. *Acta Psychiatrica Scandinavica 303:*57–67, 1983.

4. Hoffman, F. G. *A Handbook on Drug and Alcohol Abuse.* New York: Oxford University Press, 1975.

5. Glatt, M. M. Abuse of solvents "for kicks." *Lancet 1:*485, 1977.

6. Steadman, C., Dorrington, L. C., Kay, P., & Stephens, H. Abuse of a fire-extinghishing agent and sudden death in adolescents. *Medical Journal of Australia 141:*115–117, 1984.

7. Faillace, L. A., & Guynn, R. W. Abuse of organic solvents. *Psychosomatics 17:*88–189, 1976.

8. Jaffe, J. H. Drug addiction and drug abuse. In A. G. Gilman, L. S. Goodman, T. W. Rall, & F. Murad (Eds.), *The Pharmacological Basis of Therapeutics* (7th ed.). New York: Macmillan, 1985, pp. 532–567.

9. King, G. S., Smialek, J. E., & Troutman, W. G. Sudden death in adolescents resulting from the inhalation of typewriter correction fluid. *Journal of the American Medical Association 253:*1604–1606, 1985.

10. Daniels, A. M., & Latchman, R. W. Petrol sniffing and schizophrenia in a Pacific island paradise. *Lancet 1:*389, 1984.

11. O'Flynn, R. R., Murphy, E., & Waldron, H. A. Violence and solvents. *Lancet 2:*1470, 1987.

12. Cohen, S. Inhalant abuse. *Drug Abuse and Alcoholism Newsletter 6*(9). San Diego: Vista Hill Foundation, 1975.

13. Yamawaki, S., Segawa, T., & Sarai, K. Effects of acute and chronic toluene inhalation on behavior and ^{3}H-serotonin binding in the rat. *Life Sciences 30:*1977–2002, 1982.

14. Fuxe, K., Andersson, K., Nilsen, O. D., et al. Solvent abuse. *Toxicology Letters 12:*115, 1982.

15. Clark, D., & Tinstone, D. Acute inhalation toxicity of some halogenated and non-halogenated hydrocarbons. *Human Toxicology 1:*239–247, 1982.

16. Editorial: Solvents and the central nervous system. *Lancet 2:*565–566, 1981.

17. Adriani, J. Drug dependence in hospitalized patients. In P. G. Bourne (Ed.), *A Treatment Manual for Acute Drug Abuse Emergencies.* Washington, D.C.: U.S. Government Printing Office, 1974, pp. 125–136.
18. Editorial: Solvent abuse. *Lancet 2:*1139–1140, 1982.
19. Lewis, P. W., & Patterson, D. Acute and chronic effects of the voluntary inhalation of certain commercial volatile solvents by juveniles. *Journal of Drug Issues 3:*162–175, 1974.
20. Daniels, A. M., & Fazakerley, R. C. Solvent abuse in the Central Pacific. *Lancet 1:*75, 1983.
21. Lewis, J. D., Moritz, D., & Mellis, L. P. Long-term toluene abuse. *American Journal of Psychiatry 138:*368–370, 1981.
22. Crites, J., & Schuckit, M. A. Solvent misuse in adolescents at a community alcohol center. *Journal of Clinical Psychiatry 40:*63–67, 1979.
23. Hershey, C. O. & Miller, S. Solvent abuse: A shift to adults. *International Journal of Addictions 17:*1085–1089, 1982.
24. Albeson, H., Cohen, R., Schrayer, D., *et al.* Drug experience, attitudes, and related behavior among adolescents and adults. In The National Commission on Marijuana and Drug Abuse (Ed.), *The Technical Papers of the Second Report of the National Commission on Marijuana and Drug Abuse,* Vol. 1. Washington, D.C.: U.S. Government Printing Office, 1972.
25. Editorial: National survey finds continuing decline in use of illicit drugs by high school seniors. *Hospital and Community Psychiatry 36:*1011–1012, 1985.
26. Mason, T. *Inhalant Use and Treatment. NIDA Services Research Monograph Series,* U.S. Department of Health, Education and Welfare Publication No. ADM 79-793, Washington, D.C.: U.S. Government Printing Office, 1979.
27. Beavais, F., Oetting, E. R., & Edwards, R. W. Trends in the use of inhalants among American Indian adolescents. *White Cloud Journal 3:*3–11, 1985.
28. Reed, B. J. F., & May, P. A. Inhalant abuse and juvenile delinquency: A controlled study in Albuquerque, New Mexico. *International Journal of the Addictions 19:*789–803, 1984.
29. Jacobs, A. M., & Ghodse, A. H. Delinquency and regular solvent abuse. *British Journal of Addiction 83:*965–968, 1988.
30. DeBarona, M. S., & Simpson, D. D. Inhalant users in drug abuse prevention programs. *American Journal of Drug and Alcohol Abuse 10:*503–518, 1984.
31. Westermeyer, J. The psychiatrist and solvent–inhalant abuse: Recognition, assessment, and treatment. *American Journal of Psychiatry 144:*903–907, 1987.
32. Dager, S. R., Holland, J. P., Cowley, D. S., & Dunner, D. L. Panic disorder precipitated by exposure to organic solvents in the work place. *American Journal of Psychiatry 144:*1056–1058, 1987.
33. May, D. C., & Boltzer, M. J. A report of occupational deaths attributed to flurocarbon-113. *Archives of Environmental Health 39:*352–355, 1984.
34. Ross, W. D., & Sholiton, M. C. Specificity of psychiatric manifestations in relation to neurotoxic chemicals. *Acta Psychiatrica Scandinavica 303:*100–104, 1983.
35. Goldbloom, D., & Chouinard, G. Schizophreniform psychosis associated with chronic industrial toluene exposure: Case report. *Journal of Clinical Psychiatry 46:*350–351, 1985.
36. Dinwiddie, S. H., Zorumski, C. F., & Rubin, E. H. Psychiatric correlates of chronic solvent abuse. *Journal of Clinical Psychiatry 48:*334–337, 1987.
37. Elofsson, S. A., Gamberale, F., Hindmarsch, T., *et al.* Physical problems associated with solvent abuse. *Scandinavian Journal of Work and Environmental Health 6:*239, 1980.
38. Fornazzari, L., Wilkinson, D. A., & Kapur, B. M. Cerebellar, cortical and functional impairment in toluene abusers. *Acta Neurologica Scandinavica 67:*319–329, 1983.
39. Lazar, R. B., Mo, S. O., & Meien, O. Multifocal central nervous system damage caused by toluene abuse. *Neurology 33:*1337–1340, 1983.
40. Allison, W. M., & Jerone, D. W. A. Glue sniffing: A pilot study of the cognitive effects of long-term use. *International Journal of the Addictions 19:*453–458, 1984.
41. Morse, J. M. D., & Thomas, E. Hepatic toxicity from disinfectant abuse. *Journal of the American Medical Association 252:*1904, 1984.

42. Stybel, L. J. Deliberate hydrocarbon inhalation among low socioeconomic adolescents not necessarily apprehended by the police. *International Journal of the Addictions 11*:345–361, 1976.

43. Ravnskoy, U. Hydrocarbon exposure and glomerulonephritis. *Lancet 2:* 1214, 1983.

44. Fagan, D. G., & Forrest, J. B. "Sudden sniffing death" after inhalation of domestic lipid–aerosol. *Lancet 2:*361, 1977.

45. Schikler, K. N., Lane, E. E., Seitz, K., & Collins, W. M. Solvent abuse associated with pulmonary abnormalities. *Advances in Alcohol and Substance Abuse 3:*75–81, 1984.

46. Tenenbein, M., deGroot, W., & Rajani, K. R. Peripheral neuropathy following intentional inhalation of naphtha fumes. *Canadian Medical Association Journal 131:*1077–1079, 1984.

47. Holmberg, P. C. Central-nervous-system defects in children born to mothers exposed to organic solvents during pregnancy. *Lancet 2:*177–179, 1979.

48. Goodwin, J. M., Geil, C., Grodner, B., et al. Inhalant abuse, pregnancy, and neglected children. *American Journal of Psychiatry 138:*1126, 1981.

Over-the-Counter (OTC) Drugs and Some Prescription Drugs

11.1. INTRODUCTION

11.1.1. General Comments

Almost any substance has the potential for abuse (if we define abuse as the voluntary intake to the point of causing physical or psychological harm).[1,2] As discussed in Chapter 1, this potential is especially true if the drug has the capacity for altering an individual's perception of his environment. In this chapter, brief mention will be made of the misuse of some prescription drugs, including the antiparkinsonian medications, diuretics, and antipsychotics. However, the focus is on the over-the-counter (OTC) drugs.

The OTC drugs discussed below include nonprescription hypnotics (which contain antihistamines) and nonprescription antianxiety drugs (which usually contain substances similar to the OTC hypnotics) (Section 11.2), nonprescription cold and allergy products (11.3), bromides (11.4), OTC analgesics (which contain aspirin, phenacetin, and aspirinlike products) (11.5), laxatives (11.6), nonprescription stimulants (11.7), and diet pills (11.8). Because of the wide array of substances involved, each section essentially comprises a minichapter that includes such subsections of the usual chapter format as are relevant to the class of drugs.

The history of OTC medications is a long one. Controls on drug availability are relatively recent, and at the turn of the century anyone could purchase opium, cocaine, and other potent substances without a prescription.[3,4] Currently, there are many nonprescription drugs that have been incompletely evaluated and consequently are of questionable efficacy. On the other hand, many are capable of producing physical and emotional pathology when taken either in excessive doses or in combination with other medications or alcohol. Many contain substantial amounts of alcohol themselves.[4,5]

Unfortunately, health-care practitioners and the general public have limited knowledge of the dangers of these substances. Most people receive their information from advertisements or pharmacists, rather than from physicians.[6] The result is the very heavy use, and the frequent misuse, of these drugs, with resulting pathology coming to light in both emergency and general practice settings. Because of these common problems and the large variety of substances involved, the reader is encouraged to review other discussions of the OTC drugs.[7,8]

11.1.2. Epidemiology and Patterns of Misuse

There are more than 500,000 different OTC preparations.[6] At least 28% of the adult population of the United States uses these substances (not including aspirin), 12% taking caffeinated stimulants, 11% sleep medications, and 5% antianxiety drugs.[9] Many users combine OTC products with prescription drugs and alcohol.

OTC substances are used by all elements of society and must be considered a part of the differential diagnosis of emergency room problems in any patient; however, the most frequent user tends to be the white, middle-class woman.[3] Use of OTC substances is noted in 7–10% of emergency room cases, two thirds of these involving analgesics and 17%, sedatives.[3,4] The OTC drugs accounted for approximately 2% of the accidental overdose deaths and almost 3% of the suicides in one locale.[4]

11.2. ANTIHISTAMINIC DRUGS (SEDATIVES/HYPNOTICS)

11.2.1. General Comments

All the OTC sleep medications now contain 25–50 mg of an antihistamine such as diphenhydramine, pyrilamine, or doxylamine. These medications include Unisom, Sominex, Sleep-eze, Miles Nervine, and Nytol. Some of these agents (e.g., Quiet World and Unisom Dual Relief) also contain aspirin or acetaminophen. In the past, many of these drugs (e.g., Sleep-eze and Sominex) contained scopolamine (0.125–0.5 mg), but in recent years, the atropine-type drugs have been deleted from these medications.

Controlled studies indicate that OTC sleep aids and sedatives (such as Compōz) are probably no more effective than placebo or aspirin, and they are significantly less effective than the benzodiazepines, such as temazepam (Restoril).[10] However, when Compōz was compared with aspirin and placebo, patients taking Compōz had increased rates of side effects, including sleepiness and dizziness.

11.2.2. Pharmacology

The antihistamines are rapidly absorbed when taken orally and have a rapid onset of action. As the name implies, they work by antagonizing the actions of histamine released by the body during allergic reactions.[11] Their usefulness in treating anxiety and insomnia takes advantage of their sedative side effect.

11.2.3. Epidemiology

It has been estimated that 18 million Americans have used OTC hypnotics or sedatives, and at least 4 million have taken one of the substances in the preceding 6 months. The rate of use is higher in women: Two thirds of users are over age 35 and 50% over 50.[4] For the OTC tranquilizers, the average user tends to be younger, usually under 35.

11.2.4. Emergency Problems

Emergencies usually result from inadvertent overdose, deliberate misuse of the drugs in an attempt to achieve hallucinations, the combination of an antihistamine (e.g., pyrabenzamine) with a drug of abuse [e.g., pentazocine (Talwin)—a mixture known as *T's and Blue*], or multiple-drug interactions.[12] Therefore, the most frequently noted syndromes in the emergency room are toxic reactions and organic brain syndromes (OBSs). In addition, there are a few, usually reversible, medical problems.

11.2.4.1. Panic Reactions (Possibly 305.90 or 292.89 in DSM-III-R) (see Section 1.6.1)

A panic occurring at normal drug doses is unlikely, although a patient might present with complaints of muddled thinking related to these drugs. Reassurance should be enough to allay the patient's fears and to decrease the level of discomfort.

11.2.4.2. Toxic Reactions (see Sections 1.6.3, 2.2.3, 6.2.3, and 14.4)

The toxic reaction for the OTC antianxiety and hypnotic drugs is usually time-limited, disappearing in 2–48 hours. The clinical picture can be confusing to the clinician and life-threatening to the patient if multiple substances have been taken. The onset of symptoms varies from a few minutes, as seen in an overdose, to the more gradual evolution of signs of confusion and physical pathology in an elderly patient regularly consuming close to the "normal" doses of an OTC sedative. The patient, rarely a member of the "street culture," usually presents in a state of agitation or may evidence varying degrees of an OBS.

Therapy for the toxic reaction involves general support.

11.2.4.3. Psychoses (see Section 1.6.4)

Although this topic is discussed separately for ease of reference, the psychosis here is simply an intense toxic reaction. It consists of sedation and confusion.[12] The treatment and the prognosis are the same as outlined in Section 11.2.4.2.

11.2.4.4. Organic Brain Syndrome (Possibly 292.81 in DSM-III-R) (see Section 1.6.5)

A patient presenting with confusion and marked sedation could be labeled as having a toxic reaction. The entire clinical picture, course, and treatment are identical to those outlined in Section 11.2.4.2.

11.2.4.5. Medical Problems

There are reports that in animals, the chronic oral administration of antihistamines may be associated with a heightened risk for liver tumors.[13]

11.3. COLD AND ALLERGY PRODUCTS

These substances contain antihistamines, analgesics, decongestants, expectorants, and cough suppressants. The major clinical syndromes are similar to those seen with the antihistamines or, for elixirs, could be related to the effects of alcohol.[5,14] The latter can be present in concentrations of 25% or higher.[5]

Treatment is usually symptomatic. In addition, central nervous system (CNS) depression, especially respiratory impairment, may follow excessive doses of cough suppressants, as some contain codeinelike substances. In that instance, one can expect to see a mild form of some of the reactions noted for the opiates (see Section 6.2.3). Finally, many decongestants and antiasthma inhalers contain adrenalinelike substances (e.g., ephedrine), the abuse of which can exacerbate psychiatric syndromes, including depression.[15]

11.4. BROMIDES

11.4.1. General Comments

Bromides have been in use since approximately 1860, when they were among the few anticonvulsant and antianxiety drugs available. Problems of misuse have been noted since the 1920s, and in the 1940s and 1950s bromide intoxication was felt to be a major precipitant of psychiatric hospitalization.[16] Until recent years, a variety of OTC substances used as sedatives contained bromides, including Miles Nervine and Bromo Seltzer.

11.4.2. Pharmacology

With chronic bromide use, psychopathology is likely to develop slowly, reflecting a half-life of approximately 12 days. An individual taking 16.5 meq of bromide a day (the maximal amount allowable in OTC medications) could be expected to develop intoxication in 8 days, or sooner in children or patients with renal problems.

11.4.3. Emergency Problems

Although bromides have not been proved to be effective OTC sleep aids, they were widely available *until recent years*. They are no longer on the market.

11.4.3.1. Toxic Reactions (see Section 14.4)

11.4.3.1.1. Clinical Picture

1. *History:* The usual patient with bromide intoxication presents with the very gradual onset (over days, weeks, or months) of both physical and psychological impairment resulting from the chronic ingestion of OTC preparations containing bromide. Even with the phasing out of bromides in medications, cases still persist from the ingestion of drugs stored in the medicine cabinet or from contaminated water.[17]

2. *Physical signs and symptoms:* These are usually mild and consist of a fine tremor, a macular–papular skin rash, along with *neurological problems* such as slurred speech, impaired coordination, and dizziness.

3. *Psychological state:* Toxic disturbances include any of a wide variety of emotional problems. These range from irritability to all grades of confusion (culminating in an OBS), to any level of depression, and even maniclike behavior (hyperactivity and inability to organize thoughts.)

4. *Relevant laboratory tests:* As with all organicities, especially in the elderly, it is necessary to rule out physical abnormalities through the proper blood chemistries and counts (see Table 1.5) and through an adequate physical and neurological examination, as well as an evaluation of CNS and cardiac functioning. A bromide level over 10–20 meq/liter indicates probable toxicity, and definite impairment is noted at 80 meq/liter.

11.4.3.1.2. Treatment

Treatment consists of general supportive care and the intravenous (IV) administration of either sodium or ammonium chloride. One can also use normal saline at a rate of 330 ml/hour for 2 liters which, for younger healthy individuals, is then alternated with 5% dextrose in saline.[18]

11.5. OTC ANALGESICS

11.5.1. General Comments

These drugs usually contain aspirin, aspirinlike substances (such as phenacetin or acetaminophen), and caffeine. They are used for relief from minor pains, such as headache, and—in the case of aspirin and aspirin compounds—for the treatment of some chronic inflammatory disorders such as arthritis. Abuse reflects psychological dependence, as these drugs are not physically addicting and do not produce hallucinations or changes in the level of consciousness.

11.5.2. Pharmacology

Aspirin is both an analgesic and an anti-inflammatory substance that is readily absorbed orally; phenacetin and acetaminophen are analgesic but not anti-inflam-

matory. Caffeine is discussed in Section 11.7 and separately in Chapter 12. Some of the analgesics also contain antiacidic compounds such as sodium bicarbonate.

11.5.3. Epidemiology and Patterns of Misuse

Analgesic use has doubled in recent years,[19] with a resulting 33 million users in the United States, 20 million of whom take the drugs in any given month. In one survey of almost 3000 individuals, 15% of the women and 18% of the men ingested aspirin daily,[19,20] with the rate of administration exhibiting no marked age or sex pattern. In a survey of drug-involved emergency room visits, 64% of those with a major problem with analgesics were taking aspirin, and 46% of those drug-involved emergencies were suicide attempts. There are now more than 300 products containing aspirin on the OTC market.[4] In addition, misuse of phenacetin has become a major health hazard, contributing to 13% of the cases of kidney dialysis and transplantation in West Germany.[21,22] It is estimated that between 0.5 and 1% of the population may be involved in intense analgesic abuse.[21,22]

11.5.4. Emergency Problems

The major emergency problems for analgesic users are toxic overdoses and medical disorders resulting from chronic use. Older individuals are especially liable to misuse analgesics and are at high risk for adverse reactions.[23]

11.5.4.1. Panic Reactions

These are virtually nonexistent with these drugs.

1.5.4.2. Flashbacks

These are not noted with the analgesics.

11.5.4.3. Toxic Reactions (see Section 1.6.3)

11.5.4.3.1. Clinical Picture

Overdose of OTC analgesics containing aspirin usually results in a profound acid–base imbalance, ringing in the ears, and electrolyte problems. This picture is most often seen in adolescents engaging in a deliberate overdose, usually in a spur-of-the-moment reaction to a life situation.

11.5.4.3.2. Treatment

The picture tends to be relatively benign responding to general supportive measures. Diuresis (see Section 2.2.3.2) is rarely needed. However, as in any

emergency situation, unforeseen complications, such as nosocomial (hospital-acquired) infections or kidney failure, can occur and may be fatal.

11.5.4.4. Psychosis

A psychosis is rarely, if ever, seen with these drugs.

11.5.4.5. Organic Brain Syndrome (see Section 1.6.5)

An OBS occurring with OTC analgesics is usually the result of acid–base or electrolyte imbalance. It is temporary and will clear with supportive care.

11.5.4.6. Medical Problems

11.5.4.6.1. Clinical Picture

The medical problems seen with analgesics vary from acute, usually benign, reactions to more permanent responses due to chronic drug misuse. Acutely, aspirin may cause gastrointestinal (GI) upset, bleeding, gastric ulcers, minor changes in blood coagulability, asthmatic attacks, and skin reactions.[4] Theoretically, at least, acetaminophen combined with moderate to high doses of ethanol over a period of time can produce a toxic metabolite that can result in liver-cell damage.[24]

Chronic use of OTC analgesics can be associated with anemia, peptic ulcers, upper GI bleeding, renal disease, and possibly a neuropathy.[25] Phenacetin, in chronic high doses, can produce kidney failure and chronic anemia, although this picture usually develops in the context of misuse of OTC analgesics containing multiple substances.[21,22,26]

11.5.4.6.2. Treatment

The treatment is symptomatic and supportive, based on the individual clinical picture.

11.6. LAXATIVES

11.6.1. General Comments

Laxatives consist of a wide variety of substances that act through diverse methods, including increasing bulk in the colon, increasing intracolonic fluid and electrolytes, and directly stimulating bowel motility.[27] These drugs can be generally divided into dietary fiber and bulk-forming laxatives, saline and osmotic laxatives, and colonic stimulants.[27,28]

11.6.2. Pharmacology

The pharmacology, of course, differs with the specific laxative. Those most likely to cause systemic problems contain phenolphthalein, which, when absorbed, can cause cardiac and respiratory distress in susceptible individuals, as can those drugs that contain magnesium and potassium salts.[27]

11.6.3. Epidemiology and Patterns of Misuse

Laxative use, especially by elderly people, has become entrenched in Western societies.[28–30] It has been estimated that more than 30% of people over age 60 take a weekly dose of a cathartic with the goal of achieving daily bowel movements, even though there is little convincing evidence that such regularity is necessary or desirable for everyone.[27]

11.6.4. Emergency Medical Problems

Laxatives are not physically addicting, do not directly cause changes in level of consciousness, and have no direct effect on the CNS; consequently, the major problems are medical.

1. The effects of laxative misuse include diarrhea, abdominal pain, thirst, muscular weakness, cramps secondary to hypokalemia, and the characteristic radiological appearance of a distended and flaccid colon.
2. Mineral-oil laxatives may impede the absorption of some minerals and fat-soluble vitamins, thus producing a hypovitaminosis syndrome.
3. Saline cathartics can also result in dehydration and electrolyte imbalance, with important consequences for individuals with preexisting cardiac disorders. These saline and osmotic laxatives often contain magnesium salts (e.g., milk of magnesia and epsom salts) that can add to electrolyte problems.
4. Other disorders that can be seen after a chronic overuse of laxatives include melanosis coli, fecal impaction from a flaccid colon, osteomalacia, and protein loss.[29,30]
5. The stimulant-type laxatives such as bisacodyl (Dulcolax) can produce gastric irritation and burning of the rectum, especially with prolonged use.
6. Other stimulant laxatives containing anthraquinone (e.g., Senna and Cascara) can cross in mother's milk to the nursing infant and can also possibly contribute to nephritis and GI pain.[27]

11.7. STIMULANTS (see Chapters 5 and 12 and Section 11.8)

11.7.1. General Comments

These substances, which usually contain caffeine as their major active ingredient, are mostly used by people who work unusual hours, such as cross-country truck drivers and students preparing for exams. Similar emergency problems can be seen with the OTC asthma products, especially those that contain stramonium, and with OTC weight-reducing drugs.

11.7.2. Pharmacology

The properties of caffeine have been recognized for centuries.[4] Found naturally in teas, coffees, colas, and cocoa, caffeine produces mild stimulating effects. With doses in excess of 100 mg (1–2 cups of coffee contain 150–250 mg), people begin to experience a slightly increased thought flow, enhancement of motor activity, and decreased drowsiness and fatigue. Accompanying these psychological changes are increases in heart rate and blood pressure, along with GI irritability. Fatal overdosage from caffeine would require about 10 g (70–100 cups of coffee).

11.7.3. Epidemiology and Patterns of Misuse

Not counting beverages, 16 million Americans have used OTC stimulants. Two thirds of the users are male, but all races and socioeconomic groups are represented. There is an increased level of use among students and employed males.

The drugs that contain caffeine as their major ingredient are NōDōz (which has 100 mg/tablet), Tirend (100 mg), and Vivarin (200 mg/tablet).[31] Other drugs are Come Back, Enerjets, and Chaser for Hangover.[32]

11.7.4. Emergency Problems

The most frequent emergencies include panic reactions and medical problems. There is no evidence that these substances are physiologically addicting, no evidence of flashbacks, and little information to indicate that they produce psychoses. The exceptions regarding psychosis are likely to be drugs that contain ephedrine (e.g., antiasthma medications and Efed II).[33,34] Of course, in high enough doses, these changes can produce an OBS, but such an occurrence is extremely rare.

11.7.4.1. Panic Reactions (Possibly 305.90 or 292.89 in DSM-III-R)(See Sections 1.6.1 and 5.2.1)

11.7.4.1.1. Clinical Picture

Stimulants can produce an increased blood pressure, a rapid heart rate, and palpitations, which may be perceived by the individual as a heart attack.[35,36]

11.7.4.1.2. Treatment

The treatment is exactly the same as that for any panic reaction (see Sections 5.2.1.2 and 7.2.1.2):

1. Carry out a rapid physical examination, including an electrocardiogram (EKG), to rule out physical pathology.
2. Draw blood (10 cc) or collect urine (50 ml) for a toxicological screen.
3. Center treatment on gentle reassurance.

11.7.4.2. Medical Problems

The major medical disorders seen with stimulants include exacerbation of preexisting heart disease or hypertension and precipitation of pain in individuals with ulcers. Treatment is symptomatic.

11.8. WEIGHT-CONTROL PRODUCTS (see also Section 11.7 and Chapters 5 and 12)

11.8.1. General Comments

These substances are of limited value, if any, in weight control. As is true of the prescription CNS stimulants, any weight reduction that occurs tends to be temporary. Most OTC weight-control products contain either a relatively weak sympathomimetic-type drug (phenylpropanolamine), a local anesthetic (benzocaine), or a bulk producer (methylcellulose).

11.8.2. Pharmacology

Phenylpropanolamine is a sympathomimetic or adrenalinelike agent, similar to amphetamine, that produces an adrenaline-type response along with weak CNS stimulation. In the suggested dosages, it is of questionable efficacy in decreasing appetite. The drug is associated with nervousness, restlessness, insomnia, headaches, palpitations, and increased blood pressure.

Benzocaine is a local anesthetic that is included in some weight-control products in an attempt to decrease hunger. There is no evidence that this drug is effective in doing so.

Methylcellulose produces bulk and thus a feeling of fullness in the stomach. However, this substance is no more effective than a low-calorie, high-residue diet, and it does have the danger of producing esophageal obstruction.

11.8.3. Epidemiology and Patterns of Misuse

There is very little, if any, evidence available on the patterns of misuse of weight-control substances. One would estimate the most frequent users to be young to middle-aged women.

11.8.4. Emergency Problems

There are now adequate data to show that in high enough doses, phenylpropanolamine can produce emergency situations similar to those outlined for the CNS stimulants (Section 5.2).[36] Case reports indicate that the OTC stimulantlike weight-reducing products are capable of producing psychoses almost identical to the CNS stimulant psychosis described in Section 5.2.4.[33,37] In addition, syndromes of depression and manialike states and/or mania have also been noted after chronic misuse.[38,39] The clinical characteristics, diagnostic procedures, and treatments are identical to those described in Section 5.2.4.

Methylcellulose can produce esophageal obstruction, especially in individuals who already have esophageal or gastric disease. The obstruction should be treated symptomatically.

11.9. MISUSE OF SOME PRESCRIPTION DRUGS

11.9.1. Antiparkinsonian Drugs

Probably the most commonly misused of the prescription drugs not yet described in this text are the anticholinergic-type antiparkinsonian agents. These include drugs used to treat Parkinson's disease itself and those prescribed for the relief of the parkinsonian side effects of antipsychotic drugs. The most widely prescribed of these agents are trihexyphenidyl (Artane) and benztropine (Cogentin), as well as biperiden (Akineton), procyclidine (Kemadrin), and ethopropazine (Parsidol).[40] The potential misuse of these substances reflects their wide level of prescription (they are among the ten most prescribed drugs in the United States).[41] A dose of 10–15 mg of trihexyphenidyl has been reported by patients to be associated with an increased sense of well-being (i.e., euphoria), as well as increased social interactions and a transient feeling of the relief of depression.[42,43]

The mode of action is probably related to changes in the cholinergic nervous system that may tie in with the euphoria.[44–46] Evidence of the potential misuse of these substances was first presented in 1960, when a patient deliberately increased the trihexyphenidyl dose from 8 per day to 30 mg per day, with subsequent interference in functioning. Four additional cases were presented in 1974 as part of a description of individuals with toxic reactions, and cases of misuse, particularly of trihexyphenidyl and benztropine, have consistently surfaced over the last decade. It is now estimated that as many as 7–10% of mental health outpatients taking these drugs actually misuse them for a "high."[47,48]

11.9.1.1. Clinical Picture

The onset of symptoms varies from a few minutes, as seen in an overdose, to the more gradual evolution of signs of confusion and physical pathology in an elderly patient consuming close to the "normal" doses.[49,50] Agitation and anxiety may be accompanied by a very rapid heart rate and other anticholinergic signs, such as dry mouth, difficulty swallowing, abdominal distension, urinary retention, blurred vision and sensitivity to light, and a rash covering the face and the upper neck. There may also be an elevation of blood pressure.[51] The patient usually presents in a state of agitation and may evidence varying degrees of an OBS. The signs of confusion, along with the stigmata of an anticholinergic crisis (e.g., dry mouth and warm dry skin), usually establish the diagnosis.[52,53] However, a toxicological screen (10 cc of blood or 50 ml of urine) may be useful. As with any patient with unstable vital signs and a level of organic impairment, it is necessary to establish baseline levels of functioning and to rule out physical causes, such as infections, trauma, and tumors.

11.9.1.2. Treatment

Therapy for the toxic reaction involves general support; symptomatic treatment of physiological reactions, such as the elevated body temperature; and a direct attack on the anticholinergic syndrome. The factors to consider are listed below, but their order of importance may change with specific clinical situations.

1. Attention must be paid to the maintenance of an adequate airway, adequate circulation, and the control of any traumatic lesions or bleeding. This treatment is described in greater depth in Sections 2.2.3.2 and 6.2.3.2.
2. A rapid physical exam and careful monitoring of vital signs must be carried out.
3. Because these drugs are usually taken orally, saline gastric lavage might be beneficial if a toxic overdose has occurred. The procedure should be continued until a clear return from the stomach is noted. However, if the patient is comatose or semicomatose, lavage may be done safely only with an inflated cuff on a tracheal tube.
4. Relatively normal body temperature must be maintained by using a hypothermic blanket or alcohol/ice soaks, if necessary.[53]
5. The anticholinergic syndrome is best treated directly by the antidote physostigmine, given by slow IV injection of 1–4 mg (0.5–1.0 mg/kg for children).[53] The dose can be repeated in 15 minutes if the patient does not respond, and once improvement is noted, it may be repeated every 1–3 hours until the symptoms abate. With this regimen, one can expect improvement in the mental status and the physiological symptoms, although there will be no reversal in pupillary dilatation until the anticholinergic drugs wear off.
6. It is wise to avoid all other drugs, if possible. However, if the patient is exceptionally excitable, one might use diazepam (Valium) in doses of 5–20 mg given orally, or chlordiazepoxide (Librium) in doses of 10–25 mg orally. The dose may be repeated in an hour, if necessary.

11.9.2. Other Prescription Drugs

The misuse of other psychotropic medications probably occurs in the context of ''pill testing'' among young people trying to experience the effects of the substances found in the medicine cabinet. In one series of individuals treated for misuse of antipsychotic drugs [e.g., haloperidol (Haldol)], the symptoms usually occurred within hours and tended to encompass prominent parkinsonian side effects, such as muscle spasms and bruxism (grinding of the teeth), along with feelings of unreality.[1] The treatment generally consists of the IM administration of the antiparkinsonian drugs described above diphenhydramine (Benadryl, 50 mg for an adult), which generally result in a rapid clearing of the clinical picture.

An additional related but fairly unusual problem can occur in individuals who seek out and self-administer diuretics for any of a variety of reasons, frequently in an attempt to lose weight.[54] The problems are primarily those of elctrolyte and acid–base imbalance. Abuse of anabolic steroids by bodybuilders[55] and athletes can precipitate mood swings, depression, and psychoses while increasing the risk for a number of tumors.

11.10. GENERAL CONCLUSIONS

The misuse of OTC drugs, whether deliberate or inadvertent, can result in toxic reactions characterized by panic, OBS, or medical complications. These substances must be considered whenever an individual presents to an emergency room with a fairly rapid evolution of an OBS. In evaluating all patients, it is important to gather an adequate history of OTC drug preparations, being especially wary regarding older or more debilitated individuals.

REFERENCES

1. Doenecke, A. L., & Heuermann, R. C. Treatment of haloperidol abuse with diphenhydramine. *American Journal of Psychiatry 137:*487–488, 1980.
2. Brady, J. V. The reinforcing functions of drugs and assessment of abuse liability. Paper presented at the Committee for Problems of Drug Dependence Annual Meeting, Philadelphia, June 4, 1987.
3. Parker, W. A. Alcohol-containing pharmaceuticals. *American Journal of Drug and Alcohol Abuse 9:*195–209, 1983.
4. Inciardi, J. A. Over-the-counter drugs: Epidemiology, adverse reactions, overdose deaths, and mass media promotion. *Addictive Diseases: An International Journal 3:*253–272, 1977.
5. Fleckenstein, J. L. Nyquil and acute hepatic necrosis. *New England Journal of Medicine 313:*48, 1985.
6. Boatman, D. W., & Gagnon, J. P. The pharmacist as an information source for non-prescription drugs. *Journal of Drug Issues 7:*183–193, 1977.
7. Inglefinger, F. J. Those "ingredients most used by doctors." *New England Journal of Medicine 295:*616–617, 1976.
8. Caro, J. P. Sleep aid and sedative products. In American Pharmaceutical Association Project Staff (Eds.), *Handbook of Nonprescription Drugs* (5th ed.). Washington, D.C.: American Pharmaceutical Association, 1977, pp. 107–111.
9. Brecher, E. M. *Licit and Illicit Drugs.* Boston: Little, Brown, 1972.
10. Rickels, K. Use of antianxiety agents in anxious outpatients. *Psychopharmacology 58:*1–17, 1978.
11. Douglas, w. W. Histamine and 5-hydroxytryptamine (serotonin) and their antagonists. In A. G. Gilman, L. S. Goodman, T. W. Rall, & F. Murad (Eds.), *The Pharmacological Basis of Therapeutics* (7th ed.). New York: Macmillan, 1985, pp. 605–638.
12. Garey, R. E., Daul, G. C., Jr., Samuels, M. S., *et al.* Medical and sociological aspects of T's and blues abuse in New Orleans. *American Journal of Drug and Alcohol Abuse 9:*171–182, 1983.
13. Lijinsky, W. Liver tumor induced in rats by oral administration of an antihistamine. *Science 209:*817–818, 1980.
14. Cormier, J. F., & Bryant, B. G. Cold and allergy products. In American Pharmaceutical Associa-

tion Project Staff (Eds.), *Handbook of Nonprescription Drugs* (5th ed.). Washington, D.C.: American Pharmaceutical Association, 1977, pp. 112–119.

15. Whitehouse, A. M. Ephedrine psychosis rediscovered. *British Journal of Psychiatry 150:*258–261, 1987.

16. Burch, E. A., Jr. Bromide intoxication—1976 literature review and case report. *Current Concepts in Psychiatry 2:*13–20, 1976.

17. Brenner, I. Bromism: Alive and well. *American Journal of Psychiatry 135:*857–858, 1978.

18. Stewart, R. B. Bromide intoxication from a nonprescription medication. *American Journal of Hospital Pharmacology 30:*85–86, 1973.

19. Dubach, U. C., Rosner, B., & Pfister, E. Epidemiologic study of abuse of analgesics containing phenacetin. *New England Journal of Medicine 308:*357–362, 1983.

19. Gilles, M. A., & Skyring, A. P. The pattern and prevalence of aspirin ingestion as determined by interview of 2,921 inhabitants of Sydney. *Medical Journal of Australia 1:*974–979, 1972.

21. Pommer, W. Banning phenacetin to prevent analgesic nephropathy? *Lancet 2:*40, 1986.

22. Pommer, W., Bronder, E., Offerman, G., *et al.* Analgesic consumption and analgesic-associated nephropathy: Extent, prevalence, and costs: Data from the Federal Republic of Germany and Berlin (West). *Muenchener Medizinische Wochenschrift 128:*220–223, 1986.

23. George, A. Survey of drug use in a Sydney suburb. *Medical Journal of Australia 2:*233–237, 1972.

24. Lieber, C. S. Interactions of alcohol and nutrition: Introduction to a symposium. *Alcoholism: Clinical and Experimental Research 7:*2–4, 1983.

25. Robertson, C. E. Mefenamic acid neuropathy. *Lancet 2:*230–231, 1980.

26. Dubach, U. C., Rosnery, B., & Pfister, E. Epidemiologic study of abuse of analgesics containing phenacetin. *New England Journal of Medicine 308:*357–362, 1983.

27. Brunton, L. L. Chapter 43: Laxatives. In A. G. Gilman, L. S. Goodman, T. W. Rall, & F. Murad (Eds.), *The Pharmacological Basis of Therapeutics* (7th ed.). New York: Macmillan, 1985, pp. 994–1002.

28. Schuckit, M. A., & Moore, M. A. Drug problems in the elderly. In O. J. Kaplan (Ed.), *Psychopathology in the Aging.* New York: Academic Press, 1979, pp. 229–242.

29. Levine, D. Purgative abuse. *Lancet 1:*919–920, 1981.

30. Barton, J. L., Terry, J. M., & Barton, E. S. Enema abuse. *British Journal of Psychiatry 141:*621–623, 1982.

31. Baker, C. E., Jr. *Physicians Desk Reference for Nonprescription Drugs.* Oradell, New Jersey: Medical Economics, 1982.

32. Walker, C. A. Stimulant products. In American Pharmaceutical Association Project Staff (Eds.), *Handbook of Nonprescription Drugs* (5th ed.). Washington, D.C.: American Pharmaceutical Association, 1977, pp. 136–147.

33. Dietz, A. J. Amphetamine-like reactions to phenylpropanolamine. *Journal of the American Medical Association 245:*601–602, 1981.

34. Whitehouse, A. Ephedrine psychosis rediscovered. *British Journal of Psychiatry 150:*258–261, 1987.

35. Pratt, H. F. Abuse of salbutamol inhalers in young people. *Clinical Allergy 12:*203–208, 1982.

36. Waggoner, W. C. Phenylpropanolamine overdosage. *Lancet 2:*1503–1504, 1983.

37. Schaffer, C. B., & Pauli, M. W. Psychotic reaction caused by proprietary oral diet agents. *American Journal of Psychiatry 137:*1256–1257, 1980.

38. Achor, M. B., & Extein, I. Diet aids, mania and affective illness. *American Journal of Psychiatry 138:*392–393, 1981.

39. Waters, B. G. Secondary mania associated with sympatho-mimetic drug use. *American Journal of Psychiatry 138:*837, 1981.

40. Bianchine, J. R. Drugs for Parkinson's disease, spasticity, and acute muscle spasms. In A. G. Gilman, L. S. Goodman, T. W. Rall, & F. Murad (Eds.), *The Pharmacological Basis of Therapeutics* (7th ed.). New York: Macmillan, 1985, pp. 994–1002.

41. Swett, C., Jr. Patterns of drug use in psychiatric wards. *Journal of Clinical Psychiatry 40:*464–468, 1979.
42. Coid, J., & Strang, J. Mania secondary to procyclidine ("Kemadrin") abuse. *British Journal of Psychiatry 141:*81–84, 1982.
43. Kaminer, Y., Munitz, H., & Wijsenbeek, H. Trihexyphenidyl (Artane) abuse: Euphoriant and anxiolytic. *British Journal of Psychiatry 140:*473–474, 1982.
44. Smith, J. M. Abuse of antiparkinsonian drugs: A review of the literature. *Journal of Clinical Psychiatry 41:*351–358, 1980.
45. Goetz, C. G., Tanner, C. M., & Klawans, H. L. Pharmacology of hallucinations induced by long-term drug therapy. *American Journal of Psychiatry 139:*494–497, 1982.
46. Brower, K. Smoking of prescription anticholinergic drugs. *American Journal of Psychiatry 144:*383, 1987.
47. Pullen, G. P., Best, N. R., & Maguire, J. Anticholinergic abuse. *British Journal of Psychiatry 145:*671–672, 1984.
48. Pullen, G. P., Best, N. R., & Maguire, J. Anticholinergic drug abuse: A common problem? *British Medical Journal 289:*612–613, 1984.
49. Van Putten, T., Gelenberg, A. J., Lavori, P. W., et al. Anticholinergic effects on memory: Benztropine vs amantadine. *Psychopharmacology Bulletin 23:*26–29, 1987.
50. McEvoy, J. P. Effects of amantadine and trihexyphenidyl on memory in elderly normal subjects. *American Journal of Psychiatry 144:*573–577, 1987.
51. Sennhauser, F. H., & Schwarz, H. P. Toxic psychosis from transdermal scopolamine in a child. *Lancet 2:*1033, 1986.
52. McEvoy, J. P. A double-blind crossover comparison of antiparkinson drug therapy: Amantadine versus anticholinergics in 90 normal volunteers, with am emphasis on differential effects on memory function. *Journal of Clinical Psychiatry 48:*20–23, 1987.
53. Johnson, A. L., Hollister, L. E., & Berger, P. A. The anticholinergic intoxication syndrome: Diagnosis and treatment. *Journal of Clinical Psychiatry 42:*313–317, 1981.
54. Editorial: Diuretic abuse. *Lancet 1:*1066, 1980.
55. Pope, H. Body builders psychosis (related to steroids). *Lancet 1:*363, 1987.

Xanthines (Caffeine) and Nicotine

12.1. GENERAL COMMENTS

This chapter deals with the most culturally accepted legal drugs. As might be expected, these relatively mild (per usual dose) and highly attractive psychoactive substances have the widest use in our society. Despite the relatively benign effects that can be expected at low doses, the high prevalence of use results in frequent morbidity and (for tobacco) even a high level of mortality. These substances are discussed here because of the interaction between their use and various psychiatric disorders, as well as because of medical complaints that can be seen in emergency settings. The chapter first deals with the xanthines, including caffeine, and then goes on to a discussion of nicotine.

12.2. XANTHINES (CAFFEINE)

12.2.1. General Comments

Coffee, tea, and, to a lesser extent, colas and cocoa all contain these related psychoactive substances. The use of xanthines can probably be traced back to prehistoric humans, who appear to have recognized that caffeine-containing substances can yield stimulation and an elevation in mood, as well as an enhanced capacity to work.[1] The modern use of caffeine originated in the New World and the Orient and first reached Europe via Venice in the early 1600s. Probably because of the relatively mild apparent side effects and attractive psychoactive properties, by 1700 these substances were widely used on the European continent and in England.[2]

12.2.2. Pharmacology

The three substances discussed in this section are caffeine (found in coffee, tea, cocoa, colas, and chocolate), theobromine (found primarily in chocolate), and theophylline (found in most of these beverages and, because of its relatively high potency, also marketed as an antiasthmatic agent on its own and as a compound in aminophylline).[1] Most xanthine-containing beverages also have significant amounts of oils (perhaps contributing to some of the gastric irritability caused by coffee), tannin (perhaps responsible for the constipating properties of tea), and a variety of other substances.[1] Thus, it is difficult to be certain of the specific etiology of the symptoms associated with the use of coffee and tea.[2-5]

The probable levels of xanthines in the most popular beverages and some over-the-counter and prescription drugs have been established.[6] The interested reader is advised to review the information in Section 11.7 on over-the-counter stimulants, most of which contain caffeine. Among the beverages, the highest level of caffeine is in brewed coffee (85–120 mg per cup), with less caffeine in a cup of instant coffee or tea (about 70 mg) and still less in 12 oz of a cola (20 mg). There are about 5 mg of caffeine and 25 mg of theobromine (a less potent relative of caffeine) in a cup of cocoa and similar amounts in chocolate.[1,2,7]

The xanthines (also known as *xanthine derivatives* and *methyl xanthines*) are closely related alkaloids derived from plants.[1] They are readily absorbed from the gastrointestinal (GI) tract, are widely distributed in the body, and are metabolized mostly in the liver, with 1% excreted unchanged in the urine and a plasma half-life of 3–7 hours.[1,8,9] The modes of action of caffeine are relatively complex and probably involve direct and indirect increases in brain serotonin, possible central nervous system (CNS) release of norepinephrine, effects on beta-adrenergic receptors, and perhaps interactions with benzodiazepine receptors.[3,10-12] Much recent data has focused on the structural similarity between caffeine and adenosine: In animals, regular coffee administration results in an increase in a number of adenosine receptor sites, and there are additional indications that one major mechanism of functioning for caffeine in the CNS may be through antagonistic actions on adenosine receptors.[1,13-16]

12.2.2.1. Predominant Effects

The effects of caffeine and 1,3,7-trimethylxanthine (and other xanthines) are dose-related, more mild (and frequently beneficial) results coming from low doses and more troublesome effects from higher doses.[17,18] In the cardiovascular system, caffeine tends to increase cardiac contractility and to decrease vascular resistance at lower doses, but it increases resistance at higher levels.[1,3,5] In a similar dose–response relationship, lower levels of caffeine appear to decrease the heart rate secondary to vagal stimulation, but higher doses result in an increased pulse and can even cause arrhythmias.[1,10] Clinically relevant doses of caffeine might also contribute to the possibility of heart disease through an increase in free fatty acids.[1] The effects on the respiratory system include an increase in breathing rate, secondary to direct stimulatory effects in the medulla or an increased brain-stem CO_2 sensitivity, and a beneficial effect similar to that of theophylline and aminophylline on the relaxation of smooth muscle in the bronchi, which, in the case of theophylline, can be helpful in asthma.[1,3,19]

The caffeinelike substances also have important effects on the kidneys and the GI system. Increased production of urine is a predictable finding, occurring, in part, through a direct effect of the substances on the renal tubules in a manner similar to that noted for the thiazide diuretics.[1,3] GI problems are related to the increase in gastric acid secretion, perhaps through a direct effect on the system both by the oils in coffee and by caffeine, as well as indirectly, through the release of peripheral catecholamines.[1,20] Diarrhea and GI pain may be related to the direct effect of caffeinelike substances that stimulate the phasic contraction of gut muscle, as well as to a direct irritation of the mucosa and the enhancement of gastric acid secretion.[3] Although the usual effect of caffeine is an *increase* in esophageal sphincter pressure, individuals with preexisting impaired sphincter strength can experience "heartburn" after caffeinated beverage ingestion, perhaps because of increased gastric secretions of pepsin and acid.[1,20]

Additional organ-system effects include an increase in the capacity for skeletal muscle work, with a subsequent increase in muscle tension.[1] The endocrine effects can include a reactive hypoglycemia (perhaps secondary to catecholamine release).[2] As is true of most psychoactive substances, caffeine interacts with the actions and the metabolism of other substances, antagonizing the actions of the benzodiazepines, perhaps through a direct effect on relevant receptors, and increasing the metabolism of other substances via a possible induction of microsomal enzyme systems in the liver.[12,21] Of course, the reverse can also be true; smokers, for example, probably metabolize caffeine more rapidly secondary to nicotine-related induction of relevant liver enzymes.[1] Although the caffeinelike substances may antagonize the effects of opiates, they do not markedly antagonize the depressant effects of ethanol.[22]

Actions on the CNS are probably important in the attractiveness of these drugs. There appears to be a direct stimulation of the cortex, with a decrease in drowsiness and an increased flow of thought with doses as low as 80 mg of caffeine.[1,3] As already mentioned, caffeine appears to have a direct stimulatory effect in the brain stem on the respiratory, vagal, and vasomotor centers.[2] Paradoxically, caffeine appears to cause vasoconstriction in the CNS, and some xanthine derivatives might actually be useful in treating vascular headaches.[1] Through a combination of both central and peripheral actions, increasing doses of caffeine result in insomnia, restlessness, tremor, and anxiety. The interference with sleep involves a decrease in the deeper sleep levels, a possible shift of the rapid-eye-movement (REM) type of sleep to later in the evening, and a fragmentation of the usual sleep pattern.[1,8] The resulting effects on behavior are discussed in greater depth below.[22,23]

12.2.2.2. Tolerance and Dependence

As discussed in Chapter 2, tolerance is a complex phenomenon involving changes in metabolism, CNS responses, and behavioral mechanisms. Dependence is also related to the pharmacological results of chronic exposure of the nervous tissues to the substance, but it has behavioral components as well. Thus, almost by definition, most attractive psychoactive substances produce tolerance and dependence, and the xanthines, especially caffeine, are no exception.[1,8] Rapid cessation of chronic use results in a subtle but annoying pattern of discomfort that has been characterized as withdrawal, which is discussed further in Section 12.2.4.6.

12.2.3. Epidemiology

The use of caffeinated beverages is almost universal in Western societies, as these substances, even more than nicotine, are the most popular psychotropic drugs ingested in North America.[18] It has been estimated that in the 1970s, the per capita consumption in the United States was 14.3 pounds of coffee per year per adult; the resulting average was at least 200 mg of caffeine per day, 90% of which was taken as coffee.[1,8]

The use of caffeine in the form of colas begins in childhood, and the use of brewed beverages, including coffee and tea, begins in the early teens.[25] There is some evidence of a correlation between specific characteristics of the child and his or her propensity to use caffeinated beverages—with higher levels of use appearing to correlate with lower usual levels of autonomic arousal and higher levels of impulsivity.[26]

Although most caffeine consumers drink two or three cups of coffee a day or the equivalent, between one quarter and one third ingest 500–600 mg of caffeine daily.[25] The pattern of consumption appears to be higher in males, Caucasians, those with lower education, and those with lower levels of religious beliefs, and it tends to increase with age.[3] There also appears to be a direct correlation between the level of caffeine used and the use of benzodiazepines and other antianxiety medications.[27]

Most individuals appear to ingest caffeinated beverages both for their taste and for their ability to combat feelings of fatigue and lethargy.[18] As may be true of most of the substances described in this text, the desire to tolerate the side effects and to seek out the active effects of the drug appears to be familial and may be genetically influenced.[28]

12.2.4. Emergency Problems

12.2.4.1. Panic Reactions (e.g., 305.90 in DSM-III-R) (see Sections 1.6.1 and 5.2.1)

12.2.4.1.1. Clinical Picture

Caffeinated beverages (as well as the prescribed xanthines, like theophylline) can induce a classic panic picture.[29] With caffeine doses in excess of 500–600 mg per day, the symptoms of "caffeinism" resemble those of panic attacks and must be included in the differential diagnosis of all high-anxiety-level problems seen in medical settings.[18,27]

Consistent with the general dictum that substances of abuse are likely to exacerbate preexisting psychiatric problems, there is evidence that caffeinated beverages worsen preexisting anxiety syndromes. Self-reports of diagnosed psychiatric patients indicate that at least half of those with panic disorder or agoraphobia with panic report that coffee exacerbates their symptoms, with 17% relating that caffeine can actually precipitate a panic attack.[10,14,30] Research experiments have also demonstrated that administration of between 240 and 720 mg of caffeine can precipitate panic attacks in panic-disorder patients, but not controls, with one recent report relating that over two thirds of patients with panic experience symptoms similar to panic episodes with 10 mg/kg body weight of caffeine.[10,15] There is also evidence that caffeine might increase feelings of anxiety in patients with depressive disorders.[31] It is interesting to speculate on the possible relationship between intensification of symptoms of anxiety and the effects that caffeine appears to have on adenosine and benzodiazepine receptors.[16]

12.2.4.1.2. Treatment

As the half-life of many of the caffeinated substances is between 3 and 7 hours,[1] and as the symptoms are relatively mild, treatment involves observation, education, and waiting several hours until the symptoms dissipate. Antianxiety medications are rarely required.

12.2.4.2. Flashbacks

Probably because of the relatively mild effects of caffeine and the short half-life, flashbacks are not seen.

12.2.4.3. Toxic Reactions (see Sections 1.6.2, 5.2.3, 11.7 and 11.8)

12.2.4.3.1. Clinical Picture

An overdose of caffeine tends to be relatively mild, and death is exceptionally rare.[1] Very high doses of caffeine, a drug that can function as a pesticide,[32] either through excessive coffee drinking or (more likely) through the ingestion of over-the-counter and prescription substances containing caffeine, result in a potentially serious clinical pattern consistent with the pharmacological effects of the drugs (see also Sections 11.7 and 11.8). Most patients present with hyperstimulation, high levels of anxiety, dizziness, tinnitus (a ringing in the ears), and feelings of derealization, but these can progress to visual hallucinations and confusion.[1,33] The cardiovascular effects can result in high blood pressure, tachycardia, and possible extrasystoles, as well as an increased respiratory rate.[1] At least one case of death has been reported after the ingestion of between 6 and 12 g of caffeine (along with other substances), with resulting pulmonary edema, enlarged liver, probable arrhythmias, and a dilated GI tract.[7] Blood levels in lethal overdoses have been reported to vary widely, probably between 80 μg and 1 mg/ml.

12.2.4.3.2. Treatment

The treatment is symptomatic. Attention should be given to adequate respirations, control of body temperature, control of convulsions, and control of hypertension.

12.2.4.4. Psychosis

Psychotic pictures are rarely observed as a direct effect of the caffeinated beverages. However, these substances may exacerbate preexisting psychotic disorders, and there are anecdotal reports of relatively rare psychotic syndromes resulting from caffeine itself. There is also the danger that through the decreases in the diameter of cerebral vessels associated with caffeine there may be a decrease in the delivery of medications to neurons.[34]

12.2.4.4.1. Clinical Picture

A possible clinical worsening of schizophrenia-type disorders after caffeine ingestion has been described by a number of investigators.[3,8] This deterioration may be related to the direct CNS effects of these substances or, perhaps, to an antagonism of the effects of antipsychotic medications, as precipitation of these substances in solution has been observed *in vitro*.[21] Even mild stimulants like the xanthines have been noted to increase the symptoms of clinically significant mania.[18]

Thus, it appears that caffeine-type substances can worsen most psychiatric disorders. Despite this observation, between 15 and 20% of psychiatric patients consume 500–750 mg of caffeine per day.[8,27] These figures underscore the necessity of taking a careful history of caffeine intake by all psychiatric patients (in whom caffeine may exacerbate symptoms) as well as by general medical and psychiatric patients (for whom caffeinism should be considered part of the differential diagnosis of anxiety).

12.2.4.4.2. Treatment

Treatment involves the recognition of caffeinated beverages as possible exacerbating and causative factors in all psychiatric disorders. Decreasing and then stopping caffeine intake can be expected to result in improvement in a matter of hours to days.

12.2.4.5. Organic Brain Syndrome (see Sections 1.6.5)

12.2.4.5.1. Clinical Picture

It is unlikely that caffeine is a major cause of clinically significant confusion. However, it has been reported that caffeine in high doses (perhaps in excess of 500–600 mg a day) can induce periods of agitated confusion (i.e., delirium) and that these substances should be considered a part of the differential diagnosis in all such clinical pictures.[18]

12.2.4.5.2. Treatment

As is true of all the caffeine problems, treatment involves stopping the substances in the expectation of relatively rapid improvement.

12.2.4.6. Withdrawal (Possibly 292.00 in DSM-III-R) (see Section 1.6.6)

12.2.4.6.1. Clinical Picture

The withdrawal symptoms seen after the chronic intake of a relatively mild substance like caffeine are probably a mixture of direct pharmacological and behavioral effects. No matter what the etiology, the rapid cessation of heavy caffeine intake has been associated with a variety of mild but disturbing symptoms.[24] Most patients complain of headache along with increased levels of muscle tension, irritability, anxiety, and fatigue; these symptoms begin within a matter of hours.[3,5,35-37]

12.2.4.6.2. Treatment

The importance of recognizing these symptoms is to rule out caffeine withdrawal whenever the clinician is dealing with patients with muscle tension, anxiety, or related symptoms. As is true with most relatively mild withdrawal syndromes, treatment involves reassurance and the passage of time.

12.2.4.7. Medical Problems

The series of medical complaints that can be associated with a chronic and relatively high intake of xanthines are predictable, given the physical and psychological effects of these drugs. However, these difficulties may be more than just "mild," as animal models have demonstrated that moderate to high intake of caffeine can result in decreased longevity and impaired general physical condition in rodents.[38]

1. High levels of xanthines can result in increased blood pressure, tachycardia, and arrhythmias.[3] These substances should be considered a part of the differential diagnosis of all such problems. The combination of increases in heart rate, blood pressure, and free fatty acids, and other unknown mechanisms, might contribute to the recent report of a 2.5-fold increase in myocardial infarctions, angina, and cardiac sudden death in men drinking 5 or more cups of coffee per day.[39]
2. Another relatively frequent problem involves GI upset, including pain (seen in perhaps 20% of heavy coffee drinkers), diarrhea (also seen in 20%), and even peptic ulcers, as well as exacerbation of esophagitis with associated heartburn.[3,20]
3. Neuromuscular problems can include a feeling of restlessness in the legs and arms as well as persistent tremor.[2,3]
4. Both direct and indirect effects on the CNS can result in insomnia (reported by 40% of regular heavy users), headache (reported by 20–25%), and anxiety and agitation as described above.[3,40]
5. More serious and life-threatening problems can also occur. There is a

possible weak (but potentially significant) association between caffeine and cancer of the bladder, lower urinary tract, kidney, and pancreas.[1,40-42]

6. The long-held belief that caffeine is relatively safe in pregnancy has been challenged by the observation of teratogenic effects in animals, and this substance has been taken off the "generally recognized as safe" list by the Food and Drug Administration.[1,43,44]

7. Caffeine not only readily crosses the placenta to the developing fetus, but also is found in milk of lactating mothers.[1] Thus, the pediatrician must be aware of potential behavioral and physiological symptoms in nursing babies.

12.3. NICOTINE

12.3.1. General Comments

Nicotine ingestion is an ancient and widespread practice. Prior to the discovery of the New World by Europeans, nicotine was used by North American natives, usually through tobacco smoking, chewing, or salves.[45] The goal was to achieve a transcendental experience, often as part of a ceremony of offerings to the gods and of warding off evil. It is possible that the older forms of tobacco were more potent and may have contained high concentrations of psychoactive substances.[46] Tobacco ingestion was taken back to the Old World following the explorations of Columbus in the 1490s and soon spread throughout Europe and thence to Africa and Asia over the next 50–100 years.

Nicotine can be thought of as causing a prototype dependency process.[47] It resembles all the other substances of abuse in that people begin feeling that they can stop at any time, they ingest the substance despite knowledge of its serious dangers, they tend to titrate their dose, most deny problems even after the problems are obvious to those around them, there is a high rate of relapse once use ceases, and genetic factors may influence the risk for abuse.[45,48] The widespread use despite known dangers probably reflects nicotine's low cost until recent years, its high level of social acceptance, and its relatively mild immediate side effects.

12.3.2. Pharmacology

In Western cultures, nicotine is ingested primarily through smoking or chewing tobacco. In the predominant mode of administration, smoking, almost 4000 substances are inhaled, including nitrogen oxides, ammonia, and aldehydes (e.g., acetaldehyde), with the specifics depending on the temperature of burning. A smaller number of substances are ingested by chewing or intranasal administration through snuff.[45] The three major components of *Nicotinia tobacum* (named after Jean Nicot, who promoted nicotine for its medicinal value) are tars, carbon monoxide (CO), and nicotine.[45] The tars, or total particulate matter (TPM), are measured through collection by a Cambridge filter after the subtraction of moisture and nicotine, and they contain possible cancer-causing aromatic amines, nitrosamines, and polycyclic aromatic hydrocarbons, the latter of which also induce liver enzymes. These chemicals cause changes in the metabolism of other body substances.[45,48,49] The CO causes a decreased ability of the blood to carry oxygen and thus an increase in red blood cell number (polycythemia), and it is probably a major culprit in the generation of heart disease, perhaps through the promotion of atherosclerosis.[50] Additional potentially important constitutents of tobacco smoke include ammonia, hydrogen cyanide, alcohols, acetaldehyde, formaldehyde, metallic ions, and some radioactive compounds.[45] The prominent psychoactive component of tobacco ingestion, however, is nicotine, and unless otherwise specified, this chapter deals primarily with this substance.

Nicotine, first isolated in 1828, is probably the major (although not the only) reinforcer of tobacco ingestion and as such is also probably the rate-limiting substance in tobacco intake.[45] Most smokers and chewers modify their use on the basis of the nicotine content (although there is not a perfect correlation).[51,52] This alkaloid is one of the few naturally occurring liquids of its class and is rapidly absorbed through the lungs or the digestive tract; a puff of smoke results in measurable nicotine levels in the brain within seconds.[45]

The average cigarette contains between 1.5 and 2.5 mg of nicotine, with perhaps slightly lower levels for filter cigarettes, although these "low-tar" products may have heightened levels of CO.[45,50] Snuff contains 4.5–6.5 mg of nicotine per "dip," and nicotine gums contain between 2 and 4 mg per stick.[53,54] After ingestion, peak plasma concentrations are found in the range of 25–50 ng/ml, with a half-life of disappearance from the plasma of 30–120 minutes.[45]

Nicotine is oxidized primarily in the liver to the relatively inert substance cotinine with a half-life of approximately 19 hours (thus, smoking levels can be monitored through observation of plasma levels and of excretion of this metabolite).[45] Through the actions of nicotine on the liver, smokers are likely to induce enzymes with subsequent increased metabolic rates of a variety of drugs, including theophylline, warfarin, phenacetin, propranolol, imipramine, and caffeine—a consideration that is of potential importance in prescribing medications for patients.[45] Nicotine is also reported to have the possible effects of increasing the needed doses of opioids and benzodiazepines and of decreasing the antianginal effect of drugs like nifedipine (Procardia), atenolol (Tenormin), and propranolol (Inderal).

Due to the increasing popularity of smokeless tobacco in the late 1970s and early 1980s, it is important to briefly discuss these substances.[55] The most popular, snuff, is cured, ground tobacco manufactured in three varieties: dry, moist, and fine cut. The second most popular form of smokeless tobacco is chewing tobacco, which is also prepared in three ways: loose-leaf, plug, and twist chewing tobacco. These substances are usually used by placing a pinch of snuff or a plug of chewing tobacco between the gum and the cheek or chewing the leaves or the plug. The tobacco subsequently mixes with the saliva, and clinically significant levels of nicotine are absorbed through the oral mucous membrane linings. The mode of ingestion of snuff and chewing tobacco poses its own problems of irritation and increased cancer risks, as discussed in Section 12.3.4.7.[55]

12.3.2.1. Predominant Effects

Nicotine has potent effects on many body systems.[45,56,57] As is true of all the drugs discussed in this text, prominent actions are apparent in the CNS. In this site, one can demonstrate in both animal and human models enhanced alertness along with initial arousal that can be followed by feelings of calm.[58] Many smokers relate that they think the drug increases clear thinking and concentration, assertions corroborated in studies that demonstrate enhanced performance in visual surveillance, increases in rapidity of information processing, and enhanced recall.[45,59] Direct results of actions on the brain include a generalized stimulating electroencephalographic (EEG) pattern with low-voltage fast waves predominating, while in the periphery there is evidence of a decrease in muscle tone and deep tendon reflexes (DTRs) (perhaps related to the direct effects on the spinal cord.)[45,51,60]

In the *digestive* tract, there is a decrease in the strength of stomach contractions (perhaps related to appetite suppression), but intake can also result in nausea and vomiting through a direct effect on the medulla.[45,51] Research has also documented a decreased consumption of sweet-tasting substances by both humans and animals after nicotine exposure, and there is evidence that on the average smokers weigh less than nonsmokers at the same age.[61] Effects on the *respiratory* system include local irritation, the deposit of potential cancer-causing substances, and a decrease in ciliary motion.[45] Acute effects on the *cardiovascular* system include an increase in heart rate (perhaps related to a release of epinephrine), an increase in blood pressure, cutaneous vasoconstriction, an increase in the strength of heart contractions, and an elevation in platelet adherence.[50,51] The *endocrine* system reacts to nicotine with a release of epinephrine and norepinephrine, both from the adrenals and from the adrenergic axons, along with an increase in growth hormone, cortisol, and antidiuretic hormone.[45,50]

As is true of so many psychoactive substances, nicotine interacts with other drugs. The clinical observation of an increase in smoking with increased coffee intake has been substantiated experimentally, although the specific mechanism is unknown. Similarly, the interaction between alcohol intake and smoking has been observed in adolescents and in adults, leading some authors to speculate that drinkers may turn to tobacco to antagonize some of the CNS-depressant properties of ethanol.[62]

12.3.2.2. Tolerance and Dependence

Tolerance to nicotine is real and is probably a combination of behavioral and metabolic effects, as well as pharmacodynamic changes.[45,63] Tolerance does not develop uniformly to all aspects of nicotine's actions, as, for example, the most prominent changes occur for nausea, dizziness, and vomiting, with less for heart rate, tremors, and skin-temperature changes. Some aspects of tolerance begin to disappear within several days of abstinence, whereas others may be relatively long-lasting.[45,63] As discussed further in Section 12.3.4.6, both psychological and physiological withdrawal symptoms are prominent and may be in part responsible for the difficulty that smokers have in stopping.[45,64]

12.3.3. Epidemiology and Natural History

The percentage of smokers in most Western cultures increased after World War I, reaching a peak in the mid-1960s when it was estimated that 52% of American males and 32% of American females were regular smokers, consuming 600 billion cigarettes per year.[45,65] In 1964, an Advisory Commission to the Surgeon General of the United States reported that tobacco intake was a major health hazard, with almost 50% of males and 35% of females using tobacco products.[64] After this time, per capita consumption began to drop, with a marked decrease during the early 1970s.[66,67] By 1975, the percentage of regular smokers among males had decreased to 39%, although females showed only a slight drop, to 29%.[65-67] The decrease in consumption has continued into the 1980s, with the figure for 1983 for cigarette consumption being the lowest in 35 years.[66] The percentage of smokers among males has dropped to about one third in the United States, while the figures for women continue to plateau at approximately 29%.[66] In the United Kingdom, while decreases in intake have occurred, the rates for men and women in the mid-1980s were higher than in the United States, being 38 and 33%, respectively for men and women.[68] Findings in adolescents (age 12–18) have also showed moderate decreases over the years. While 70% of boys and girls have tried cigarettes by the end of high school, by 1982, this figure included only 20% of high school seniors who were reported to be regular smokers, compared to a figure of 29% in 1977.[45,66,69]

It is possible, however, that the intake of smokeless tobacco in the United States has increased in the early 1980s, especially in the South, West, and Northeast.[55] Reflecting patterns of intake in all age groups, the amount of moist snuff marketed in the United States increased from 10.7 million kilograms in 1978 to 16.7 million kilograms in 1984, with similar increases of between 36 million kilograms and 39 million kilograms for chewing tobacco during the same period.[55] Considering the medical problems posed by smokeless tobacco described in Section 12.3.4.7, these findings are cause for some alarm.

Regular tobacco smoking is likely to be higher in certain subgroups than in the general United States population. One such group described by Hughes *et al.*[70] is psychiatric patients. In their survey, 52% of 227 psychiatric outpatients were considered smokers, with especially high rates of 88% for those carrying diagnoses of schizophrenia and 70% for those diagnosed as manic. A second subgroup at a theoretically high risk for smoking is children of regular smokers.[71,72] Family studies revealed a 2- to 4-fold increased risk for smoking among individuals whose parents or siblings are smokers, twin investigations have demonstrated a significantly higher level of similarity in smoking histories for identical rather than fraternal twins, and an adoption study has demonstrated a significantly higher level of correlation in the number of cigarettes smoked per day between adopted-out children and their biological parents than is observed between such children and their adoptive parents.

Even with the decrease in consumption, the tobacco industry continues to have a great deal of financial impact. For example, a 1984 report listed tobacco as a $16 billion per year industry, generating $8 billion in tax revenues in the United States.[73] On the other hand, in the United States alone, over a similar time frame, $16 billion in costs of health care and an additional $37 billion in lost productivity and associated problems were estimated to have occurred because of tobacco use— figures that translate into an annual per capita loss of at least $200 per year per smoker and $100 per year per nonsmoker through public programs and increases in health insurance.[66] In addition, it is estimated that $500 million per year in property loss, medical costs, and other losses were incurred because of fire and smoke damage and injuries.

The natural history or usual course of smoking has not appeared to change much in recent decades. Smoking usually begins in early adolescence, and most young people experiment by age 12 or 13.[74] The characteristics of smokers parallel those of ingesters of other substances—indeed, few young people begin using marijuana or other substances of potential abuse unless they are smokers. Thus, the chance of smoking tobacco in youth increases with increasing signs of adjustment problems (e.g., academic failure), increased evidence of risk-taking, and increased characteristics of extraversion.[51]

When asked, the majority of smokers (anywhere from one half to two thirds) say they want to stop.[75] Whether it is a true desire to stop or just an attempt to tell investigators what the subjects think they want to hear, these findings still reflect the recognition by most smokers that tobacco is socially undesirable and dangerous to health.[75] Thus, it is not surprising that the natural history of smoking is one of frequent attempts to abstain, but there is (unfortunately) as high a rate of relapse with tobacco intake as there is with illicit drugs.[51]

12.3.4. Emergency Problems

Although 20 years ago nicotine was likely to be seen as a benign substance, this drug and its associated chemicals taken in through tobacco are responsible for a great amount of morbidity and mortality.

12.3.4.1. Panic Reactions (Possibly 305.90 or 292.89 in DSM-III-R) (see Sections 1.6.1 and 7.2.1)

With the exception of the toxic reactions described below, it is unlikely that nicotine intake results in a full-blown panic in individuals not so predisposed. However, for a person under stress or with preexisting anxiety disorders, the increased blood-pressure and heart-rate changes caused by nicotine could precipitate attacks.[51] Treatment is symptomatic, and it includes reassurance and informing the patient that his tobacco intake is exacerbating his existing problems.

12.3.4.2. Flashbacks

Flashbacks are not a problem known to exist with nicotine.

12.3.4.3. Toxic Reactions (see Section 1.6.3)

12.3.4.3.1. Clinical Picture

A fatal overdose of nicotine in adults can occur with 60 mg (as might be seen with an ingestion of some insecticides). Lesser amounts (even from tobacco) are dangerous for children. In a less severe reaction, the symptoms can include nausea, salivation, abdominal pain, diarrhea, vomiting, headache, dizziness, decreased heart rate, and weakness.[53] In higher doses, these problems are followed by feelings of faintness, a precipitous drop in blood pressure, a decrease in respirations, onset of convulsions, and even death from respiratory failure.[53]

12.3.4.3.2. Treatment

The treatment of nicotine overdose is symptomatic. In addition to general support of respiration and blood pressure, as well as the administration of oxygen, a number of maneuvers can be used to try to rid the body of the substance. Gastric lavage can be useful, as emptying is often delayed, and a slurry of activated charcoal can also help.[53] The excretion of nicotine is probably enhanced by acidifying the urine through the use of ammonium chloride (500 mg orally every 3–4 hours).[53]

12.3.4.4. Psychosis

No known clinically significant psychotic state has been reported with nicotine in modern times. This topic is of historical value, however, in light of the possibility that in ancient times, more potent tobacco forms may have been used by North American natives to achieve transcendental states along with visual hallucinations.[46]

12.3.4.5. Organic Brain Syndrome

With the exception of the toxic reaction described above, nicotine is not expected to precipitate an OBS. However, a number of states of confusion are associated with the chronic effects of this substance through the destruction of the lung architecture, as is seen in chronic obstructive lung disease, or emphysema.

12.3.4.6. Withdrawal (292.00 in DSM-III-R) (see Section 1.6.6)

12.3.4.6.1. Clinical Picture

There is little doubt in the mind of any smoker that sudden cessation or attempts to "cut down" cause a withdrawal syndrome. The actual symptoms tend to be disturbing but relatively mild, and the intensity varies greatly among people.[45] It has been hypothesized that most heavy smokers get to the point where they continue to administer nicotine to avoid withdrawal symptoms rather than actually to enjoy the substance itself.[51,53]

The symptoms tend to begin within hours of stopping intake, increasing over the first half day.[45] The discomfort is often worse in the evening.[45,51,53] The most prevalent withdrawal symptoms were recently analyzed in an evaluation of 50 heavy smokers who were observed over 4 days of abstinence. Consistent with the descriptions of this syndrome given in DSM-III-R, most patients complained of increased tobacco craving, irritability, anxiety, difficulty concentrating, and restlessness.[76] While there appears to be a relationship between prior evidence of tolerance to nicotine and the subsequent intensity of withdrawal symptoms, more than three quarters of regular smokers report four or more of such symptoms. Additional difficulties reported in other investigations include an EEG slowing with a decreased arousal pattern, a feeling of dullness or drowsiness, as well as feelings of hostility, headache, and sleep problems accompanied by an increase in rapid-eye-movement (REM) latency and total REM time.[51,75] Similar symptoms can be seen after abrupt cessation of nicotine gum—indicating that the syndrome observed by smokers is closely related to the development of physical dependence on nicotine.[76–78] Constipation and/or diarrhea may also occur early, and there may be a significant weight gain, frequently 5 kg or more.[64] In some individuals, these changes can be observed for 30 days or longer, and the psychological symptoms of craving may persist for many months after that.[64]

Nicotine withdrawal has an interesting associated phenomenon not seen with most other drugs. It appears that tapering off may result in even more intense symptoms of craving than precipitous stopping. When tapering off, the symptoms last over a longer period of time; thus, tapering off may be inferior to "cold turkey" stopping and may be associated with a higher level of relapse.

12.3.4.6.2. Treatment

Most tobacco users attempt to stop on their own (perhaps as many as 95% of people who quit successfully do so in this way). Treatment of the withdrawal symptoms may be an important part of "rehabilitation" and may require general supports, counseling (so the smoker knows he is not going through it alone), and perhaps the administration of nicotine gum in decreasing quantities over 3 weeks or more.[79] These approaches are described in greater depth in Section 15.6.

12.3.4.7. Medical Problems

With the possible exception of alcohol, tobacco has the highest cost to society of any abused substance. It has been estimated that 12% or more of deaths annually are related to smoking and that tobacco intake increases the mortality rate 3-fold while also significantly enhancing morbidity.[65,80–82] The highest levels of morbidity and mortality are seen with cigarette smoking. The levels are probably lower for cigars and even lower for smoking a pipe, chewing, and using snuff. Tobacco consumption has been estimated to be one of the most important causes of preventable morbidity and mortality in the United States, with deaths exceeding actuarial expectations in the general population by more than 350,000 per year.[66] This figure is greater than the number of Americans lost in World War I, Korea, and Vietnam combined and is approximately equal to the number of Americans who perished in World War II. The overall mortality risk for smokers is approximately 2.0 if consumption averages two packs per day or more.[45]

1. There is little doubt that tobacco substances, especially through smoking, are associated with a significantly elevated rate of cancer, especially of the lung, the oral cavity, the pharynx, the larynx, and the esophagus.[50,80,83] At least 30% of cancer deaths in the United States are related to smoking, including 80% of cancers of the lung.[66] It is also estimated that 84% of cancers of the larynx are related to smoking (a relative risk of between 2.0 and 27.5 in heavy smokers vs. nonsmokers) and that there is a 13-fold increased risk for oral cancer, a 2- to 3-fold increased risk for bladder cancer, a 2-fold increased risk for pancreatic cancer, and the possibility of a 5-fold increased risk for cancers of the kidney or uterine cervix.[66] Heightened cancer risks are also obvious for snuff and chewing tobacco users, up to 64% of whom have some precancerous cellular changes of the mouth (leukoplakia), with overall cancer risks similar to those noted for smokers, or perhaps even higher.[55] Paradoxically, the decreased estrogen levels observed in female smokers might decrease their risk for endometrial uterine cancers by as much as 50%.[84]

2. High levels of morbidity and mortality are also associated with both cerebrovascular and cardiovascular problems, including strokes, heart attacks, and angina.[50,81,82,85] It is estimated that 33–40% of coronary deaths in the United States are related to smoking,[66] with evidence that the chances for a myocardial infarction increase approximately 3-fold in smokers.[86] This may relate to an increased arterial-wall stiffness that could contribute to atherosclerosis as well as increases in blood pressure and other difficulties with vascular disease.[45,87] Consistent with these factors is the 2- to 3-fold increased risk for abdominal aortic aneurysms among heavy smokers as well as the 2- to 3-fold increased risk for both thrombo embolic and hemorrhagic stroke in heavy smokers.[66,88] Beneficial effects are to be expected with cessation of smoking, through either actual decreased risk or arrest of the increasing risk noted with increasing years of smoking.[86,89] Although low-tar cigarettes appear to lower the level of cancer risk, they have little beneficial effect on the increased risk for heart disease.

3. An area of concern is the effect of nicotine and other tobacco substances on the developing fetus and the neonate. Many of these substances (especially nicotine) easily cross the placenta to the baby and are also found in breast milk. An increase in the fetal heart rate can be seen for 90 minutes after the mother has smoked a cigarette .[66,90–92] Mothers who smoke heavily have almost a 2-fold increased risk of spontaneous abortion, are likely to deliver babies who are small for their gestational age, and have offspring with over a 2-fold increased risk of congenital abnormalities, including patent ductus arteriosis, tetralogy of Fallot, and cleft palate and lips.[91,93] Although fewer data are available, the children of mothers who smoke heavily may demonstrate a higher risk of symptoms of hyperactivity in childhood

and adolescence and may demonstrate higher risks for cancer later in life.[90,91] Smoking is also associated with abnormal sperm forms and evidence of chromosomal damage in lymphocytes.[94]

4. The problems in the respiratory system do not stop with cancer. There is evidence of acute effects of tobacco smoke on decreased ciliary action, which may help explain the increased risk of bronchitis and other infections in smokers.[80] Once these problems persist, chronic obstructive lung disease (*COLD*) can be expected.[66,80,95] In fact, it is estimated that 80–90% of cases of COLD are related to smoke, with a relative risk of between 2.2 and 24.7 vs. the general population, depending on the number of packs smoked per day and the number of years the user has smoked.[66] Although this discussion of associated morbidity may be bad news for the smoker, the good news is that abstinence for 5–10 years returns the risk for most of these problems to normal levels.[45]

5. Other difficulties include an enhanced risk for the development and recurrence of GI ulcers,[96,97] with a relative risk of at least 2-fold for peptic ulcer disease.[66] Smokers run enhanced risk for periodontal disease, as do users of snuff and chewing tobacco.[55,66]

6. An additional difficulty comes from the effects of nicotine on sex hormones. The overall antiestrogen properties of this drug in women, a problem relating to increased rates of metabolism of this hormone, contribute to early menopause and high risks for osteoporosis.[84,98]

7. Finally, recent evidence has documented the importance to the nonsmoker of smoke in the ambient air. This phenomenon of passive smoking involves nicotine, tars, and carbon monoxide both from exhaled smoke (mainstream) and from smoke emanating from the tip of the cigarette (sidestream smoke).[66,92] Problems in adults from passive smoking include eye irritation, headaches, and cough and nasal symptoms, as well as more serious problems of allergic attacks, an increase in angina symptoms, an increase in asthma risk, and even an increase in lung cancer for spouses of smokers who smoke one pack per day or more.[66] Problems extend as well to children of smokers, as these young people carry a higher risk for bronchitis, pneumonia, middle-ear infections, and worsening of an asthma condition.[66]

12.3.5. Treatment and Prevention

Rehabilitation efforts offered to smokers are important attempts to decrease the serious morbidity and mortality described above. The usual approach focuses on education, attempts to increase and maintain high levels of motivation, and behavior modifications. Pharmacological agents of potential importance in rehabilitation of smokers include the recent development of nicotine-containing gum.[77,99] Because these efforts represent yet another special case for rehabilitation, the reader is referred to Section 15.6.

A special word regarding prevention is in order. Considering the relatively wide use of tobacco substances and its high cost to society, as well as the difficulty many users have in stopping, it is worthwhile to discuss briefly the apparent success of prevention strategies. This may be a lesson of importance for prevention of abuse of other substances, as few areas of public health can boast changes in the national patterns of a deleterious problem such as those described in Section 12.3.3. No one is certain why consumption in the Western countries (especially the United States) has decreased. It may be because the approach to prevention has involved a combination of factors, including increasing the price of tobacco products through taxation and through extensive public education and antismoking campaigns targeted at youth. Health problems may have also decreased slightly through the development of less harmful cigarettes that filter out some of the tars and nicotine.[83,100]

REFERENCES

1. Rall, T. W. Central nervous system stimulants: The methylxanthines. In A. G. Gilman, L. S. Goodman, T. W. Rall, & F. Murad (Eds.), *The Pharmacological Basis of Therapeutics* (7th ed.). New York: Macmillan, 1985, pp. 589–603.
2. Lutz, E. G. Restless legs, anxiety and caffeinism. *Journal of Clinical Psychiatry 39:*693–698, 1978.
3. Victor, B. S., Lubetsky, M., & Greden, J. F. Somatic manifestation of caffeinism. *Journal of Clinical Psychiatry 42:*185–188, 1981.
4. Krnjevic, K. Metabolism of theophylline to caffeine in human fetal liver. *Science 206:*1319–1322, 1979.
5. Kalsner, S. A coronary vasoconstrictor substance is present in regular and "decaffeinated" forms of both percolated and instant coffee. *Life Sciences 20:*1689–1696, 1977.
6. Nagy, M. Caffeine content of beverages and chocolate. *Journal of the American Medical Association 229:*337–339, 1974.
7. Diamo, V. J. M., & Garriott, J. C. Lethal caffeine poisoning in a child. *Forensic Science 3:*275–278, 1974.
8. Mikkelsen, E. J. Caffeine and schizophrenia. *Journal of Clinical Psychiatry 83:*732–735, 1978.
9. Mitchelle, M. C., Hoyumpa, A. M., Schenker, S., et al. Inhibition of caffeine elimination by short-term ethanol administration. *Journal of Laboratory and Clinical Medicine 101:*826–834, 1983.
10. Uhde, T. W., Boulenger, J. P., Jimerson, D. C., & Post, R. M. Caffeine: Relationship to human anxiety, plasma MHPG, and cortisol. *Psychopharmacology Bulletin 20:*426–430, 1984.
11. Fernstrom, M. H., Bazil, C. W., & Fernstrom, J. D. Caffeine injection raises brain tryptophan level, but does not stimulate the rate of serotonin synthesis in rat brain. *Life Sciences 35:*1241–1247, 1984.
12. Procter, A. W., & Greden, J. F. Caffeine and benzodiazepine use. *American Journal of Psychiatry 139:*32, 1981.
13. Gould, R. J., Murphy, K. M. M., Katims, J. J., & Snyder, S. H. Caffeine actions and adenosine. Paper presented at the American College of Neuropsychopharmacology Annual Meeting, San Juan, Puerto Rico, December 12–16, 1983.
14. Boulenger, J. P., Uhde, T. W., Wolff, E. A., & Post, R. M. Increased sensitivity to caffeine in patients with panic disorders. *Archives of General Psychiatry 41:*1067–1071, 1984.
15. Charney, D. S., Heninger, G. R., & Jatlow, P. I. Increased anxiogenic effects of caffeine in panic disorders. *Archives of General Psychiatry 42:*233–243, 1985.
16. Marangos, P. J., & Boulenger, J. P. Anxiety, caffeine and the adenosine receptor. Paper presented at the American College of Neuropsychopharmacology Annual Meeting, San Juan, Puerto Rico, December 1984.
17. Judd, L. Effects of psychotropic drugs on cognition and memory. In H. Y. Meltzer (Ed.), *Psychopharmacology: The Third Generation of Progress.* New York: Raven Press, 1987, pp. 1467–1476.
18. Neil, J. F., Himmelhock, J. M., Mallinger, A. G., et al. Caffeinism complicating hypersomnic depressive episodes. *Comparative Psychiatry 19:*337–385, 1978.

19. Becker, A. B., Simons, K. J., Gillespie, C. A., & Simons, F. E. R. The bronchodilator effects and pharmacokinetics of caffeine in asthma. *New England Journal of Medicine 310:*743–746, 1984.

20. Cohen, S. Pathogenesis of coffee-induced gastrointestinal symptoms. *New England Journal of Medicine 303:*122–124, 1980.

21. Kulkanek, F., Linde, O. K., & Meisenberg, G. Prescription of antipsychotic drugs in interaction with coffee or tea. *Lancet 2:*1130, 1979.

22. Boublik, J. H., Quinn, M. J., & Clements, J. A. Coffee contains potent opiate receptor binding activity. *Nature (London) 301:*246–248, 1983.

23. Elins, R. N., Rapoport, J. L., Zahn, T. P., *et al.* Acute effects of caffeine in normal prepubertal boys. *American Journal of Psychiatry 183:*178–182, 1981.

24. Gilliland, K., & Andress, D. Ad lib caffeine consumption, symptoms of caffeinism, and academic performance. *American Journal of Psychiatry 138:*512–514, 1981.

25. Tennant, F. S., & Detels, R. Relationship of alcohol, cigarette, and drug abuse in adulthood with alcohol, cigarette and coffee consumption in childhood. *Preventive Medicine 5:*70–77, 1976.

26. Rapoport, J. L., Berg, C. J., Ismond, D. R., *et al.* Behavioral effects of caffeine in children. *Archives of General Psychiatry 41:*1073–1079, 1984.

27. Greden, J. F., Fontaine, P., Lubetsky, M., *et al.* Anxiety and depression associated with caffeinism among psychiatric inpatients. *American Journal of Psychiatry 135:*963–966, 1978.

28. Abe, K. Reactions to coffee and alcohol in monozygotic twins. *Journal of Psychosomatic Research 12:*199–203, 1968.

29. Schuckit, M. A. Anxiety treatment: A commonsense approach. *Postgraduate Medicine 75:*52–63, 1984.

30. Breier, A., Charney, D. S., & Heinger, G. R. Agoraphobia with panic attacks. *Archives of General Psychiatry 43:*1029–1036, 1986.

31. Lee, M. A., Fiegel, P., Greden, J. F., & Cameron, O. G. Caffeine as an anxiogenic agent: Comparison of panic and depressed patients. Paper presented at the 41st Meeting of the Society of Biological Psychiatry, Washington, D.C., May 7–11, 1986.

32. Dimaio, V., & Garriott, J. Lethal caffeine poisoning. *Forensic Science 3:*275–278, 1974.

33. Sours, J. A. Case reports of anorexia nervosa and caffeinism. *American Journal of Psychiatry 140:*235–236, 1983.

34. Mathew, R. J., Barr, D. L., & Weinman, M. L. Caffeine and cerebral blood flow. *British Journal of Psychiatry 143:*604–608, 1983.

35. Gibson, C. J. Caffeine withdrawal elevates urinary MHPG excretion. *New England Journal of Medicine 304:*363, 1981.

36. White, B. C., Lincoln, C. A., Pearce, N. W., *et al.* Anxiety and muscle tension as consequences of caffeine withdrawal. *Science 209:*1547–1548, 1980.

37. Kozlowsky, L. T. Effect of caffeine on coffee drinking. *Nature (London) 264:*354–355, 1976.

38. Bauer, A. R., Rank, R. K., & Kerr, R. The effects of prolonged coffee intake on genetically identical mice. *Life Sciences 21:*63–70, 1977.

39. LaCroix, A. Z., Mead, L. A., Liang, K. Y., *et al.* Coffee consumption and the incidence of coronary heart disease. *New England Journal of Medicine 315:*977–982, 1986.

40. Roth, T., Zorick, F., Roehrs, T., *et al.* Insomnia treatment: A new pharmacological approach. Paper presented at the American Psychiatric Association Annual Meeting, Toronto, Ontario, Canada, May 1982.

41. Heuch, I., Kvale, G., Jacobsen, B. K., & Bjelke, E. Use of alcohol, tobacco, and coffee, and risk of pancreatic cancer. *British Journal of Cancer 48:*637–643, 1983.

42. Binstock, M., Krakow, D., Stamler, J., *et al.* Coffee and pancreatic cancer: An analysis of international mortality data. *American Journal of Epidemiology 118:*630–640, 1983.

43. Vaughn, R. Coffee in pregnancy. *Lancet 1:*554, 1981.

44. Hoff, W. V. Caffeine in pregnancy. *Lancet 1:*1020, 1982.

45. Jaffe, J. H. Drug addiction and drug abuse. In A. G. Gilman, L. S. Goodman, T. W. Rall, & F. Murad (Eds.), *The Pharmacological Basis of Therapeutics* (7th ed.). New York: Macmillan, 1985, pp. 554–558.

46. Janiger, O., & deRios, M. D. Suggestive hallucinogenic properties of tobacco. *Medical Anthropology Newsletter 4:*1–6, Aug. 1973.

47. Krasnegor, N. A. Introduction. In N. A. Krasnegor (Ed.), *Cigarette Smoking as a Dependence Process: Research Monograph 23*. Rockville, Maryland: National Institute on Drug Abuse, 1979, pp. 1–3.

48. Pechacek, T. F. An overview of smoking behavior and its modification. In N. A. Krasnegor (Ed.), *Behavioral Analyses and Treatment of Substance Abuse: Research Monograph 25*. Rockville, Maryland: National Institute on Drug Abuse, 1979, pp. 92–113.

49. Dilsaver, S. C., Majchrzak, M. J., & Alessi, N. E. Chronic treatment with amitriptyline produces supersensitivity to nicotine. *Biological Psychiatry 23:*169–175, 1988.

50. Meade, T. W., Imeson, J., & Stirling, Y. Effects of changes in smoking and other characteristics on clotting factors and the risk of ischaemic heart disease. *Lancet 2:*986–988, 1987.

51. Kozlowsky, L. T., Jarvik, M. E., & Gritz, E. R. Nicotine regulation and cigarette smoking. *Clinical Pharmacology and Therapeutics 17:*93–97, 1975.

52. Schachter, S., Silverstein, B., Kozlowsky, L. T., *et al*. Studies of the interaction of psychological and pharmacological determinants of smoking. *Journal of Experimental Psychology: General 106:*3–40, 1977.

53. Taylor, P. Ganglionic stimulating and blocking agents. In A. G. Gilman, L. S. Goodman, T. W. Rall, & F. Murad (Eds.), *The Pharmacological Basis of Therapeutics* (7th ed.). New York: Macmillan, 1985, pp. 215–221.

54. Tonnesen, P., Fryd, V., Hansen, M., *et al*. Effect of nicotine chewing gum in combination with group counseling on the cessation of smoking. *New England Journal of Medicine 318:*15–18, 1988.

55. Connolly, G. N., Winn, D. M., Hecht, S. S., *et al*. The reemergence of smokeless tobacco. *New England Journal of Medicine 314:*1020–1027, 1986.

56. Jarvik, M. E. Nicotine as a psychoactive drug—Panel summary. *Psychopharmacology Bulletin 22:*882–883, 1986.

57. Rose, J. E. Cigarette smoking blocks caffeine-induced arousal. *Alcohol and Drug Research 7:*49–55, 1986.

58. Pomerleau, O. F. Nicotine as a psychoactive drug: Anxiety and pain reduction. *Psychopharmacology Bulletin 22:*865–869, 1986.

59. Domino, E. F. Nicotine as a unique psychoactive drug: Arousal with skeletal muscle relaxation. *Psychopharmacology Bulletin 22:*870–873, 1986.

60. Rosecrans, J. A. Nicotine as a discriminative stimulus. In N. A. Krasnegor (Ed.), *Cigarette Smoking as a Dependence Process: Research Monograph 23*. Rockville, Maryland: National Institute on Drug Abuse, 1979, pp. 58–69.

61. Grunberg, N. E. Nicotine as a psychoactive drug: Appetite regulation. *Psychopharmacology Bulletin 22:*875–881, 1986.

62. Mintz, J. Alcohol increases cigarette smoking. *Addictive Behaviors 10:*203–207, 1985.

63. Abood, L. G., Lowy, K., & Booth, H. Acute and chronic effects of nicotine. In N. A. Krasnegor (Ed.), *Cigarette Smoking as a Dependence Process: Research Monograph 23*. Rockville, Maryland: National Institute on Drug Abuse, 1979, pp. 136–149.

64. Hughes, J. R., Gust, S. W., & Pechacek, T. F. Prevalence of tobacco dependence and withdrawal. *American Journal of Psychiatry 144:*205–208, 1987.

65. Davis, R. Current trends in cigarette smoking and marketing. *New England Journal of Medicine 316:*725–732, 1987.

66. Fielding, J. E. Smoking: Health effects and control. *New England Journal of Medicine 313:*491–498, 1985.

67. Warner, K. E. Cigarette smoking in the 1970's. The impact of the anti-smoking campaign on consumption. *Science 211:*729–731, 1981.

68. Chapman, S. Stop-smoking clinics: A case for their abandonment. *Lancet 1:*918–920, 1985.

69. Smart, R. G., Goodstadt, M. S., Adlaf, E. M., *et al*. Trends in the prevalence of alcohol and other drug use among Ontario students: 1977–1983. *Canadian Journal of Public Health 76:*157–161, 1985.

70. Hughes, J. R., Hatsukami, D. K., Mitchell, J. E., & Dahlgren, L. A. Prevalence of smoking among psychiatric outpatients. *American Journal of Psychiatry 143*:993–997, 1986.

71. Hughes, J. R.: Genetics of smoking: A brief review. *Behavioral Therapy 17*:335–345, 1986.

72. Crumpacker, D. W., Cederlof, R., Friberg. L., *et al.* A twin methodology for the study of genetic and environmental control of variation in human smoking behavior. *Acta Geneticae Medicae et Gemellologiae 28*:173–195, 1979.

73. Henningfield, J. E. Pharmacologic basis and treatment of cigarette smoking. *Journal of Clinical Psychiatry 45*:24–34, 1984.

74. O'Donnell, J. A. Cigarette smoking as a precursor of illicit drug use. In N. A. Krasnegor (Ed.), *Cigarette Smoking as a Dependence Process: Research Monograph 23*. Rockville, Maryland: National Institute on Drug Abuse, 1979, pp. 30–43.

75. Kozlowsky, L. T., Herman, C. P., & Frecker, R. C. What researchers make of what cigarette smokers say: Filtering smokers' hot air. *Lancet 1*:699–700, 1980.

76. Hughes, J. R., & Hatsukami, D. Signs and symptoms of tobacco withdrawal. *Archives of General Psychiatry 43*:289–294, 1986.

77. Hughes, J. R., Hatsukami, D. K., & Skoog, K. P. Physical dependence on nicotine in gum. *Journal of the American Medical Association 255*:3277–3279, 1986.

78. Hughes, J. R., Arana, G., Amori, G., *et al.* Effect of tobacco withdrawal on the dexamethasone suppression test. *Biological Psychiatry 23*:96–98, 1988.

79. Lichtenstein, E. Social learning, smoking and substance abuse. In N. A. Krasnegor (Ed.), *Behavioral Analysis and Treatment of Substance Abuse: Research Monograph 25*. Rockville, Maryland: National Institute on Drug Abuse, 1979, pp. 114–127.

80. Quellet, B. L., Romeder, J. M., & Lance, J. M. Premature mortality attributable to smoking and hazardous drinking in Canada. *American Journal of Epidemiology 109*:451–463, 1979.

81. Willett, W. C., Green, A., Stampfer, M. J., *et al.* Relative and absolute excess risks of coronary heart disease among women who smoke cigarettes. *New England Journal of Medicine 317*:1303–1309, 1987.

82. Kaufman, D. W., Palmer, J. R., Rosenberg, L., & Shapiro, S. Cigar and pipe smoking and myocardial infarction in young men. *British Medical Journal 294*:1315–1316, 1987.

83. Blot, W. J., McLaughlin, J. K., Winn, D. M. *et al.* Smoking and drinking in relation to oral and pharyngeal cancer. *Cancer Research 48*:3282–3287, 1988.

84. Michnovicz, J. J., Hershcopf, R. J., Naganuma, H., *et al.* Increased 2-hydroxylation of estradiol as a possible mechanism for the anti-estrogenic effect of cigarette smoking. *New England Journal of Medicine 315*:1305–1309, 1986.

85. Kaufman, D. W., Helmrich, S. P., Rosenberg, L., *et al.* Nicotine and carbon monoxide content of cigarette smoke and the risk of myocardial infarction in young men. *New England Journal of Medicine 308*:409–413, 1983.

86. Rosenberg, L., Kaufman, D. W., Helmrich, S. P., & Shapiro, S. The risk of myocardial infarction after quitting smoking in men under 55 years of age. *New England Journal of Medicine 313*:1511–1514, 1985.

87. Caro, C. G., Parker, K. H., Lever, M. J. & Fish, P. J. Effect of cigarette smoking on the pattern of arterial blood flow: Possible insight into mechanisms underlying the development of arteriosclerosis. *Lancet 2*:11–14, 1987.

88. Abbott, R. D., Yin, Y., Reed, D. M., & Yano, K. Risk of stroke in male cigarette smokers. *New England Journal of Medicine 315*:717–720, 1986.

89. Cook, D. G., Pocock, S. J., Shaper, A. G., & Kussick, S. J. Giving up smoking and the risk of heart attacks. *Lancet 2*:1376–1378, 1986.

90. Everson, R. B. Individuals transplacentally exposed to maternal smoking may be at increased cancer risk in adult life. *Lancet 2*:123–126, 1980.

91. Christiansen, R. Gross deficiencies observed in the placentas of smokers and nonsmokers. *American Journal of Epidemiology 110*:178–187, 1979.

92. Greenberg, R. A., Haley, N. J., Etzel, R. A., & Loda, F. A. Measuring the exposure of infants to tobacco smoke. *New England Journal of Medicine 310*:1075–1078, 1984.

93. Fabia, J., & Drolette, M. Twin pairs, smoking in pregnancy and perinatal mortality. *American Journal of Epidemiology 112:*404–408, 1980.

94. Evans, H. J., Fletcher, J., Torrence, M., *et al.* Sperm abnormalities and cigarette smoking. *Lancet 1:*627–629, 1981.

95. White, J. R., & Froeb, H. F. Small-airways of dysfunction in nonsmokers chronically exposed to tobacco smoke. *New England Journal of Medicine 302:*720–723, 1980.

96. Sontag, S., Graham, D. Y., Belsito, A., *et al.* Cimetidine, cigarette smoking, and recurrence of duodenal ulcer. *New England Journal of Medicine 311:*689–693, 1984.

97. Boyko, E. J. Risk of ulcerative colitis among cigarette smokers. *New England Journal of Medicine 316:*707–710, 1987.

98. Jensen, J., Christiansen, C., & Rodbro, P. Cigarette smoking, serum estrogens, and bone loss during hormone-replacement therapy early after menopause. *New England Journal of Medicine 313:*873–875, 1985.

99. Lam, W., Sacks, H. S., Sze, P. C. & Chalmers, T. C. Meta-analysis of randomized controlled trials of nicotine chewing-gum. *Lancet 2:*27–30, 1987.

100. Atkinson, A. B., & Townsend, J. L. Economic aspects of reduced smoking. *Lancet 2:*494–492, 1977.

CHAPTER 13

Multidrug Abuse

13.1. INTRODUCTION

13.1.1. General Comments

The format of this chapter differs slightly from that of the rest of the text; it emphasizes some major types of drug interactions. Because the focus is on the relationships among types of drugs of abuse, careful reading of this chapter will give you an opportunity to review much of the material already presented. In other words, chapter 13 reviews the general lessons given in this text about drug interactions.

Few members of our society who abuse drugs take only one substance. There is a strong correlation between the abuse of heroin and alcohol problems, abusers of stimulants frequently also abuse depressants, and alcoholics may be at higher risk for the abuse of both other depressants and stimulants. However, as I observe the treatment programs available in most communities, I'm struck by the relative absence of "polydrug" or "multidrug" programs; that is, the multidrug abuser must usually convince treatment personnel that his major problem includes alcohol or opiates before he will be admitted. With that in mind, I hope that clinicians working with methadone maintenance programs and those interested in alcoholism treatment will read this chapter carefully and go back and review the information presented on specific classes of drugs [e.g., central nervous system (CNS) depressants and CNS stimulants] to find the best way to meet the needs of the patients entering their programs.

13.1.2. Problems of Definition and Classification

The first issue is the importance of distinguishing between use, abuse, and physical dependence. As documented in each of the relevant chapters of this text, a majority of young people in our society have had some experience with at least one illicit drug at some time during their lives. It is likely that men and women who demonstrate legal difficulties as well as those who appear for help in mental-health settings may have more experience with substances of abuse than the general population. Therefore, in dealing with patients of any kind, it is important to take a history of *exposure* to other drugs, and to differentiate *use* (which may be no different from the experience in the general population), possible *temporary problems* related to other substances, actual *abuse,* and *dependence* that meets the criteria in DSM-III-R. In the latter case, possible issues related to the abstinence syndrome must be addressed, at least for brain depressants, stimulants, and opiates.

Even after making these important distinctions, it is advantageous to develop some scheme for classifying *polydrug* and *multidrug* use. Polydrug involvement, by convention, indicates the use of more than one psychoactive substance, *not including opiates,* whereas multidrug use involves two psychoactive substances other than alcohol, nicotine, caffeine, or prescribed medications.[1] Although most polydrug clinics exclude individuals who have difficulties related to opiates,[1] the recognition that many people who primarily use multiple drugs may also casually use opiates leads me to use the less restrictive term *multidrug* here.

For the sake of completion, it is of interest to note that abuse of multiple drugs can be further classified from a variety of clinical perspectives (none of which has been proved to be better than the others):

1. First, it is possible to divide users by the *type of drug* taken:
   a. Those who regularly abuse *narcotics,* who can be subdivided into:
      i. Those who use only narcotics.
      ii. Those who use narcotics and alcohol, as well as other psychoactive substances when available.
      iii. Those who use other drugs, but only during methadone maintenance or when narcotics are unavailable.
   b. Those who primarily abuse *alcohol* and occasionally turn to other drugs of abuse.
   c. Those who abuse *hallucinogens, stimulants,* and/or *depressants,* with or without alcohol, and do not take narcotics.
2. Another somewhat overlapping subdivision is based on *patterns of drug use*[2,3]:
   a. Those who are dependent on one drug and use other drugs only when they are easily available.
   b. Those who are dependent on one drug and use other drugs only when the primary substance is not available.
   c. Those who prefer one drug but take others to decrease the side effects of the first.
   d. Those who abuse different drugs at different times of the day—for example, stimulants in the morning, antianxiety drugs during the day, and hypnotics at night.
   e. Last, those who have no drug preference but take whatever is available.
3. Of course, within any of these patterns, one must also consider:
   a. The *influence of prior psychiatric disorders* (primary versus secondary

drug abuse as described for alcohol in Section 3.1.2.3).[4,5] Men and women with the antisocial personality (see Section 3.1.2.3.1) are likely to abuse multiple substances, but they are best labeled primary antisocial personalities and secondary multidrug abusers. Similarly, primary alcoholics may begin "treating" their lethargy or depression with stimulants and their anxiety with depressants, such as the benzodiazepines, in which instance they are best labeled primary alcoholics (their first-appearing major disorder) and secondary polydrug abusers. As discussed in depth elsewhere, the proper assignment of primary and secondary labels is essential if the clinician wishes to predict the probable course and to select the most effective treatment.

b. The *frequency and amount* of drug abuse.
c. Whether drugs are taken *intravenously* or orally (as the former often yields higher risk of problems).
d. Whether the person is a middle-class individual who usually obtains substances from a physician or is more actively involved in a *street culture*.

In summary, there are almost an infinite number of ways to divide and further subdivide the characteristics of people who abuse multiple drugs. In the long run, each approach has some assets and liabilities, so that each clinician is likely to have his or her own preference. Personally, I prefer to distinguish between the primary and secondary abuse of multiple substances, placing primary alcoholics, primary antisocial personalities, and primary opiate abusers in a category separate from primary multidrug abusers. However, I assume that many patients will also have had experience with other drugs, and some will have even developed secondary abuse or dependence. I remind myself to always ask about problems with multiple drugs and to consider such exposure and possible physical dependence while carrying out the physical examination and detoxification procedures (if needed). Many of these issues are discussed further in Chapter 15.

13.1.3. Natural History of Multidrug Abuse

The ages of first use and abuse and the pattern of drug intake vary among groups.[4-8] For example, a person with an antisocial personality[4] utilizes drugs as part of a larger antisocial picture—drugs are almost "incidental" to his life pattern.[5] One recent long-term follow-up of a group of inner-city youth demonstrated that the antecedent life-styles and stresses are probably different for antisocial personalities and alcoholics, implying that the same might be true of multidrug abusers vs. antisocial personalities.[9] When substance abuse and the delinquency coexist, it is most often the case that the delinquency antedated the drug-use pattern, a fact that indicates the probability that the patient may demonstrate an antisocial personality.[10]

Also, natural histories differ with the immediate environment, as exemplified by the greater access to drugs like heroin in urban ghettos as compared to middle-class suburbs. In addition, the changing views of society might be expected to have a great impact on use and abuse patterns of marijuana.

With these caveats in mind, it is still possible to make some generalizations about likely patterns of abuse. In Western society, youth begin drug experiences with caffeine, nicotine, and alcohol. If they go on to use other substances, the next drug is likely to be marijuana, followed in frequency by one of the hallucinogens, depressants, or stimulants, usually taken on an experimental basis, ingested orally, and with few immediately serious consequences. Individuals who go on to heavier intake may graduate to intravenous drug use, with a progression to opiates.[10–12]

This patterning of abuse has been viewed by some investigators as an age-related clustering of drugs reflecting the use of whatever substance is most available and culturally acceptable at a given age. Here the drug pattern is not viewed as a continuum or a ''stepping-stone'' from one particular drug to another.[11] Other researchers, however, have outlined a sequential pattern of misuse, from nonuse to beer or wine, progressing to cigarettes and/or hard liquor, and then to marijuana, which may presage the use of other drugs.[12,13] The available data do not defini-tively rule out either the clustering or the stepping-stone theory.

13.1.4. Pharmacology

13.1.4.1. General Comments

The effects of a drug may be either increased or decreased through interactions with other drugs:

1. The effect of a drug is *decreased* when it is administered to an individual who, while *not* taking any other drug at the same time, has in the recent past developed cross-tolerance to a similar drug. This can occur through metabolic tolerance (usually reflecting the increased production of the relevant metabolic enzymes in the liver) or pharmacodynamic mechanisms (by which the effect of the substance on brain cells has been decreased). Thus, higher levels of the substance are needed to generate the expected clinical effects. A relevant example is the need for higher levels of anesthetics, hypnotics, antianxiety drugs, or analgesics in re-cently sober alcoholics.

2. The results are the opposite, however, when two drugs with similar effects are administered *concomitantly*. In this instance, both drugs must compete for the same enzyme and protein systems, both in the liver and at the target cell, the latter usually located in the brain. One likely result is an increased half-life in the body for the drugs when both are administered acutely, although this adaptation may be lost after continued exposure to both agents.[14,15] The overall effect with concomitant acute administration of agents can be *potentiation,* through which, for example, the amount of depression of brain activity that results from the conjoint administration of two depressant drugs is more than would be expected from the actions of either drug alone. The effect can be an unexpected lethal overdose for the individual who

has had too much to drink and decides that a few extra sleeping pills will help him rest through the night.

13.1.4.2. Some Specific Examples

Thus, the clinician should think twice before administering more than one drug to a patient. Because of the opposing effects, specific drug–drug interactions are somewhat unpredictable, underlining the dangers in multidrug abuse. However, it is possible to make some generalizations about combinations of particular types of drugs.

13.1.4.2.1. Depressants–Depressants

The mechanisms of actions of most brain depressants are not completely understood. This is true even for the benzodiazepines (Bz's), which, as outlined in Section 2.1.1.4.3, have been shown to exert a substantial portion of their effects through an interaction between Bz receptors and gamma-aminobutyric acid (GABA) receptor complexes in the central nervous system (CNS). Of course, there is ample evidence of cross-tolerance among the brain depressants, including documentation of this phenomenon regarding alcohol and Bz's.[16] Much interesting information in the last few years has shown that at least part of the effect of alcohol occurs either directly or indirectly via GABA, and there are additional data indicating that the number of Bz receptors in the frontal cortex may be depleted in chronic alcoholics.[17,18] Consistent with this data is a recent investigation of a Bz antagonist showing that this substance blocks part of the anxiolytic and intoxicating actions of ethanol, at least in animals.[17,19] As exciting as these findings are, the interaction between Bz antagonists and beverage alcohol appears to be only part of the clnical picture of the effects of ethanol, and the interactions may not be as specific and selective as was first hoped.[17,20,21] These new discoveries, however, underscore the potential clinical as well as research importance of interactions between two or more depressants.

Consistent with the preceding discussion, if the two depressants are not used at the same time, one would expect a decreased potency of the second depressant when administered to an individual who has already developed tolerance to the first. If, however, the two depressants (e.g., alcohol and sleeping pills) are given at the same time, potentiation of respiratory depression develops, with resulting morbidity and even mortality.[22] In one clinical example, a lethal overdose of barbiturates might require blood levels of 1.0–1.5 mg/100 ml (1.0–1.5 mg/dl) if taken alone, but in the presence of 100 mg/dl of ethanol, the lethal barbiturate blood level may be as low as 0.5 mg/dl.[22]

13.1.4.2.2. Depressants–Opiates

Interest in the relationship between alcohol-related problems and opiate-related difficulties has a long history.[23] Over the last 100 years, clinicians have touted the possible benefits of substituting alcohol for opiates among drug addicts and the possibility of using opiates as a substitute for alcohol among alcoholics.[23] These speculations are based in part on the partial "cross-tolerance" between the two classes of drugs, at least for analgesic effects of ethanol.[24] There is information, related in Section 4.2.3.2 (item 3), concerning a possible ability of opiate antagonists to ameliorate severe alcohol intoxication (although this appears to be unrelated to the direct effects of the alcohol and may be more closely tied to aspects of "shock"), as well as a theory that ethanol might exert at least some of its important effects through endogenous opiate peptides or opiate receptors.[25-27] Other investigators have attempted to establish a familial tie between opiate abuse and alcoholism, but the evidence is unimpressive once one excludes the potential impact of a primary diagnosis of the antisocial personality disorder (in which abuse of many substances can be expected) and when one observes the drug-intake pattern of offspring of non-alcohol-abusing opiate addicts.[28]

Even though the depressants and opiates do not have true cross-tolerance, one frequently sees a decreased efficacy of one drug when administered to an individual who has developed tolerance to the second class. Of greater clinical importance, however, is the fact that both opiates and depressants have depressing effects on the CNS, so that each potentiates the actions of the other in overdose, increasing the likelihood of death.

Reflecting this evidence, it is not surprising that alcohol and opiates are the first two leading causes of death among methadone maintenance patients both in treatment and during follow-up, with abuse of ethanol significantly decreasing the 10-year survival among these men and women.[29] In addition to the obvious deleterious effects of ethanol itself, there is also the possibility that concomitant administration of ethanol with methadone could result in increased brain concentrations of the latter (at least in animals).[14] Misuse of alcohol also appears to contribute heavily to the termination of treatment among opiate abusers.[29] Thus, independent of the possible mechanisms involved, use, abuse, and dependence on ethanol must be carefully considered among all opiate abusers, misuse of both types of substances is highly likely in individuals with the antisocial personality disorder, and, although much less prevalent, the use of opiates has been reported in perhaps 10% of primary alcoholics.[6]

13.1.4.2.3. Depressants–Stimulants

The brief discussion of epidemiology in Section 13.1.5 highlights the likelihood that alcoholics are likely to abuse stimulants. Similar generalizations can be made about opiate abusers, where, in one recent study, 74% of heroin addicts had experience with cocaine, although additional data on the percentage of individuals with actual dependence or abuse need to be developed.[30]

The concomitant use of depressant and stimulant drugs can decrease the level of the side effects encountered with one drug alone. For example, the depressant-drug abuser or the alcoholic may seek out stimulants to help him feel less sleepy from abusing his favorite drug, or the CNS-stimulant abuser may use alcohol or other depressants to help him feel less anxious and demonstrate less tremor while taking his preferred drug. The dangers rest with the unpredictability of the reaction, as the CNS and metabolic systems attempt to maintain equilibrium (homeostasis) in the presence of multiple drugs with opposite effects.

13.1.4.2.4. Hallucinogens–Stimulants

The similarities in clinical action and chemical structure of these two classes of drugs frequently lead to a potentiation of side effects. Therefore, in treating a hallucinogen-related toxic reaction (Section 8.2.3.2), stimulants are to be avoided, as they may worsen, not improve, clinical symptoms.

13.1.4.2.5. Hallucinogens–Atropinic Drugs

The same generalizations hold for this type of combination as for the hallucinogen–stimulant interaction. This makes it unwise to use antipsychotic medications, with their anticholinergic side effects, in treating patients with a hallucinogen-induced toxic reaction.

13.1.4.2.6. Marijuana–Other Drugs

Marijuana has been shown to potentiate the CNS-depressing effect of alcohol,[31] and it may increase the likelihood of a flashback from hallucinogen-type drugs. Although these relationships require more research, it is unwise to take marijuana concomitantly with other substances, especially alcohol, because of the resulting motor incoordination and CNS depression, a problem with serious implications for driving abilities.[32,33]

13.1.5. Epidemiology and Patterns of Abuse

Chapter 7 documents that almost 60% of high school seniors have used marijuana at least once, and Chapter 5 reminds us that almost 20% have had experience with amphetamines or cocaine. Reflecting this high rate of drug use in the general population, it is not surprising that in a recent evaluation carried out on 171 primary alcoholics in our own treatment program, 76% of this predominantly blue-collar population had at some point used marijuana (including only 21% who had smoked in the preceding 3 months), but none met actual criteria for marijuana abuse. Of our population, 28% had taken cocaine (8% in the preceding 3 months) and 17% had used hallucinogens (only 3% in the preceding 3 months).[34] In another study, *use* of some illicit substance was reported by 79% of 102 United States Army personnel entering an alcohol treatment program, including 48% who had "more than experimentation with these other drugs," but an unknown percentage who would have fulfilled criteria for actual abuse or dependence. These figures included 32% with experience with marijuana, 16% who had taken hallucinogens, almost 20% who had used amphetamines or cocaine, and 7% who had taken brain depressants other than alcohol.[7] In data gathered from another standpoint, urine samples among 103 patients admitted to a nonmedical detoxification facility in Canada indicated that 10% had recently taken cannabinols, 7% barbiturates, and 32% a benzodiazepine.[8] These data underscore the need to consider use of drugs other than alcohol by alcoholics. They also emphasize that a history of having used a substance one or more times does not imply current use, that use does not equate with abuse or dependence, and that figures for experience with drugs among patients entering alcohol treatment programs are not always strikingly higher than drug-history experiences that might be expected in comparable groups in the general population or in other treatment settings.

Although the exact extent of multidrug abuse is not known, it certainly is a rather common phenomenon among drug abusers. There is also anecdotal evidence that multiple substance abuse has increased over the years.[3,34−36] Over one half of the people presenting to a polydrug clinic reported the use of three or more substances.[37,38] Certain individuals appear to be at especially high risk for multidrug abuse, including those with a history of psychiatric problems,[38] those "denied" access to their favorite drug (e.g., subjects in methadone maintenance programs),[39] and those who deliberately use the more "exotic" substances, such as phencyclidine (PCP)[40] (see Chapter 9). A fourth special group live in high-stress situations while separated from their families, such as young soldiers who were using drugs, 70% of whom, according to one survey, persistently administer multiple substances.[41]

In general, multidrug abusers tend to be young and from middle-class backgrounds, and they often show some evidence of preexisting life maladjustment, sometimes severe enough to be labeled a personality disorder.[42]

13.1.6. Establishing a Diagnosis

It is important to remember that substance abuse is a relatively common phenomenon in our society and must be considered in the differential diagnosis of a wide variety of medical and psychological problems. To review briefly, in evaluating an individual who, by past history, fits the criteria for the antisocial personality, one must note the likelihood that he or she is abusing multiple drugs. This is also probable for those on methadone maintenance programs and those living in high-stress situations. On another level, any individual presenting to the emergency room with a drug overdose must be evaluated for the *possibility* of multidrug abuse, particularly any person who does not show the usual response to emergency room interventions.

13.2. EMERGENCY ROOM SITUATIONS

The most important clinical pictures seen with multiple drugs include toxic reactions (usually overdoses), drug withdrawal pictures, psychoses, and organic brain syndromes (OBSs). The discussion here is brief, the reason being that once multidrug problems are indicated, treatment involves combining the procedures used for each substance alone.

13.2.1. Panic Reactions (see Section 1.6.1)

The clinical picture, course, and treatment for panic reactions resemble those seen for any one of the substances, including marijuana, the hallucinogens, the stimulants, and the atropinic drugs. The treatment is as outlined in the specific drug chapters. Good examples are given in Sections 5.2.1, 7.2.1, 11.7.4.1, 11.8.4, 11.9.1.1, and 14.2.

13.2.2. Flashbacks

Flashbacks are seen with the hallucinogens or marijuana, and the clinical course and treatment for recurrences after the use of these drugs in combination with others are the same as outlined in Sections 7.2.2 and 8.2.2 for the individual drugs.

13.2.3. Toxic Reactions (see Sections 1.6.3 and 14.4)

13.2.3.1. Clinical Picture

Toxic reactions, of great clinical significance, most often result from the concomitant administration of two depressant-type drugs or of opiates along with depressants.

13.2.3.1.1. Multiple Depressants (see Sections 2.2.3 and 4.2.3)

Multiple-depressant overdosage is complex because the depth of respiratory depression and the length of severe toxicity are difficult to predict. However, the clinical manifestations are those described for the CNS depressants and for alochol.

13.2.3.1.2. Depressants–Opiates (see Sections 2.2.3, 4.2.3, and 6.2.3)

The concomitant administration of opiates and depressants results in unpredictable vital signs, reflexes, and pupillary reactions, along with fluctuation between stupor and semialertness.[2] The specific symptoms are combinations of those reported for the CNS depressants and the opiates.

13.2.3.2. Treatment

13.2.3.2.1. Multiple Depressants

For mixed-depressant toxic reactions, the treatment is that outlined in Section 2.2.3.2, including acute life-preserving steps and the use of general life supports, relying on the body to detoxify the sbustances. Dialysis or diuresis should be reserved for extremely toxic cases. The major unique caveat is the unpredictability of the length of drug effects when multiple depressants are involved.

13.2.3.2.2. Depressants–Opiates

In the instance of combined opiate and CNS-depressant overdose, acute emergency procedures (e.g., airway and cardiac status) are again followed. Naloxone

(Narcan) is administered at doses of 0.4 mg intramuscularly (IM) or intravenously (IV), with repeat doses given every 5 minutes for the first 15 minutes and every several hours thereafter, as needed, for control of the respiratory depression and the degree of stupor. General supports are then continued until the body is able to destroy the drugs. These procedures are outlined in Sections 2.2.3.2 and 6.2.3.2.

13.2.3.2.3. Other Combinations

The treatment of other drug combinations is symptomatic in nature and follows the procedures outlined in the relevant drug chapters. It is worthwhile to note the importance of physostigmine when atropinic drugs [e.g., the antiparkinsonian drugs, such as benztropine (Cogentin)] are involved (Section 11.9.1.2).

13.2.4. Psychoses (see Section 1.6.4)

The drug-induced psychoses seen with stimulants (Section 5.2.4) or CNS depressants (Sections 2.2.4 and 4.2.4) are evanescent pictures, disappearing with general supportive care. Little, if any, information is available on the psychoses produced by the multiple administration of these substances.

13.2.5. Organic Brain Syndrome (see Section 1.6.5)

Any drug in high enough doses can cause confusion and disorientation, the hallmarks of an OBS. In drug combinations, one can expect this clinical picture to be evanescent, and the general treatment plans outlined in the individual chapters should be followed. However, it is wise to remember that with multiple drugs, the course is unpredictable, and it is probable that the patient will be impaired for a longer time than would be expected with either drug alone.

13.2.6. Withdrawal from Multiple Drugs (see Section 1.6.6)

The most common multidrug withdrawal pictures are those seen following the concomitant abuse of multiple depressants, depressants and stimulants, or multiple addictions to opiates and depressant drugs.

13.2.6.1. Clinical Picture

13.2.6.1.1. Multiple Depressants

The depressant withdrawal syndrome, described in Section 2.2.6, is similar for all CNS-depressant drugs; however, a higher incidence of convulsions is seen with benzodiazepines or barbiturates than with alcohol. The latency of onset and the length of the acute withdrawal syndrome roughly parallel the half-life of the drugs, ranging from relatively short periods of time for alcohol to much longer withdrawals for drugs such as chlordiazepoxide (Librium) and phenobarbital. It is probably safest to treat withdrawal from the longer-acting drug most aggressively, assuming that the second depressant will be adquately "taken care of" through this approach, but keeping an open eye for any unusual symptoms.

13.2.6.1.2. Depressants–Stimulants (see Sections 2.2.6, 4.2.6, and 5.2.6)

The withdrawal from depressants and stimulants more closely follows the CNS-depressant withdrawal paradigm, but probably includes greater levels of sadness, paranoia, and lethargy than would be expected with depressants alone.

13.2.6.1.3. Depressants–Opiates (see Sections 2.2.6, 4.2.6, and 6.2.6)

The individual withdrawing from depressants and opiates usually demonstrates an opiate-type withdrawal syndrome (Section 6.2.6) along with heightened levels of insomnia and anxiety and a depressant-related risk for convulsions and confusion (see Sections 2.2.6 and 4.2.6).

13.2.6.1.4. Other Combinations

Withdrawal reactions for other classes of drugs either have not been proved to exist or have low levels of clinical significance. Therefore, multiple withdrawal syndromes for drugs other than depressants, stimulants, and opiates will not be discussed here.

13.2.6.2. Treatment

13.2.6.2.1. Multiple Depressants

Adequate therapy for physical addiction to multiple depressants follows the guidelines outlined in Section 2.2.6.2, with the added caveat that the time–course of withdrawal is unpredictable.

1. Thus, it is unwise to decrease the level of administered CNS depressant at a rate faster than 10% a day, taking special care to reinstitute the last day's dose if there are increasing signs of serious withdrawal.
2. It is usually possible to carry out a smooth withdrawal from multiple CNS depressants by administering only one of the depressant drugs to the point where the symptoms are markedly decreased on Day 1.

13.2.6.2.2. Depressants–Stimulants

In the case of multiple addiction to depressants and stimulants, it is the depressant withdrawal syndrome that produces the greatest amount of discomfort and is the most life-threatening (Section 2.2.6). Thus, although there may be an intensification of some of the symptoms, it is best to proceed with the mode of treatment for depressant withdrawal.

13.2.6.2.3. Depressants–Opiates

1. In the case of addiction to CNS depressants and to opiates, it is advisable to administer both an opiate and a CNS depressant, as outlined in Sections 2.2.6.2 and 6.2.6.2, until the withdrawal symptoms have been abolished or greatly decreased.
2. Most authors then recommend stabilization with the opiate (Section 6.2.6.2), while the depressant is withdrawn at 10% a day (Section 2.2.6.2).
3. After the depressant withdrawal is completed, opiate withdrawal can then proceed (Section 6.2.6.2).[2,43,44]

13.2.7. Medical Problems

The concomitant administration of two substances over an extended period of time very likely does increase the risk of the development of medical consequences. However, the specific problems depend on the specific drugs involved, as well as the individual's age, preexisting medical disorders, and concomitant nutritional status and experience of stress. When treating a patient who is abusing multiple drugs, the clinician should review the sections on medical problems in each of the relevant chapters.

One special problem is seen in those individuals whose drug abuse has occurred secondary to attempts at controlling pain, usually by abusing depressants or analgesics on a doctor's prescription. Pain syndromes that are unresponsive to the usual measures (frequently back pain and chronic headache) are very difficult to treat and not at all well understood. It is important to gather a history of any addiction and of concomitant medical complaints in evaluating any drug abuser. Following withdrawal, these identified individuals can be included as part of a polydrug or individual drug program, but they will probably also require additional care, such as that offered in specialized pain clinics.[45,46]

REFERENCES

1. Kaufman, E. The abuse of multi drugs. 1. Definition, classification, and extent of problem. *American Journal of Drug and Alcohol Abuse 3:*272–292, 1976.
2. Cohen, S. Polydrug abuse. *Drug Abuse and Alcoholism Newsletter 5:*1–5, 1976. San Diego: Vista Hill Foundation.
3. National Clearinghouse for Drug Abuse Information. *Polydrug Use: An Annotated Bibliography.* Rockville, Maryland: National Institute on Drug Abuse, 1975.
4. Goodwin, D. W., & Guze, S. B. (Eds.). *Psychiatric Diagnosis* (4th ed.). New York: Oxford University Press, 1988.
5. Schuckit, M. A. Alcoholism and sociopathy—Diagnostic confusion. *Quarterly Journal of Studies on Alcohol 34:*157–164, 1973.
6. Schuckit, M. A. Alcohol and drug interactions with antianxiety medications. *American Journal of Medicine 82:*27–32, 1987.
7. Hawkins, M. R., Kruzich, D. J., & Smith, J. D. Prevalence of polydrug use among alcoholic soldiers. *American Journal of Drug and Alcohol Abuse 11:*27–35, 1985.
8. Ogborne, A. C., & Kapur, B. M. Drug use among a sample of males admitted to an alcohol detoxification center. *Alcoholism: Clinical and Experimental Research 11:*183–185, 1987.

9. Vaillant, G. Natural history of male alcoholism. V. Is alcoholism the cart or the horse? Paper presented at the American Psychiatric Association Annual Meeting, Toronto, Ontario, May 1982.
10. Kraus, J. Juvenile drug abuse and delinquency: Some differential associations. *British Journal of Psychiatry 139:*422–430, 1981.
11. Hamburg, B. A., Kraemer, H. C., & Jahnke, W. A hierarchy of drug use in adolescence: Behavioral and attitudinal. *American Journal of Psychiatry 132:*1155–1164, 1975.
12. Kandel, D. Antecedents of adolescent initiation into stages of drug use. In D. Kandel (Ed.), *Longitudinal Research on Drug Use.* Washington, D.C.: Hemisphere Publishing, 1978, pp. 73–100.
13. Gould, L. C., & Kleber, H. D. Changing patterns of multiple drug use among applicants to a multimodality drug treatment program. *Archives of General Psychiatry 31:*408–413, 1974.
14. Lane, E. A., Guthrie, S., & Linnoila, M. Effects of ethanol on drug and metabolite pharmacokinetics. *Clinical Pharmacokinetics 10:*228–247, 1985.
15. Guthrie, S. K., & Lane, E. A. Reinterpretation of the pharmacokinetic mechanism of oral benzodiazepine ethanol interaction. *Alcoholism: Clinical and Experimental Research 10:*686–690, 1986.
16. Chan, A. W., Langan, M. C., Leong, F. W., et al. Substitution of chlordiazepoxide for ethanol in alcohol-dependent mice. *Alcohol 3:*309–316, 1986.
17. Suzdak, P. D., Glowa, J. R., & Crawley, J. N. Is ethanol antagonist Ro15-4513 selective for ethanol? *Science 239:*648–650, 1988.
18. Freund, G., & Ballniger, W. E.: Decrease of benzodiazepine receptors in frontal cortex of alcoholics with normal brains at autopsy. *Alcoholism: Clinical and Experimental Research 10:*110, 1986.
19. Suzdak, P. D., Glowa, J. R., & Crawley, J. N. A selective imidazobenzodiazepine antagonist of ethanol in the rat. *Science 234:*1243–1248, 1986.
20. Britton, K. T., & Koob, G. F. Ethanol antagonist Ro15-4513 is not selective for ethanol. *Alcoholism: Clinical and Experimental Research 11:*225, 1987.
21. Nutt, D. J., & Lister, R. Studies of the putative alcohol antagonist Ro15-4513. *Alcoholism: Clinical and Experimental Research 11:*218, 1987.
22. Cohen, S. Psychotropic drug interactions. *Drug Abuse and Alcoholism Newsletter 6(6).* San Diego: Vista Hill Foundation, 1977.
23. Siegel, S. Alcohol and opiate dependence: Re-evaluation of the Victorian perspective. In S. Siegel (Ed.), *Research Advances in Alcohol and Drug Problems,* Vol. 9, 1986, pp. 279–314.
24. Fidecka, S., Tamborska, E., Malec, D. & Langwinski, R. The development of cross tolerance between ethanol and morphine. *Polish Journal of Pharmacology and Pharmacy 38:*277–284, 1986.
25. Nyers, R. D., Borg, S., & Mossberg, R. Antagonism by naltrexone of voluntary alcohol selection in the chronically drinking macaque monkey. *Alcohol 3:*383–388, 1986.
26. Cheong Ton, J. M., & Amit, Z. Stereospecific interaction between alcohol and opiates mediated by the Mu high-affinity binding receptor. *Alcohol 2:*333–337, 1985.
27. Trachtenberg, M. C., & Blum, K. Alcohol and opioid peptides: Neuropharmacological rationale for physical craving of alcohol. *American Journal of Drug and Alcohol Abuse 13:*365–372, 1987.
28. Kosten, T. R., Rounsaville, B. J., & Kleber, H. D. Parental alcoholism in opioid addicts. *Journal of Nervous and Mental Disease 173:*461–468, 1985.
29. Joseph, H., & Appel, P. Alcohol and methadone treatment: Consequences for the patient and program. *American Journal of Drug and Alcohol Abuse 11:*37–53, 1985.
30. Kosten, T. R., Gawin, F. H., Rounsaville, B. J., & Kleber, H. D. Cocaine abuse among opioid addicts: Demographic and diagnostic factors in treatment. *American Journal of Drug and Alcohol Abuse 12:*1–16, 1986.
31. Siemens, A. J., Kalant, H., & Khanna, J. M. Effects of cannabis on pentobarbital induced sleeping time and pentobarbital metabolism in the rat. *Biochemical Pharmacology 23:*477–489, 1974.

32. Janowsky, D. S., Meacham, M. P., Blane, J. D., *et al.* Simulated flying performance after marihuana intoxication. *Aviation, Space, and Environmental Medicine 47:*124–128, 1976.
33. Whitehead, P. C., & Ferrence, R. G. Alcohol and other drugs related to young drivers' traffic accident involvement. *Journal of Safety Research 8:*65–72, 1976.
34. Schuckit, M. A., & Irwin, M. The clinical characteristics of 171 primary alcoholics. Paper presented at the American College of Neuropsychopharmacology Annual Meeting, San Juan, Puerto Rico, December 5, 1987.
35. Simpson, D. D., & Sells, S. B. Patterns of multiple drug abuse: 1969–1971. *International Journal of the Addictions 9:*301–314, 1974.
36. Blackford, L. Student drug use surveys—San Mateo County, California, 1968–1975. San Mateo, California: Department of Public Health and Welfare, June 6, 1975.
37. Cook, R. F., Hostetter, R. S., & Ramsay, D. A. Patterns of illicit drug use in the Army. *American Journal of Psychiatry 132:*1013–1017, 1975.
38. Fischer, D. E., Halikas, J. A., Baker, J. W., *et al.* Frequency and patterns of drug abuse in psychiatric patients. *Diseases of the Nervous System 36:*550–553, 1975.
39. Green, J., & Jaffe, J. H. Alcohol and opiate dependence: A review. *Journal of Studies on Alcohol 38:*1274–1293, 1977.
40. Schuckit, M. A., & Morrissey, E. R. Propoxyphene and phencyclidine (PCP) use in adolescents. *Journal of Clinical Psychiatry 39:*7–13, 1978.
41. Callan, J. P., & Patterson, C. P. Patterns of drug abuse among military inductees. *American Journal of Psychiatry 130:*260–264, 1973.
42. Prichep, L. S., Cohen, M., Kaplan, J., *et al.* Psychiatric evaluation services to court referred drug users. *American Journal of Drug and Alcohol Abuse 2:*197–213, 1975.
43. Sapira, J. D., & Cherubin, C. E. *Drug Abuse: A Guide for the Clinician. Excerpta Medica, Amsterdam.* New York: American Elsevier, 1975.
44. Smith, D. E., & Wesson, D. R. Phenobarbital technique for treatment of barbiturate dependence. *Archives of General Psychiatry 24:*56–60, 1971.
45. Reuler, J. B., Girard, D. E., & Nardone, D. A. The chronic pain syndrome: Misconceptions and management. *Annals of Internal Medicine 93:*588–596, 1980.
46. Sternbach, R. A. *Pain: Psychophysiologic Analysis.* New York: Academic Press, 1968.

Emergency Problems: A Quick Overview

14.1. INTRODUCTION

14.1.1. Comments

If you have come to this section of the book after having read (or at least skimmed) Chapters 1 through 13, you should be ready to use this chapter as a review. If you are here because you feel that an overview of emergency problems is the most important task for you, I bid you welcome and hope that you will have a chance to go back and review the other topics in greater depth. This single chapter *cannot* review each topic in depth, and it is hoped, for instance, that you will *not* approach the toxic reaction or overdose patient without also looking at the material in the relevant subsections of the chapters on central nervous system (CNS) depressants, opiates, and so on (e.g., see Sections 2.2.3 and 6.2.3).

The goal of this chapter is to teach some general guidelines for drug emergencies. The material is presented from a perspective different from that in the rest of the text. I have approached the problem from the standpoint of *patient symptoms,* assuming a situation in which you do not know the specific drug involved. The chapter is divided into topic areas similar to those in other chapters, with emergent situations ranging from panic to medical problems.

14.1.2. Some General Rules

1. You would, of course, by common sense, first address life-threatening problems, then gather a more substantial history and carry out other patient-care procedures, and, finally, plan disposition and future treatment.[1,2] The first priority is to support respirations, maintain adequate blood pressure, aggressively treat convulsions, and establish an intravenous (IV) line.[3]

2. Avoid giving additional medications whenever possible.[1] The administration of additional drugs to an individual with a drug-related problem can result in unpredictable drug–drug interactions, which can be made all the worse by the high

level of arousal usually demonstrated by the patient. However, when there is good reason for administering medications, it is important that they be given in doses adequate to produce clinical effects.

3. It is always important to establish a complete history by gathering information from the patient *and from an additional resource person,* usually the spouse. The belongings of a patient who is stuporous or out of contact with reality might contain the names of individuals able to provide accurate information.

4. Your general *attitude* and demeanor can be important, especially if you are dealing with a panicked, confused, or psychotic patient. While carrying out your evaluations, it is important that you first clearly identify yourself, and consistently behave in a self-assured and (as much as possible) calm manner.[3] Reassurance can be provided through both verbal and nonverbal support, the latter including frequent eye contact.

5. Finally, it is important to review briefly how to determine the relevant drug-problem category (see Section 1.6):

First: Any patient who has taken enough of a drug to show a serious compromise in vital signs should be regarded as having a toxic reaction. In the midst of this, he may demonstrate hallucinations or delusions or may show high levels of confusion, but all of these can be expected to return to normal once the toxic reaction has been adequately treated.

Second: Patients with basically stable vital signs but showing symptoms of withdrawal are labeled as drug withdrawal *even if* they show confusion and/or signs of a psychosis, as these can occur as part of withdrawal.

Third: Any patient with basically stable vital signs and no obvious withdrawal, but with clinically significant levels of confusion, is regarded as having an organic brain syndrome (OBS). In the midst of this, he may demonstrate hallucinations or delusions, but these will be expected to return to normal once the OBS is adequately treated.

Fourth: An individual with stable vital signs and no clinically significant confusion or withdrawal, but showing hallucinations and/or delusions without insight, would be regarded as having a psychosis.

Thus, as is true in medicine in general, it is not only the specific signs or symptoms that are used to arrive at a diagnosis, but also the constellation or grouping of symptoms along with their time course.[4]

14.1.3. An Overview of Relevant Laboratory Tests

There is no perfect laboratory panel that should be covered for every drug-emergency patient. You are best advised to follow the general rule of allowing your medical knowledge and common sense to dictate which of the specific tests must be ordered—always making an effort to avoid unnecessary costs, on one hand, but trying to be certain that the patient's condition is adequately evaluated, on the other.

Table 1.5 lists a variety of blood chemistries and blood counts that are important in many drug-related situations. In addition, you should consider a urinalysis

Table 14.1
A Brief List of Relevant Blood Toxicologies

Drug	Toxic blood level	Units
Bromide	10–20	mq/liter
Chlordiazepoxide (Librium)	0.6–2.0	mg/dl
Diazepam (Valium)	0.5	mg/dl
Ethchlorvynol (Placidyl)	1.5–10.0	mg/dl
Glutethimide (Doriden)	1.0–3.0	mg/dl
Meperidine (Demerol)	100–500	μg/dl
Meprobromate (Miltown, Equanil)	5.0–10.0	mg/dl
Morphine	0.1–0.5	mg/dl
Oxazepam (Serax)	0.5–1.5	mg/dl
Phenobarbital	3–10	mg/dl

(you will be collecting urine for a toxicological screen anyway) to look for evidence of kidney damage or infections; a screening for the hepatitis-related Australia antigen for patients who have misused drugs IV[5]; in similar patients, the need to rule out acquired immune deficiency syndrome (AIDS)[6]; a chest x ray for all patients who have not received one in the last 6 months; a Pap smear for women who have not had one in the last 6 months; a baseline electrocardiogram (EKG) for patients over the age of 35 and/or those who have any evidence of heart disease; a serology evaluation for syphilis; and a possible culture for gonorrhea for patients who have a history of sexual promiscuity or prostitution. A word of warning is needed regarding Table 1.5, however, because the normal values for most blood tests differ among laboratories, and the reader is encouraged to check with his own facility.[7]

A toxicological screen on blood and/or urine should be considered in all relevant patients. Some representative toxic levels are shown in Table 14.1. Take care in interpreting negative results, however, as signs of withdrawal, OBS, psychosis, and so on may persist for up to 2 weeks or longer after blood and urine levels return to zero by most techniques.

14.1.4. An Introduction to Specific Emergency Problems[8]

Table 14.2 gives some helpful symptoms and signs that can be used in making an educated guess as to which drug was taken and the future course of problems. I must emphasize that this table allows you to establish only a *guesstimate*. It has not been tested in controlled investigations and therefore can be used as nothing more than a guideline.

For example, if an individual comes to you with decreased respiration and pinpoint pupils, one of the first things to be considered is a toxic opiate overdose. A second example is an individual who comes with an elevated temperature; warm, dry skin; and fixed, dilated pupils: This is probably a toxic reaction involving an atropinelike anticholinergic drug.

Table 14.2
A Rough Guide to Symptoms and Signs in Drug Reactions

Symptom or sign	Reaction type	Possible drugs
Vital signs		
Blood pressure		
Increase	Toxic	Stimulants or lysergic acid diethylamide (LSD)
	Withdrawal	Depressants
Pulse		
Increase	Toxic	Stimulants
	Withdrawal	Depressants
Body temperature		
Irregular	Toxic	Solvents
Increase	Toxic	Atropine-type, stimulants, or LSD
Decrease	Withdrawal	Opiates or depressants
Respirations		
Decrease	Toxic	Opiates or depressants
Head		
Eyes		
Pupils		
Pinpoint	Toxic	Opiates
Dilated		
Reactive	Toxic	Hallucinogens, withdrawal, opiates
Sluggish	Toxic	Glutethimide or stimulants
Unreactive	Toxic	Atropine-type
Sclera		
Injected (bloodshot)	Toxic	Marijuana or solvents
Nystagmus	Toxic	Depressants
Tearing	Withdrawal	Opiates
Nose		
Runny (rhinorrhea)	Withdrawal	Opiates
Dry	Toxic	Atropine-type
Ulcers in membrane or septum	Chronic use	Cocaine
Skin		
Warm		
Dry	Toxic	Atropine-type
Moist	Toxic	Stimulants
Needle marks	Chronic use	Opiates, stimulants, or depressants
Gooseflesh	Toxic	LSD
	Withdrawal	Opiates
Rash over mouth or nose	Toxic	Solvents
Speech		
Slow		
Not slurred	Toxic	Opiates
Slurred	Toxic	Depressants
Rapid	Toxic	Stimulants
Hands		
Fine tremor	Toxic	Stimulants or hallucinogens
	Withdrawal	Opiates

Table 14.2
(Continued)

Symptom or sign	Reaction type	Possible drugs
Coarse tremor	Withdrawal	Depressants
Neurological		
Reflexes		
Increased	Toxic	Stimulants
Decreased	Toxic	Depressants
Convulsions	Toxic	Stimulants, codeine, propxyphene, methaqualone
Lungs		
Pulmonary edema	Toxic	Opiates or depressants

I will now proceed with a discussion of each of the major emergency-room situations, first giving a definition, then making some generalizations about the drug state and reviewing some of the drugs that might be involved. The reader is encouraged to return to the chapters that deal with specific drugs for more in-depth discussions.

14.2. PANIC REACTIONS (See Section 1.6.1)

14.2.1. Clinical Picture

The panic reaction is identified by a patient's presenting with a high level of anxiety, usually expressing fears that he is losing control, is going crazy, is having a heart attack, or has done damage to his body. He may give a drug history and is able to maintain contact with reality in a highly structured environment. The history usually demonstrates that the patient is a naive user and that other individuals have taken the same amount of drug with no serious effects. This state is usually a benign, self-limited, emotional overreaction to the usual drug effects.[9]

14.2.2. Differential Diagnosis

Panic reactions most frequently occur with drugs that stimulate the user and change the level of consciousness: *hallucinogens, cannabis,* or *stimulants.* It is important to rule out physical disease (e.g., a genuine heart attack or a hyperthyroid state) and to consider possible psychiatric pictures, such as panic disorder, obsessive–compulsive disease, or phobic disorders.[4,10]

14.2.3. Treatment

The cornerstone of treatment is reassurance, education about the drug effects, and time.

1. Carry out a quick physical examination.
2. Gather a history of recent events.
3. Give reassurance, talk to the patient as frequently as possible, and help him to orient to time, place, and person. It is best to place the patient in a quiet room, with friends or relatives available to help "talk him down."
4. For individuals who show lability in vital signs, bed rest is important, with carefully monitored blood pressure and pulse.
5. Avoid additional medication, but where needed, I would suggest a benzodiazepine [e.g., diazepam (Valium) at doses of 15–30 mg] given either orally or, if absolutely necessary, intramuscularly (IM). These doses can be repeated every 1–2 hours as needed, the dose being kept as low as possible.
6. In the midst of a panic, some patients may not only be frightened but also demonstrate violence [e.g., with PCP (see Chapter 9)]. There are a number of general guidelines that you can follow in approaching a patient who has recently demonstrated either verbal or physical violence or who is threatening to do so[3]:
   a. Do not approach a violent patient alone; it is much better to have several staff personnel and all carefully approach the patient at one time in as nonthreatening a manner as possible.
   b. Avoid any aggressive actions (e.g., sudden moves toward the patient) unless there is an immediate possibility of serious injury to the patient or to those around him. When approaching the individual, be sure that he knows who you are, reassure him that you will not harm him, and inform him of each movement you are about to make and its purpose.
   c. When making physical contact to control the patient, try to limit all movements to those that do not represent possible direct physical harm to him. Thus, you should use defensive manipulations such as holding the patient's arms and legs and rolling him in a blanket if needed.
   d. Do *not* approach an armed and aggressive patient. Under these circumstances, it is usually best to call hospital security or the police. More thorough discussions of approaching and working with violent patients are offered elsewhere.[3,11]

14.3. FLASHBACKS (see Section 1.6.2)

14.3.1. Clinical Picture

This drug-induced state involves a recurrence of feelings of intoxication some time after the initial drug effects have worn off. This is a benign, self-limited condition that rarely, if ever, represents a serious physical threat.

14.3.2. Differential Diagnosis

Flashbacks are seen primarily with *marijuana* and the *hallucinogens*. However, it is also important to take time to rule out the possibility of underlying psychiatric disorders, especially schizophrenia or affective disorder,[4] or an OBS.

14.3.3. Treatment

The approach to this condition is straightforward reassurance and education.[9] If the person does not respond to reassurance, he may be administered an antianxiety drug such as diazepam (Valium) in doses of 10–20 mg orally, repeated as needed.[9]

14.4. TOXIC REACTIONS (see Section 1.6.3)

14.4.1. Clinical Picture

In this instance, the individual has ingested more than the usual amount of a substance and presents with an overdose. To allow for generalizations, I have in this text distinguished somewhat arbitrarily among a *toxic overdose,* with unstable vital signs predominating; a *psychosis,* with hallucinations and delusions in an alert individual; and an *organic brain syndrome,* in which the major symptomatology is confusion and disorientation. However, the high level of overlap among these syndromes must be noted.

14.4.2. Differential Diagnosis

The serious overdoses are most likely to be seen with drugs that depress the CNS, such as *opiates,* and *depressants.* Because the treatments for the toxic reactions of these drugs differ slightly, it is important to identify the drug involved.

There are no major psychiatric syndromes that mimic the overdose, with the possible exception of a catatonialike stupor seen with serious depression[4], but medical disorders that can cause coma (e.g., hypoglycemia or severe electrolyte abnormalities) must be considered.

14.4.3. Treatment

The definitive treatment of shocklike states is complex and requires precise knowledge that is beyond the scope of this text. Briefly, it is necessary to address acute life supports and then to provide general patient care, allowing the body to metabolize the drug ingested.

14.4.3.1. Acute Life-Saving Measures (see references 11–18)

1. Establish the vital signs.
2. Assure adequate ventilation:
   a. Straighten the head.
   b. Remove any obstructions from the throat.
   c. Carry out artificial respiration, if necessary.
   d. Do tracheal intubation, if necessary (use an inflatable cuff tube, if at all possible, to allow for safer gastric lavage).
   e. Establish the patient on a respirator, if necessary. Use 10–12 respira-

tions per minute, avoiding oxygen, as this may decrease spontaneous respirations.

   f. Maintain an adequate circulatory state. Very briefly:

      i. If the heart is stopped, use external chest massage and administer intracardiac adrenaline.

      ii. If there is evidence of cardiac fibrillation, use a defibrillator.

      iii. If inadequate circulation is evident, use an intravenous drip of 50 ml of sodium bicarbonate (3.75 g) to treat the acidic state.

3. Carry out a quick physical examination to rule out serious bleeding, life-threatening trauma, and so on.

4. Start an IV:

   a. Use a large-gauge needle.

   b. Use restraints, if necessary, to make sure that the needle will stay in place.

   c. Use a slow IV drip until the need for IV fluids has been established.

5. Aggressively control convulsions, protecting the patient from aspiration by placing him on his side with (if possible) his head slightly extended over the side of the table. Maintain ventilation, be certain that an adequate IV line has been started, and loosen clothes. In most instances, a single seizure or a limited number of seizures will occur, but repeated convulsions (i.e., status epilepticus) require aggressive treatment with IV diazepam (e.g., slow infusion of 10 mg, which can be repeated in 20 minutes if necessary) or (less preferred) with phenytoin, 600–1000 mg IV, given in 100-mg boluses, or even with general anesthesia.[3] The proper control of convulsions is not covered in detail here, and the reader is referred to general medical texts and emergency manuals.[14]

6. Draw blood for chemical analysis:

   a. 10 cc, at a minimum, is needed for a toxicological screen.

   b. 30–40 cc is necessary for the usual blood count, electrolytes, blood sugar, and blood urea nitrogen (BUN).

7. If there is any chance that the individual is hypoglycemic, administer 50 cc of 50% glucose IV.

8. An EKG or rhythm strip is especially important because of the cardiac irregularities that may be seen with nonbarbiturate hypnotics.[14]

9. For recent ingestions, induce vomiting or carry out gastric lavage[3,14]:

   a. Do not do this until the heart rate is stable, to avoid inducing a clinically significant vagal response and subsequent cardiovascular problems.

   b. For the awake and cooperative patient, emesis can be induced with syrup of ipecac, which is given as 10–30 mg orally and repeated once in 15–30 minutes if vomiting does not occur. Some patients require one glass of fluids (e.g., water or saline) to distend their stomachs slightly to allow them to vomit. Take care not to give ipecac and activated charcoal at the same time, as the latter will block the effects of ipecac.

c. If the patient is not awake and cooperative or if emesis does not work, carry out gastric lavage. For sleepy or comatose patients, lavage only after tracheal intubation. Use an inflatable cuff to prevent aspiration.

d. Gastric lavage should be carried out only on individuals who have taken drugs orally within the last 4–6 or, at most, 12 hours. The longer period of time is especially important with PCP, as this drug may be recycled and excreted in the stomach for more than 6 hours after the actual ingestion. Lavage should *not* be carried out after individuals have also ingested corrosives, kerosene, strychnine, or mineral oil.

e. For adults, a nasogastric tube is usually used, and the patient is placed on his or her left side with the head slightly over the edge of the table.

f. After evacuating the stomach, administer an isotonic saline lavage until the returned fluid looks clear. It is preferable to use small amounts of fluid so as to not distend the stomach and increase the passage of the drug into the upper intestine. Lavage may be repeated 10–12 times, and it is best to save the washings for drug analyses.

g. Consider administering activated charcoal or castor oil (60 ml) to help stop absorption. The castor oil is especially important for lipid-soluble substances such as glutethimide (Doriden).

10. Collect urine if possible—which may require catheterizing the bladder. Send 50 ml of the urine for a toxicological screen.[8]

11. If the patient's blood pressure has not responded, you may use plasma expanders or pressors as for any shocklike state, taking care to titrate the needed dose and being aware of any potentially life-threatening drug interactions.

12. If there is a chance that the overdose includes an opiate, administer a test dose of naloxone (Narcan)[14] in doses of 0.4–0.8 mg (1–2 ml) IM or IV, as discussed in Section 6.2.3.2. However, it is important to beware of precipitating a severe opiate withdrawal syndrome—which would usually be treated with reassurance and readministration of a mild analgesic, such as propoxyphene (Darvon), or with methadone (Section 6.2.6.2).

13. If the overdose appears to involve an atropinelike (anticholinergic) drug as indicated by a rapid heart rate, dry skin and mouth, a rash, and so on, consider giving physostigmine, 1–4 mg, by slow IV injection.

14.4.3.2. Subacute Treatment

1. Establish the vital signs every 15 minutes for at least the first 4 hours; then monitor carefully (perhaps every 2–4 hours) over the next 24–48 hours, even if the patient's condition is improved. Many of the substances [e.g., the fat-soluble hypnotics like glutethimide (Doriden) or ethchlorvynol

(Placidyl)] clear from the plasma temporarily and are then rereleased from fat stores, causing severe reintoxication after the patient has apparently improved. Also, for opiate overdoses, the antagonists are active for only a relatively short period after administration.

2. Carry out a thorough physical examination, with special emphasis on the status of and changes in neurological signs.[12]

3. Gather an intensive history from the patient and a resource person, such as the spouse.

4. Establish a flow sheet to monitor vital signs, medications, fluid intake, fluid output, and so on.

5. Establish a baseline weight that can be used as a guide to fluid balance.

6. Dialysis or diuresis is rarely needed:

   a. If you choose to carry out diuresis, you may use furosemide (Lasix) in doses of 40–100 mg, administered regularly to maintain a urinary output of approximately 250 ml/hour. Of course, it is very important to replace electrolytes and fluids.

   b. Diuresis can also be carried out through the careful administration of enough IV fluids to maintain a urinary output in excess of 200 ml/hour using half-normal saline with potassium supplementation (Section 2.2.3.2).

   c. Dialysis is effective for almost all nonbarbiturate sedatives. If available, hemodialysis is preferable to peritoneal dialysis, as the former tends to be more efficient and has less chance of decreasing respiration.

   The indications for dialysis include severe intoxication with markedly abnormal vital signs, report of the probable ingestion of a highly lethal dose of the drug, blood levels of the drug in the lethal dose range, impaired excretion or metabolism of the drugs due to liver or kidney damage, progressive clinical deterioration, prolonged coma, and underlying lung disease. Once again, it is important to emphasize that most overdose patients will recover completely without dialysis or diuresis.

7. Avoid administering any medications unless absolutely necessary.

8. If the patient is comatose, take the steps necessary for adequate care, including careful management of electrolytes and fluids, eye care, frequent turning of the patient, and careful tracheal toilet.

14.5. PSYCHOSIS (see Section 1.6.4)

14.5.1. Clinical Picture

Psychosis is a loss of contact with reality, which occurs, as discussed in this text, in the midst of a clear sensorium. The patient usually presents with hallucinations (most frequently auditory) and/or delusions (usually persecutory). Although clinically very dramatic, this is usually a self-limited problem, running its course within a matter of days to a week for most drugs (an exception is STP).

14.5.2. Differential Diagnosis

Any psychiatric disorder capable of producing a psychotic picture, especially schizophrenia, mania, an OBS, or depression, must be considered a part of the differential diagnosis.[4] The drugs most frequently involved in psychoses are *alcohol*, the other *CNS depressants*, and *stimulants*. When patients on PCP develop hallucinations and/or delusions, it is usually part of an OBS. Unless they are part of a toxic reaction, hallucinogen-induced visual hallucinations usually occur with insight.

14.5.3. Treatment

The major goal is to protect the patient from harming himself or others or from carrying out acts that would be embarrassing or would cause later difficulties. At the same time, it is important to review the problems adequately, so as to rule out other serious medical and psychiatric disorders. The patient who presents with a hallucinating/delusional state therefore usually requires hospitalization until the delusions clear.

14.6. ORGANIC BRAIN SYNDROME (see Section 1.6.5)

14.6.1. Clinical Picture

The organic state can be caused by high doses of any drug and consists of confusion and disorientation along with decreased general mental functioning. This reaction may be accompanied by illusions (misinterpretations of real stimuli, such as shadows or machinery sounds), hallucinations (usually visual or tactile), or delusions.

14.6.2. Differential Diagnosis

Any drug can cause an OBS, but in clinical practice this problem is most likely to be seen with *CNS depressants, atropine-type drugs, solvents, stimulants,* and *phencyclidine* (PCP).[19,20]

Whenever organicity is observed, it is important to consider the possibility of acute or chronic brain damage, trauma, vitamin deficiency, or serious medical problems that might disrupt electrolyte balance. If these medical disorders are overlooked, a life-threatening condition can ensue.

14.6.3. Treatment

The treatment consists of general life supports. Because this problem is either a minor toxic reaction or the early stage of a serious overdose, the treatment is identical to that outlined in Section 14.4.3 for the relevant toxic reaction. Although most organicities disappear within a matter of hours to days, some secondary OBS pictures caused by vitamin deficiencies or traumas can take many months to clear (see Section 4.2.5).

14.7. DRUG WITHDRAWAL STATES (see Section 1.6.6)

14.7.1. Clinical Picture

A sudden cessation or a rapid decrease in the intake of any of the drugs capable of producing physical dependence can result in the withdrawal state. This, simplistically, is manifested by anxiety, a heightened drive to obtain the drug, a flulike syndrome, and physiological symptoms that are usually in the direction opposite to those expected with intoxication.

Withdrawal from drugs is rarely life-threatening (with the possible exception of the CNS depressants) unless the patient is allowed to go through it in a seriously impaired physical state.

14.7.2. Differential Diagnosis

It is important to determine whether the withdrawal state is related to *stimulants, depressants,* or *opiate analgesics,* as the specific treatments differ greatly. It is also necessary to rule out the physiological disorders that can result in a flulike syndrome and to implement proper medical treatment.

14.7.3. Treatment

In addition to recognizing and treating all concomitant medical disorders, offer reassurance, rest, and good nutrition.

1. Carry out a good physical examination, taking special care to rule out infections, hepatitis, AIDS, subdural hematomas, heart failure, and electrolyte abnormalities. A patient entering withdrawal with impaired physical functioning has a markedly increased chance of dying during the withdrawal. Also, if any physiological abnormality is overlooked at the inception of withdrawal, it may be difficult, as the abstinence syndrome progresses, to tell whether abnormal vital signs are a response to the withdrawal or represent other physical pathology.

2. Specific treatment of the withdrawal depends on recognition that the symptoms have developed because the drug of addiction has been stopped *too quickly.* Therefore, the basic paradigm of treatment is to give enough of the drug of addiction (or one to which the individual has cross-tolerance) to greatly diminish the withdrawal symptoms on Day 1. This drug is then decreased by 10–20% of the initial day's dosage each day over the subsequent 5–10 days or more.

REFERENCES

1. Schuckit, M. A. Alcoholism and other psychiatric disorders. *Hospital and Community Psychiatry* *34:*1022–1027, 1983.

2. Chapel, J. L. Emergency room treatment of the drug-abusing patient. *American Journal of Psychiatry 130:*257–259, 1973.
3. Lewis, D. C., & Senay, E. C. *Treatment of Drug and Alcohol Abuse.* New York: State University of New York, 1981.
4. Goodwin, D. W., & Guze, S. B. *Psychiatric Diagnosis* (4th ed.). New York: Oxford University Press, 1988.
5. Lettau, L., & McCarthy, J. Outbreak of severe hepatitis due to delta and hepatitis B viruses in drug abusers. *New England Journal of Medicine 317:*1256–1262, 1987.
6. Piot, P., Plummer, F. A., Mhalu, F. S., *et al.* AIDS: An international perspective. *Science 239:*573–579, 1988.
7. Cohen, S., & Gallant, D. M. *Diagnosis of Drug and Alcohol Abuse.* New York: State University of New York, 1981.
8. Dimijian, G. G. Differential diagnosis of emergency drug reactions. In P. G. Bourne (Ed.), *A Treatment Manual for Acute Drug Abuse Emergencies.* Washington, D.C.: U.S. Government Printing Office, 1974, pp. 1–7.
9. Ungerleiter, J. T., & Frank, I. M. Management of acute panic reactions and flashbacks resulting from LSD ingestion. In P. G. Bourne (Ed.), *A Treatment Manual for Acute Drug Abuse Emergencies.* Washington, D.C.: U.S. Government Printing Office, 1974, pp. 73–76.
10. American Psychiatric Association. *Diagnostic Criteria from the DSM III-R.* Washington, D.C., American Psychiatric Press, 1987.
11. Tuason, V. B. The psychiatrist and the violent patient. *Diseases of the Nervous System 32:*764–768, 1971.
12. Setter, J. G. Emergency treatment of acute barbiturate intoxication. In P. G. Bourne (Ed.), *A Treatment Manual for Acute Drug Abuse Emergencies.* Washington, D.C.: U.S. Government Printing Office, 1974, pp. 49–53.
13. Gentile, J. *Compendium of Drug Therapy.* New York: McGraw-Hill, 1987.
14. Knoben, J., & Andersen, P. *Handbook of Clinical Drug Data* (5th ed.). Hamilton, Illinois: Drug Intelligence Publications, 1983, pp. 194–207.
15. Schuckit, M. A. Alcohol and alcoholism. In E. Braunwald, K. J. Isselbacher, R. G. Petersdorf, *et al.* (Eds.), *Harrison's Principles of Internal Medicine* (11th ed.). New York: McGraw-Hill, 1986, pp. 2106–2110.
16. Campbell, J., & Frisse, M. (Eds.), *Manual of Medical Therapeutics* (24th ed.). Boston: Little, Brown, 1983.
17. Kleber, H. D., & Gawin, F. H. Cocaine. In *American Psychiatric Association Annual Review,* Vol. 5, *Drug Abuse and Drug Dependence,* 1986, pp. 160–185.
18. Greene, M. H., & DuPont, R. L. The treatment of acute heroin toxicity. In P. G. Bourne (Ed.), *A Treatment Manual for Acute Drug Abuse Emergencies.* Washington, D.C.: U.S. Government Printing Office, 1974, pp. 11–16.
19. Westermeyer, J. The psychiatrist and solvent–inhalant abuse. *American Journal of Psychiatry 144:*903–907, 1987.
20. McCarron, M. Acute PCP intoxication. *Annals of Emergency Medicine 10:*6–9, 1981.

Rehabilitation

15.1. INTRODUCTION

This chapter serves as an introduction to the concept of rehabilitation for alcoholism and drug abuse rather than a definitive discussion of all aspects of care. Rehabilitation is a lengthy and complex topic and the subject of numerous and diverse texts on its own. Therefore, this chapter can be read for general knowledge, for guidelines to the appropriate referral of patients, as a framework for the critical evaluation of programs, or as a basis for developing your own treatment efforts. It is hoped that you will want to turn to some of the cited readings for more information.

I will first present a series of general rules that (with modifications) fit rehabilitation for all substance misusers. These rules are followed by a discussion of guidelines specifically tailored to particular drug approaches.

15.1.1. Some General Rules

The same basic guidelines apply to all types of rehabilitation efforts with substance misusers. Each is stated only briefly below, and most are discussed in more detail in the subsections on rehabiltation of abusers of alcohol (Section 15.2) and of other drugs (Sections 15.3 through 15.6).

15.1.1.1. Justify Your Actions

Coming to see us in the midst of crises, our patients may be prepared to "do almost anything" to make things improve. However, massive efforts are not always needed because substance abuse problems tend to fluctuate naturally in intensity, with the result that one can see improvement with time alone.[1] There is also a considerable rate of "spontaneous remission" with no intervention at all. The key questions to be addressed in judging any treatment are "Did the improvement occur *because of* the treatment?" and "Were the therapeutic efforts those with the greatest chance of success?"[2] The therapist must constantly justify his actions, both within a financial cost–benefit framework and in a manner that considers patient and staff time, physical or emotional dangers to the patient, and the trauma of separation from job and family.

15.1.1.2. Know the Natural Course of the Disorder

It is only through knowledge of the probable course of drug abuse that one can make adequate treatment plans.[3,4] The usual course of alcoholism is discussed in Chapter 3.

15.1.1.3. Guard against the Overzealous Acceptance of New Treatments

Most treatment efforts "make sense" in some theoretical framework, and most patients improve, and many get "well," no matter what treatment is used. This improvement can be the result of the fluctuating nature of the disorder and of spontaneous remission. Therefore, demand good, controlled investigations before accepting newer treatment approaches as valid.

15.1.1.4. Keep It Simple

In evaluating treatment efforts or adopting new therapies, a sensible approach is to stay with the least costly, potentially least harmful, and simplest maneuvers until there are good data to justify more complex procedures.

15.1.1.5. Apply Objective Diagnostic Criteria

It is not enough to accept a patient into a program because he or she appears at the door of a treatment center. To make use of knowledge of the natural course and to predict future problems, as well as to justify treatment efforts, standard diagnostic criteria must be applied to each patient.[5] An individual may, however, be labeled "ill but undiagnosed" and given a tentative set of working diagnoses, may be given a "probable" diagnosis and treated as if he or she had a definite disorder but with extra care taken to reevaluate the label at a future date, or may be given a definite diagnosis. Of course, all patients must be evaluated for major preexisting psychiatric disorders that require treatment or affect the prognosis (e.g., primary affective disorder or primary antisocial personality, as described in Section 3.1.2.3).

15.1.1.6. Establish Realistic Goals

In treating substance misuse, we rarely achieve "dramatic cures." I attempt to maximize the chances for recovery, to encourage abstinence at an earlier age than that at which it might have been achieved with no therapeutic intervention, to offer good medical care, to help the people close to the patient better understand what is going on, and to educate patients so that they can make their own decisions about treatment goals. Although health-care practitioners can and must offer their best efforts, the patient's motivation and level of "readiness" for recovery have a great impact on outcome.

Different therapeutic interventions have different goals. For instance, a detoxification facility established in a skid row area attempts to offer the best possible medical care and general supports. However, although the treatment personnel will try to encourage abstinence, the probable rate of 10% abstention for skid row alcoholics 12 months later does not justify abstinence as the primary goal of treatment. On the other hand, an alcoholic rehabilitation program established in industry or with married and working patients does focus on rehabilitation, as two thirds of the patients are likely to be dry a year later, and most abstinent alcoholics will be functioning as well as their nonalcoholic peers.[2,5,6]

15.1.1.7. Know the Goals of Your Patients

In establishing patient goals, it is important to understand the patient's reasons for entering treatment: Was it to detox only? To meet a crisis? Or actually to aim at long-term abstinence?

15.1.1.8. Make a Long-Term Commitment

Because there is no "magic cure" in these areas, recovery is usually a long-term process that requires some counseling and therapeutic relationship for at least 6 months to a year.

15.1.1.9. Use All Available Resources

The patient's substance-abuse problem does not occur in a vacuum. Part of the therapeutic effort should be directed at encouraging the family and, if appropriate, the employer to increase their level of understanding of the problem; to be available to help you whenever necessary; to make realistic plans for themselves as they relate to the patient; and, in specific instances, to function as "ancillary therapists," helping to carry out your treatment efforts in the home or job setting.

15.1.1.10. When Appropriate, Notify All Involved Physicians and Pharmacists

When dealing with a substance misuser who is obtaining drugs from physicians or pharmacists, it is my *bias* to make all possible efforts to cut off the patient's supply. This must be done with tact, understanding, and empathy for the ego of the prescribing physician or the dispensing pharmacist involved, and with the patient's permission, to avoid infringing on his legal rights.

15.1.1.11. Do Not Take Final Responsibility for the Patient's Actions

Although I do everything within my power to help, in the final analysis the decision to achieve and maintain abstinence is the patient's responsibility. If I do not follow this rule and the patient allows me to assume the responsibility or stops only to please me, he will soon find an excuse to get angry with me and return to alcohol and/or drugs.

15.1.2. A "General" Substance-Abuse Treatment Program

Given that there are patients in need and that money is available for care, there is usually a great deal of pressure to "do something now," but that is not necessarily the best course. With some forethought, it is possible to establish a rehabilitation program that will *probably* do the most good with the least harm. I emphasize the probable nature of my recommendations, as adequately controlled investigations have rarely been carried out to test even the most basic assumptions in rehabilitation. The *usual* rehabilitation program would[2]:

1. Attempt to accomplish three basic goals:
   a. Maximize physical and mental health, as patients will find it difficult to achieve abstinence if chronic medical problems have not been adequately treated.
   b. Enhance motivation toward abstinence through educating the patient and his family about the usual course of the disorder, employing appropriate medications to stop the patient from returning to substance misuse on the spur of the moment—e.g., opiate antagonists like noroxymorphone [naltrexone (Trexan)] for drug addicts—and using such behavior modification approaches as aversive conditioning.
   c. Help the patient to rebuild a life without the substance through vocational and avocational counseling, family counseling, helping him develop a substance-free peer group, showing him how to use free time, and so on.

2. Whenever possible, use outpatient rehabilitation rather than inpatient, as the former costs less and teaches the patient how to adjust to a life without the substance while he is functioning in the "real world."[7] Candidates for inpatient rehabilitation include patients who have not responded to outpatient counseling, those with medical or psychiatric problems serious enough to warrant hospitalization, people who live a great distance from the hospital, and patients whose lives are in such chaos that it is difficult or impossible to deal with them on an outpatient basis.

3. If inpatient rehabilitation is used, keep it as short as possible (usually 2–4 weeks), as longer inpatient care and other more intensive interventions have not been demonstrated to be more effective than short-term care for the average patient if the shorter course is followed by 6- to 12-month aftercare.[1,8−11]

4. Avoid using most medications in the treatment of substance abuse after withdrawal is completed. Possible exceptions are disulfiram for alcoholism (see Section 15.2.4.1.5) and methadone or naltrexone for opiate abuse.

5. Use group more than individual counseling, as the former costs less and is probably equally effective.

6. Use self-help groups such as Alcoholics Anonymous (AA) and Narcotics Anonymous, as they can be quite helpful and they cost nothing. They offer the patient a model that may be important in his achieving and maintaining recovery.

7. Recognize that there is no evidence that any one specialized and expensive form of psychotherapy (e.g., gestalt or transactional analysis) is any more

effective than general "day-to-day" life counseling for the substance misuser.[12]

8. Maintain continued contact with the patient for at least 6–12 months. All efforts should be used to decrease attrition; for example, letters and/or phone calls noting your desire to continue to help should be used to try and get patients to come back after they have missed even one aftercare or outpatient counseling session.[13]

9. Use nondegreed (paraprofessional) counseling staff supervised by people with more formal training in counseling, as there is little evidence that treatment can be successfully carried out only by individuals with advanced degrees.

15.2. A SPECIAL CASE: ALCOHOLISM (303.90 or 305.00 in DSM-III-R)

Because alcohol is the most common substance of abuse, I have used rehabilitation of the alcoholic as the prototype for my discussion of all other types of rehabilitation. The discussion was written from a viewpoint that assumes you have already reviewed Chapter 3 and recognize that the average alcoholic is a middle-class man or woman with a family, who comes into your office with general complaints and is unlikely to appear in a state of intoxication or withdrawal. The diagnosis is made by recognizing that one in five patients is alcoholic and through observing the pattern of medical problems (e.g., mild hypertension; cancers of the esophagus, stomach, or head and neck; or impotence) and the pattern of psychological problems (e.g., depression, anxiety, or insomnia) most closely associated with alcoholism. Diagnosis will be aided by carefully observing the pattern of laboratory results, especially mild elevations in the mean corpuscular volume (MCV), uric acid, triglycerides, and gamma-glutamyl transferase (GGT).[6,14,15] With these points in mind, this section reviews general treatment philosophy, confrontation, and rehabilitation.

To maximize the resources available and thereby reach the greatest possible number of patients, I emphasize outpatient rehabilitation. This costs 5–10 times less than inpatient care and may be just as effective.[7]

Even within inpatient approaches, the types of intervention offered should follow the general rules offered in Section 15.1.2, as the most direct and least complex schemes may be as good as or even superior to the more costly.[8,16] Figure 15.1 gives a *simplified* flow of patient problems. The diagnosis is established from the history given by the patient and his family as well as from the physical examination and the laboratory tests. Once you decide that the patient is an alcoholic, you face the decision about detoxification, remembering that if you miss potentially important withdrawal signs, the patient may lose faith because of the rigors of withdrawal and drop out of treatment. Detoxification can be carried out in either an inpatient or an outpatient mode, with inpatient care preferred for individuals who demonstrate any type of serious medical difficulties and those who have had withdrawal seizures in the past, as well as for elderly or debilitated patients (see Section

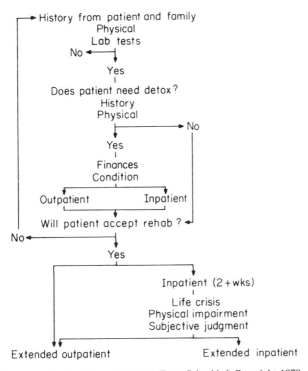

Is the problem alcohol related ?

Figure 15.1. Discussions in alcoholism treatment. From Schuckit.[6] Copyright 1979. Reprinted with permission of the McGraw-Hill Book Company.

4.2.6). Finally, rehabilitation in either an inpatient or an outpatient mode must be followed up with extended aftercare for 6–12 months for all patients.

15.2.1. Confronting the Alcoholic

The pattern of laboratory tests, physical findings, history of life problems, and information gathered from family members may help you to recognize the alcoholic. Once this is accomplished, the next step is to confront the patient in an attempt to help him or her recognize the problem and to act on that recognition.

The patient is responsible for his actions; your responsibility is to do all that is possible to raise his level of motivation. Whether your efforts "take" or not may be beyond your control.

A first step in confrontation is to utilize the patient's area of concern and to demonstrate to him how alcohol ties in. For instance, you can confront an individual coming in complaining of just "not feeling well" or of insomnia, impotence, high blood pressure, and so on by telling him that he has good reason for concern. You might then go on to share the relevant laboratory tests and physical findings, and to state: "There is one way I have of pulling all of these findings together. I believe you have reached a point in life where alcohol is causing more trouble than it's worth."

Next, you might teach him about the difficulties he can expect in the future unless he stops drinking. It may not be necessary at this point to use the term *alcoholism;* rather, in this initial confrontation, alcohol-related life problems can be the focus.

Next, discuss the probable future course of the alcohol-related problems and explore possible avenues for treatment. If he accepts help, determine if detoxification is required, and either begin counseling or refer him to an adequate alcohol-treatment facility (either outpatient or inpatient) or use AA.

Many patients will not respond to your initial confrontation with glee. Most individuals recognize somewhere deep inside that they are having alcohol-related problems, but they have been aggressively denying it both to themselves and to others. You might best tell the individual who refuses to respond to your first confrontation that you understand his disagreement but that you need to evaluate some things further and that he should return to you in several weeks (hoping that in the interim he will decrease his level of denial and be more likely to cooperate). If he refuses to come back or continues to deny problems at the next visit, I do all I can to "leave the door open," telling him that I am willing to continue to treat him for general problems and will do all I can to help him maximize his functioning despite his alcohol-related difficulties. I do warn him, however, that I will not be able to treat his medical and psychological problems adequately until he stops drinking. I thus hope that he will see me as a reasonable and caring physician and that he will return to me as his alcohol problems escalate. To try to maximize the chance that he will come back, I generally arrange with the patient for a "checkup" at least every 3 months.

Some patients respond to the initial (or 17th) confrontation by admitting that alcohol might be a problem and that they should "cut down." As is apparent in the natural history of alcoholism outlined in Section 3.4, cutting down is not usually a problem: It is staying cut down that becomes so difficult.[17] I do all I can to persuade the patient, not just to cut down, but to abstain. If he or she resists, I set up a meeting with the patient and the patient's significant other (e.g., usually the spouse). Here, I continue to try to discourage "controlled drinking," pointing out that it is not likely to work for any period of time, but I will yield if the patient insists. Next, I establish a regimen that, if followed, will stop the patient from ever becoming intoxicated. For instance, the patient's intake of alcohol should be limited to two drinks per 24 hours; a drink is defined as 12 oz of beer, 4 oz of nonfortified wine, or 1½ oz of 80-proof beverage. The 24 hours is also defined as a magical clock that begins ticking the moment the first sip of a beverage is taken. Almost inevitably, drinking escalates, problems occur, and I hope that the patient will come back to me for help.

It can be seen that confrontation is rarely a "one-shot" phenomenon. Rather, my attempts to increase motivation frequently involve multiple contacts with the patient (always keeping the responsibility for his behavior with him and not with me), outreach to the family, and various stages of general support, until the patient finally decides not to drink. Once the patient has agreed to abstinence, I then evaluate the need for detoxification (see Section 4.2.6) and enter him in either an outpatient or an inpatient rehabilitation program. Attempts to rehabilitate alcoholics consist of long-term contact aimed at enhancing motivation and increasing the ease of readjustment to life without alcohol.

15.2.2. Enhancing the Alcoholic's Motivation

These maneuvers are used during confrontation and on through rehabilitation in either the outpatient or the inpatient mode. The steps in this area include:

1. Educating the patient and the patient's family about the natural course of alcoholism and the problems they can expect in the future. The role of the family can be very important, and there is evidence that involvement of the spouse and other family members can favorably impact on the patient's success with continued abstinence.[16]

2. Emphasizing the patient's responsibility for his own actions. For example, the family should never protect the patient from the actions of his drinking by putting him to bed when he is drunk (they should let him fall asleep in front of the television set and go up to bed themselves) or rescuing him from jail (he should spend the evening in jail if necessary). In your interactions, any "Yes, but . . ." should be met with "You can make decisions about what you wish to do and the consequences you wish to accept."

3. Motivating the patient toward abstinence can be enhanced through the use of drugs that make it difficult for him to return to drinking on the spur of the moment (e.g., disulfiram, as described in Section 15.2.4.1.5). Motivation is also helped through establishing a conditioned reflex that causes the smell or taste of an alcoholic beverage to precipitate nausea or vomiting (as described in Section 15.2.4.1.4).

15.2.3. Helping the Alcoholic Readjust to a Life without Alcohol

By the time you have established a diagnosis, the average alcoholic has been having serious life problems for 10–20 years or more. Once he has entered rehabilitation, he has recognized (on some level) that alcohol is causing more troubles than it is worth and has agreed that he should stop drinking. However, because alcohol has been such a central part of his life for so long, there are many life situations that decrease his chance of continued abstinence. These must be carefully addressed.

Alcohol treatment programs utilize group counseling for the patient *and for the family,* vocational rehabilitation for the patient, sessions that center on the proper use of free time, and the establishment of a group of peers who are abstinent.[6,18] They also do everything else they can to enhance a smooth readjustment to life without alcohol. These programs may be begun in an inpatient setting, but the day to-day emphasis on group counseling should continue for many months in an outpatient or aftercare mode, so that the patient can receive support and counseling while he is actually attempting to function in his real-life situation.

15.2.4. Treatment Programs

15.2.4.1. Inpatient Treatment

If patients fulfill the criteria for inpatient rehabilitation outlined in Section 15.1.2, you will choose either to hospitalize them yourself or to refer them to an established program. Either way, there is no single best way to treat the alcoholic. Rather, because of the general helping nature of rehabilitation, most patients are offered programs with many components aimed at enhancing motivation and increasing the ase of readjustment to a life without drinking.

The selection of an inpatient or an outpatient treatment mode is based on the preferences of the patient or client and his family, financial considerations, and your prior experiences. Although there are no absolute indications for hospitalization after detoxification, patients with serious medical or emotional problems, or those who face severe crises, will probably function best in a structured environment. Also, many health-care deliverers feel that a short "time-out" from life stresses is an important part of treating the average alcoholic.

There are no data to support hospitalization of more than 2–4 weeks for the *average* patient.[9,10,18,19] Of course, common sense dictates that individuals with severe medical problems or persistent organic brain syndromes (OBSs) and those with very unstable life situations might require longer care. It is important, however, to recognize the potential dangers associated with inpatient care, which include risks of treatment-center-acquired infections, physical or emotional harm by patients or staff, loss of income or loss of job, embarrassment among peers, and family dissolution through separation at a time of crisis. In addition, the patient is treated in an artificial environment where the lessons learned may not readily generalize to everyday living.[7,18] Although inpatient care is a potentially important part of the rehabilitation spectrum, final decisions should depend on a calculated balance between the negative and positive aspects of any program.

15.2.4.1.1. The Facility

Good alcoholic detoxification and rehabilitation can be carried out in an established alcoholic program or on a general medical ward, the latter being especially important when you are dealing with a patient who has serious medical problems or who refuses care from anyone other than his primary physician. In such instances, the primary treatment is medical, but the counselor can work with the treatment staff to carry out adequate detoxification, if needed, and to enhance the patient's receptivity to rehabilitation.

In a similar manner, the relatively rare patients with primary affective disorder and secondary alcoholism (see Section 3.1.2.3.) are best treated by a psychiatrist. If these patients have active suicidal ideation, care should be given in a psychiatric facility, where suicide precautions can be observed. After detoxification, active pharmacological treatment of the affective disorder can be carried out. For patients presenting with depressions who have no history of mania, this usually entails the same treatment given any patient with unipolar affective disorders, usually tricyclic type antidepressants. Patients who have both mania and depression respond best to lithium. The reader is referred to some excellent reviews of the proper use of medications in primary affective disorders.[20,21] Some interesting data have recently appeared from projects now in progress investigating the possibility that lithium might help decrease the drive to drink.[22] The data to date, however, are not strong enough to justify the routine use of antidepressants or lithium for the average primary alcoholic.

The very rare secondary alcoholic with process schizophrenia[20] will require relatively high doses of antipsychotic medications such as chlorpromazine (Thorazine). The clinician must take special care not to misdiagnose alcoholic psychosis as schizophrenia (see Section 4.2.4).

For patients without serious medical or psychiatric problems, the treatment facility can be chosen with other considerations in mind. As it is the characteristics of the patient rather than of the treatment program that best predict outcome, a particular facility can be chosen considering the eventual financial cost, convenience to the patient, and other patient-care-related issues. Usually, a treatment program established in a freestanding facility located near a hospital can offer many of the same benefits as a hospital-based inpatient program and may be carried out at less cost (because of decreased overhead).

15.2.4.1.2. The Daily Schedule

Rehabilitation includes offering good education, counseling for the patient *and family,* and a long-term commitment to help with life adjustment. The usual inpatient schedule offers daily educational lectures and/or films, along with daily counseling and "rap" sessions and, in some centers, behavior modification therapy. Most programs favor a busy daily schedule.

15.2.4.1.3. Counseling or Psychotherapy

The patient usually meets daily with a counselor in a group setting to clarify life adjustment issues and to set the stage for outpatient follow-up visits. The family should be included in some sessions to help them deal with the life problems and to increase their level of understanding of alcoholism.

Therapy generally centers on the "here and now" of the patient's life, giving him a chance to discuss his adjustment to a life without alcohol and to the stresses of job, friends, and family. The focus is on the reactions of those around him and on how to handle the situations in which he is most likely to return to drinking.[23] In addition, lecture/discussion sessions can emphasize the dangers of alcohol and help the patient understand the course and effects of his disease. Along with other forms of therapy, patients should be encouraged to take part in AA.

Comparisons of group and individual psychotherapy for alcoholism reveal that group therapy is as effective as individual therapy.[23,24] Some authors may feel that group therapy has specific *advantages,* such as allowing the patient to share his feelings with a number of other people and teaching him social skills.[25] However, there is little hard evidence to back up this belief. The group session is an excellent place to begin an interdisciplinary approach,[26] with the psychiatrist or psychologist functioning primarily as supervisor of other therapists.

15.2.4.1.4. Behavioral Approaches

Some alcoholism treatment programs use a behavioral approach in dealing with their patients. This may include the offering of supports like biofeedback to help with anxiety and sleep problems, teaching the patient how to relax and handle stress. Another behaviorally oriented intervention, assertiveness training, is based on the premise that in the midst of their alcoholism (or perhaps because of some original problem existing before the alcoholism began), most patients do not learn how to express their desires and frustrations.[27] The training sessions usually involve education about recognizing situations in which resentment occurs and practicing a variety of methods for handling them.

Behavioral approaches can also form a core resource in the treatment of alcoholism. The behavioral modification procedures are usually added to the regular education and counseling as previously described.[18,24] Most often, this treatment involves attempts to "teach" the patient *not* to drink, by coupling the sight, scent, or taste of alcohol with an unpleasant event, such as vomiting or receiving a mild electric shock to the skin.[27,28] Chemical aversion treatments, aimed at inducing vomiting in the presence of alcohol, usually utilize such substances as emetine or apomorphine and are generally felt to be more effective than electrical aversion. These treatments are usually offered in hospitals that have special experience with them, and controlled studies seem to indicate that this approach is as effective as any other in dealing with alcoholism. Although it is possible that a specific type of patient responds preferentially to behavioral interventions, there are no data to help us choose the appropriate patients.

One modification of the electrical aversion treatment attempts to teach alcoholics how to drink in a moderate, controlled manner. This approach may have some potential, but at present, there are *no* data to justify its use in any clinical setting.[17,28,29] Any use outside the experimental laboratory must await clear demonstration that the assets of such a treatment outweigh the liabilities.

15.2.4.1.5. Medications

1. It is important to remember that any treatment (especially medications), when given as part of uncontrolled clinical evaluations, can appear effective; in reality, it may be no better than placebo.[2,30] Therefore, with the possible exception

of disulfiram (Antabuse) and vitamins, I tend to use *no* medications in treating the detoxified alcoholic.

2. Sleeping pills and antianxiety drugs, even though the patient may demand them, have *no place* in alcoholic *rehabilitation* (after withdrawal is completed). These drugs have dangers of addiction, adverse reactions with other depressant drugs such as alcohol, and, for some hypnotics, the potential for overdosage.

I use a special approach in dealing with complaints of insomnia and/or anxiety in alcoholics. First, I let them know that I understand the intensity of their discomfort and that I will try to help them. Second, I tell them that many of their problems are a physiological response to the long-term self-administration of a brain-depressing drug and that these physical changes will persist for up to 6 months or longer, although at decreasing intensity. Third, I emphasize that sleeping pills or antianxiety drugs might help them for a week or two but will then make their problems worse, and that we will inevitably have to face the day when their bodies must adjust to living without central nervous system (CNS)-depressing medications.

To help them deal with their sleep difficulties, I prescribe a regimen of going to bed at the same time every night (reading or watching television, if necessary) and awakening at the same time every morning, even if they have had only 15 minutes of good sleep. This regimen is coupled with a rule against caffeinated beverages after noon and against naps during the day. All these measures combine to force the patient's sleep cycle into a more normal pattern after several days. Problems with anxiety are handled with similar types of explanation and a search, carried out jointly with the patient, to find nonmedicinal avenues for release of tension. Possibilities range from church work, to developing a hobby, to learning to play a musical instrument, to yoga, to physical exercise, and so on.

3. Disulfiram (Antabuse) is a traditional drug for the treatment of the alcoholic, but this substance has dangers and cannot be given to patients with serious medical disorders, including diabetes that requires medications, cirrhosis, hypertension, severe heart disease, and so on.[31] These problems are likely to be exacerbated during an alcohol–disulfiram reaction. In addition, even without alcohol, disulfiram carries potential dangers of precipitating a serious neuritis (including optic neuritis), possibly exacerbating a peripheral neuropathy, inducing a life-threatening and possibly irreversible hepatitis, and, through its active metabolite, carbon disulfide, might increase the risk of atherosclerotic heart disease, although the risk for these problems is probably quite low.[32–34]

Disulfiram is given orally, usually at a daily dose of 250 mg, over an extended period of time, perhaps up to 1 year. The drug works by causing an irreversible destruction of aldehyde dehydrogenase, the enzyme responsible for the metabolism of acetaldehyde, the first major breakdown product of ethanol (see Section 3.2). As a result, after drinking, acetaldehyde builds up in the blood. The intensity of the disulfiram–ethanol reaction depends on the blood-alcohol level (and thus on the amount and rapidity of drinking), as well as on some as yet poorly understood individual characteristics of patients. Although disulfiram does not decrease the "drive" to drink, the hope is that the patient's knowledge of a possible severe physical reaction following drinking while on Antabuse will be associated with an improved recovery rate.[18,31]

In the midst of a reaction, the most frequent symptoms include facial flushing, palpitations and a rapid heart rate, difficulty breathing, a possibly serious drop in blood pressure, and nausea and vomiting. The most usual reaction begins within minutes to a half hour after drinking and may last 30–60 minutes. Once it has begun, no specific mode of treatment is available, and most authors advocate general supportive care, antihistamines (to block the effects of acetaldehyde-medicated histamine release), vitamine C (to possibly enhance acetaldehyde oxidation), and possibly 4-methylpyrazole (to stop the production of acetaldehyde) in doses of 7 mg/kg intravenously (IV).[35] Although a relatively healthy person is likely to tolerate the ethanol–disulfiram interaction well, it could be quite dangerous for individuals with a history of serious heart disease, stroke, serious hypertension, or diabetes. Disulfiram should not be prescribed for these individuals.

As is true of all treatments of alcoholism, the efficacy of this approach is difficult to prove. Controlled studies comparing disulfiram prescription with no drug prescription show a higher rate of abstinence with disulfiram. However, other studies comparing disulfiram with a placebo have not shown a convincing superiority of the active drug.[36,37] Thus, the clinician is placed in a dilemma, because if a placebo is prescribed to all alcoholic patients, eventually no one will believe that he is getting the active drug, and any placebo effect (i.e., fear of a reaction when he drinks) will be lost.

Another difficulty with disulfiram is the need to take the drug daily. Investigators are currently working on the development of a long-lasting implant, but present methods have not been successful in maintaining adequate blood levels of the drug.[38] Finally, disulfiram is *not* an effective agent for aversive conditioning, because the time lag between the ingestion of alcohol and the reaction is often up to 30 minutes, and the intensity of the reaction is unpredictable.

Because there was no single powerful therapeutic approach to alcoholism available when the first and second volumes of this text were published, I concluded that disulfiram was a viable approach for the average alcoholic. However, the recent collaborative Veterans Administration investigation of over 600 alcoholics followed for at least 12 months, taken in the context of the prior literature, casts serious doubt on the effectiveness of this drug.[36] Because of these factors as well as the continued documentation of potentially serious side effects, I *no longer recommend* disulfiram for the average alcoholic. However, I recognize the possibility that there may be a subgroup of alcoholics who are more responsive to this drug (e.g., those with high levels of functioning and enhanced levels of motivation or those who in the past have maintained abstinence only with disulfiram[37]).

4. *Other drugs of possible use in alcoholic rehabilitation:* A number of other medications show potential promise for alcoholic rehabilitation *in the future*. The key word here is "potential," because there are inadequate data at present to justify the inclusion of any of these approaches in clinical treatment until more extensive

studies document that their assets outweigh their liabilities. Perhaps more precise data will be available for inclusion in a future edition of this volume.

Animal studies indicate that drugs that can increase the amount of the brain neurotransmitter *serotonin* or inhibit angiotensin-converting enzymes may be associated with a decrease in ethanol intake.[39-41] These results are bolstered by limited clinical studies with serotonin-enhancing antidepressants [e.g., zimelidine (Zelmid), citalopram, and alaproclate], demonstrating similar changes among alcoholics.[40,41] The serotonin-enhancing drugs might decrease the drive to drink alcohol, but they also carry potentially serious side effects, and at present none is available for routine prescription for alcoholism.

A second type of promising nonmedicinal approach might incorporate one of the new *nonbenzodiazepine antianxiety agents.* Alcoholics are likely to demonstrate high levels of anxiety during withdrawal and for at least 3–6 months after the achievement of abstinence, as discussed in Chapter 3. This reflects both a probable protracted abstinence syndrome along with the exacerbation of life problems by alcoholism and the readjustments inherent in recovery. It has been hypothesized that the intense feelings of nervousness not only contribute to the alcoholic's discomfort but also might increase the risk for return to drinking. On the other hand, the traditional antianxiety agents such as the benzodiazepines [e.g., diazepam (Valium) and chlordiazepoxide (Librium)] cannot be given to the average alcoholic during rehabilitation, both because the patient is likely to develop tolerance and because after having established a pattern of abusing one brain depressant, alcohol, patients might be at enhanced risk for abusing other brain depressants, the benzodiazepines. The new nonbenzodiazepine anxiolytics such as buspirone (Buspar) appear to be as effective in dealing with anxiety syndromes as the benzodiazepines and in addition, according to studies generated to date, are less likely to be abused, do not appear to interact with brain depressants, and do not *appear* as yet to produce physical dependence.[42,43] While I look forward to the possibility of being able to recommend nonbenzodiazepine anxiolytics during alcoholic rehabilitation in a future edition, at present there are no published controlled studies of adequate size, and the use of these medications in alcoholic rehabilitation must be considered experimental.

15.2.4.2. Outpatient Programs

It is difficult to generate data to prove inpatient or outpatient rehabilitation superior.[16] Inpatient programs have the assets of enhanced intensity of intervention, while outpatient approaches carry the advantage of decreased cost and the ability to treat patients in their real-life settings. In fact, the distinction between inpatient and outpatient approaches is somewhat specious because most inpatient approaches are followed by a minimum of 3–6 months of outpatient aftercare, and many patients originally approached with outpatient care are likely over the next 12–24 months to find themselves alcoholic inpatients.[16,19]

If you do choose outpatient therapy, you may offer such rehabilitation directly or refer to any of a variety of available outpatient programs. These range from private care, to clinics, to the outpatient extensions of inpatient programs. One valuable information resource is the National Council on Alcoholism (NCA) (usually listed in the telephone book), which in most urban areas will act as a referral source. Many communities also have state- or county-operated evaluation centers that can be reached through government-run health services.

In addition, many alcoholics have life crisis problems or vocational rehabilitation needs. Referral to a social service agency, a visiting nurses' association, or state vocational rehabilitation offices can be most helpful.

Another special type of outpatient "intervention" is found in job-based rehabilitation efforts. These usually reach out to troubled employees, a large percentage of whom have substance-related problems. To be optimally effective, these troubled-employee programs require a trusting working relationship between employees and unions, with the counselor as a key element in the formula.[44,45] In the workplace, the counselor is frequently able to make an accurate diagnosis and refer for outpatient or inpatient therapy, dealing with patients who usually have assets that include a more stable living situation and, by definition, a job. The interested reader may consult a number of resources on employee assistance programs[44-46] for further reference.

As discussed in more detail elsewhere,[6] the same general approach applies both to patients who have never been hospitalized and to those beginning an aftercare program. The patient is counseled about day-to-day life adjustments and is helped to deal with crisis situations. After a period of time, life adjustment tends to stabilize, and the patient incorporates enough of the messages being presented by the counselor to stop formal treatment.

Usually, counseling is begun at a frequency of once a week, but then it is slowly decreased, so that by the end of a year, the patient is seen about once a month. If problems with drinking or life adjustment occur, the frequency of meeting can be increased to meet the acute need.

For the *secondary alcoholic* (see Section 3.1.2.3) who does not require inpatient care, referral to a mental-health specialist should be considered.[47] If the diagnosis is primary affective disorder, but the patient is *not* felt to be severely incapacitated or suicidal (if suicidal, he should be hospitalized), outpatient treatment with antidepressants is possible. In such instances, the patient should be referred either to a psychiatric clinic or to a psychiatrist for evaluation, in addition to his alcoholic rehabilitation.

In delivering care to the secondary alcoholic with a primary *antisocial personality,* it is necessary to recognize the high rates of concomitant drug abuse and the elevated risk for the commission of serious crimes by these individuals.[48,49] There is no highly effective treatment known, but some authors favor heavily structured group sessions following a therapeutic community model. Outpatient referral to an experienced health specialist is advisable, as there is no evidence that inpatient care is routinely justified.

Some individuals are not ready to return to their day-to-day life after inpatient treatment. If the problem is either a chronic medical one or psychiatric impairment, a nursing home or halfway house should be considered. For those with more serious problems, a nursing home is probably required, but whenever possible, this should be integrated with continued outpatient treatment and AA.

These nursing or halfway settings usually offer continued group meetings, supervision of medications, and help in dealing with emotional problems and crises. As is true of any of the modes of treatment, it is important that the clinician carefully evaluate each program before actual referral.

15.2.4.3. Role of Alcoholics Anonymous

AA is an excellent resource for treatment.[50,51] This group, composed of individuals who are themselves recovering alcoholics (many of whom have been "dry" for years), establishes a milieu in which help is available 24 hours a day, 7 days a week.[6] At meetings, members share their own recovery experiences, demonstrating to the patient that he is not alone and that a better life-style is possible. AA also offers additional help in the form of groups that discuss the special problems of the children of alcoholics (Alateen) and of their spouses (Alanon). Each AA group has its own personality, and the patient might want to experiment with different groups before choosing the one in which he is most comfortable.

AA can be used as a referral resource where no other outpatient service is either available or acceptable to the patient. It can also be utilized as an adjunct to outpatient or inpatient treatment efforts.

15.2.4.4. An Overview

In summary, alcoholic rehabilitation consists of a series of general helping maneuvers aimed at increasing and maintaining the highest level of motivation toward abstinence, helping the individual to reestablish a life-style without alcohol (and giving outreach to the family), and maximizing physical and mental functioning. Inpatient rehabilitation has not been shown to be essential, although individuals with specific needs may be best reached in the more sheltered setting.

Whether in an inpatient or an outpatient mode, most patients are offered group counseling sessions centering on day-to-day living and covering such problems as reestablishing meaningful relationships with the spouse and other family members, handling oneself at parties and with friends when alcohol is offered, reestablishing free-time activities and peer groups free of ethanol, adjusting job or avocational activities so that they are consistent with abstinence, and so on. Much of this work can be done by the average clinician with the help of AA and the judicious use of disulfiram.

Thus, therapy involves a commonsense approach to group counseling, long-term follow-up, working with the patient and the family together, and avoiding most medications. Specifically, there is no place in alcoholic rehabilitation for antianxiety drugs or hypnotics.

15.3. A SPECIAL CASE: OPIATE ABUSE (304.00 or 305.50 in DSM-III-R)

The primary opiate abuser and the primary alcoholic differ in that the opiate abuser tends to be younger and to have more antisocial problems, comes from different referral sources (e.g., jail or probation), and more often abuses ancillary drugs. The high level of crime associated with the illicit use of opiates has helped motivate the development of a "maintenance" program that is purported to result in lowered levels of antisocial activities,[52] but that does not deal with the basic addiction. Even with these differences, however, the same general rules for rehabilitation apply to the opiate abuser as to the alcoholic. These "basics" include detoxification, the need to reach out to the family, the need to carefully evaluate efforts, establishing patient goals and a program of counseling giving drug education, and making a long-term commitment to the patient. I will therefore concentrate on specific aspects of rehabilitation of the opiate abuser that have not already been covered.

The best predictors of the outcome of any form of opiate treatment are similar to those discussed for alcohol. Men and women entering care with a job or a legitimate source of income, relatively good health, a stable address, and fewer and less serious legal problems are much more likely to complete treatment and to be found to be abstinent several years later.[53] Such individuals are likely to show lower levels of drug abuse, lower arrest rates, and increased psychological functioning.[54,55] The worst prognosis is to be expected for those who have supported their "habit" almost solely by criminal activities.[54]

15.3.1. Methadone and Methadyl Acetate Maintenance

Methadone and methadyl acetate maintenance can be given only in licensed clinics established to ensure adequate care and to minimize the flow of methadone into illegal channels.[56]

15.3.1.1. Goals

Methadone does not "cure" opiate addiction. The program substitutes addiction to a legal and longer-acting drug (e.g., methadone) for the addiction to a shorter-acting drug such as heroin. Methadone maintenance is used to help the addict to develop a life-style free of street drugs in order to improve functioning within the family and job, to decrease problems with the law, and to improve health.[55-58]

Methadone should be given only as part of a holistic patient approach, incorporating all the other aspects of rehabilitation thus far described.[59] Specifically, in addition to outreach to families, job counseling, legal advice, referral to Narcotics Anonymous, and so on, there is also evidence that cognitive and supportive psychotherapies may be important. In this therapy, it is hoped that if the addict receives a drug legally (orally, to avoid the "rush" felt with IV drugs), at little or no cost, he will not return to the costs and problems inherent in obtaining street drugs.[60] At the same time, methadone is felt to decrease drug craving and to (at least partially) block the "high" experienced with heroin.

15.3.1.2. Treatment Program

Methadone is a long-acting opiate that shares almost all the physiological properties of heroin, including addiction, sedation, respiratory depression, and effects on heart and muscle. The addict who has been carefully screened to rule out prior psychiatric disorders may be maintained on a relatively *low*-dose (30–40 mg/day) or a higher-dose (100–120 mg/day) methadone schedule, the former giving fewer side effects but not the same degree of hypothetical "blockade" against the effects of heroin.[61] Although the results are not definite, there is some evidence that the use of higher doses of methadone may result in higher levels of retention in treatment and in consequent lower levels of arrest, readdiction to street drugs, and criminal behavior.[62]

The drug is administered in an oral liquid given once a day at the program center, with weekend doses taken by the patient at home. An approach similar to methadone maintenance utilizes a longer-acting methadone congener such as LAAM or methadyl acetate.[63,64] The dosage of the latter is usually 20–30 mg, given three times a week in the beginning, then increased to 80 mg three times a week, if necessary. Available evidence indicates that the results are similar to those with methadone.

After the period of maintenance (usually 6 months to a year, or longer), the clinician should work closely with the patient to regulate the rate of drug decrease.[65] Anecdotally, while on one hand some authors recommend very long-term use,[66] on the other most studies suggest that the dose be lowered within a limited period of time, but as slowly as 3% a week.[66,67]

Methadone-type drugs have been taken by some individuals for over 10 years and are *felt* by clinicians to be relatively safe and effective.[58,59,68,69] However, the dangers associated with these drugs include the relatively benign side effect of constipation (seen in 17%),[70] the danger of addicting the fetus when the drug is given during pregnancy, a potentially serious depression.[71–75] and the possibility that the drug will find its way into illegal channels. Another special problem (seen in as many as one quarter of methadone maintenance patients) is abuse of drugs like cocaine and alcohol, especially for those individuals who abused other substances before using the opiates or who took alcohol or drugs concomitantly with their opiate abuse.[76] These problems are discussed in greater depth in Section 6.1.2.1.2.

As is true of treatments for abuse of almost all drugs, there are few carefully controlled studies demonstrating that methadone maintenance is definitely superior to other modes of care or placebo. Most studies demonstrate that good outcome correlates significantly with the length of time in treatment (with maintenance for 3 months or less hardly being superior to detoxification alone)[77] and with the characteristics of the patients before they enter care.[78] Several recent investigations shed some light on efficacy. In the first, the authors compared individuals enrolled in two similar methadone maintenance clinics, one of which was phased out because of fiscal constraints and the other of which continued.[62,79] After a rather thorough 2-year follow-up, readdiction to heroin was observed in 55% of the men and women whose program was closed, but in only one third of those being seen in the continuing program, with similar figures of 75% vs approximately 40% for arrests, 45–65% vs. 20–40% for signs of alcohol abuse, and 40–60% vs. 30% for a history of selling drugs on the street during the subsequent 2 years. Although this study noted no differences between the two groups in the incidence of committing crimes against property, employment rates, or history of having been on welfare during the 2-year follow-up, the results do point out the possible importance of methadone maintenance to the opiate abuser. Another study was a 2.5-year follow-up demonstrating a 30% rate of continued abstinence and 47% rate of recent abstinence at follow-up as well as improvement in family and psychological functioning.[73,75] However, there was less impressive change in employment and legal problems. Finally, data from 617 addicts revealed a reduction in IV drug use, a less impressive decrease in use of other drugs, and a marked decrease in criminality.[57]

15.3.2. Opiate Antagonists

These drugs occupy opiate receptors in the brain and block the effects of heroin and other opiates.[59] Concomitant administration of an antagonist with heroin may stop the development of physical dependence, but does not block the drug hunger.[70]

15.3.2.1. Goals

The use of antagonists is not limited to rehabilitation. They help in the treatment of opiate toxic reactions and can be used to test addicts who say that they are drug-free (the antagonist will precipitate withdrawal if dependence on opiates has developed).[59] In rehabilitation, however, these drugs are administered over an extended period so that the patient experiences less of a "high" if he takes opiates.

15.3.2.2. Specific Antagonists

There are a variety of opiate antagonists, most of which are themselves addicting. They include the following:

1. *Cyclazocine* was the first antagonist tested in the early to mid-1960s.[80] Doses of 4 mg by mouth per day are effective in blocking up to 15 mg of heroin for 24 hours. However, the blockade is not complete, and most patients complain of cyclazocine side effects of sleepiness and a drunken feeling. A decrease in respirations may also be noted. Thus, this drug has not been widely used.[59]

2. *Naloxone* (Narcan) is an excellent narcotic antagonist that has no known morphinelike (agonistic) properties. Unfortunately, it is not well absorbed orally, and its action lasts no more than 2–3 hours, so that up to 3 g/day may be needed to block 15 mg of heroin for a 24-hour period.[80]

3. *Nalorphine* (Nalline) was at one time primarily used to test addiction to

opiates, for which purpose it is administered in a dose of 2–5 mg in a dark room. If the individual is addicted, pupillary dilatation is seen within 15 minutes to half an hour, whereas if no addiction is present, pupillary constriction is seen.[59] If no reaction at all is noted, 5 mg and then 7 mg can be given at half-hour intervals. This drug is now not usually used as a rehabilitative agent and has probably been replaced by naltrexone as a challenge agent.

4. *Naltrexone* (Trexan) is a widely used narcotic antagonist that can be given orally, has a length of action of approximately 24 hours, and *has few side effects.*[81–84] A dose of 50 mg/day is effective in blocking 15 mg of heroin for 24 hours, and higher doses (125–150 mg) of naltrexone are capable of blocking 25 mg of IV heroin for 72 hours.[80,85] This drug is free of agonistic properties, and there are no known withdrawal symptoms when the medication is stopped.[86] The side effects tend to be relatively mild gastrointestinal (GI) distress, anxiety, and insomnia, all of which tend to disappear over a period of days. However, many patients report a sadness, or dysphoria, especially if doses are increased relatively abruptly, and some demonstrate a reversible hepatitis, especially at doses exceeding 300 mg/day, the latter making it unwise to consider the use of naltrexone in patients who already demonstrate symptoms of acute hepatitis.[82,87,88]

In the usual approach, patients to be started on this antagonist should be relatively healthy, as demonstrated by laboratory blood tests (e.g., liver function tests) and physical examination, and should be free of opiates for a minimum of 5 days. They can then be challenged with 0.8 mg of naloxone to be certain that they will be able to tolerate the longer-acting antagonist naltrexone.[86–88] If patients have not been properly screened and administration of naltrexone precipitates relatively severe withdrawal symptoms, which can last up to 48 hours, it may be necessary to select a fairly fast-acting opiate agonist with minimal respiratory depression and minimal histamine release.[87]

Assuming that the challenge dose results in few if any withdrawal symptoms, a 10-mg dose of naltrexone can be given, and over the next 10 days, the daily dose should be increased to 100 mg on Mondays and Wednesdays and 150 mg on Fridays.[85,89] Most programs then carry out periodic blood or urine screens for opiate use.

Of course, treatment with an antagonist alone is inadequate.[80,85] Patients will benefit when they develop a close rapport with treatment personnel and may also gain from behavioral techniques that help them to learn how to handle anxiety and to cope with life situations.[80,85] However, for unknown reasons, most addicts are reluctant to begin and stay with narcotic antagonist treatment; only 60% or so completed the 6 days of noroxymorphone induction in one study.[78,85,90] Of the 153 remaining patients, 30 dropped out within 2 days of completing the induction, one third had dropped by 1 month and one half by 2 months, and slightly fewer than 10% were left at the end of 6 months.[85] Although this rate of dropout is greater than that observed with methadone maintenance in similar patients, those who do remain in treatment with antagonists are less likely than methadone patients to take other drugs—in one study, 10 versus 30%.

In summary, narcotic antagonists are not uniformly successful. Although theoretically they are very helpful, and although naltrexone has many assets (e.g., no agonistic effects, low levels of side effects, ease of oral administration, and acceptability for administration three times a week), it is probable that fewer addicts stay in treatment with antagonists than remain in methadone maintenance treatment approaches.

15.3.3. Other Drugs Used in Treatment

For any disorder with a natural history that includes periods of improvement with a relatively high rate of spontaneous remission runs, there is the danger of there being a variety of touted but ineffective treatments. Uncontrolled experiments have extolled such misleading cures as carbon dioxide inhalation, atropine coma, and lysergic acid diethylamide (LSD).[30,67,91] I will mention only a few of the more promising approaches here.

1. *Propoxyphene* (Darvon) has cross-tolerance with other opiates and has been used as a method of detoxification from opiate addiction. Because of the belief that this drug has less appeal on the street and lower side effects than some other medications, short-term ''maintenance'' with this medication (approximately 3 weeks) has been used, but has not been shown to be uniquely effective.[92]

2. *Propranolol* (Inderal) in doses of 5–120 mg/day has been administered in an attempt to block the immediate ''rush'' or ''high'' seen with heroin.[93] Uncontrolled studies indicate a decrease in drug craving, but better-controlled evaluations are necessary before this drug is used in general settings.

3. *Heroin* itself has been administered as part of a maintenance program.[94,95] The rationale is similar to that offered for methadone; that is, it is used to decrease the necessity for getting the drug on the street and to cut down on the medical complications such as acquired immune deficiency syndrome (AIDS) or hepatitis from adulterated drugs and contaminated needles.[95] It has been used primarily in Britain, where the magnitude of opiate problems is very small compared with that in the United States (it is estimated that there were only 500 addicts in Britain when heroin maintenance was begun). After it became legal to prescribe heroin, the number of addicts doubled, necessitating the establishment of clinics similar to methadone maintenance programs. It is now uncommon to find a drug clinic in Britain that prescribes heroin and only heroin, as most are turning toward methadone maintenance.

15.3.4. Drug-Free Programs

Most inpatient treatment models offered to the opiate abuser utilize modifications of the therapeutic community (TC) concept first proposed by M. Jones.[96] This is an exception to the general rule of short-term inpatient rehabilitation; while some programs last a month or less,[97] some last up to a year while the addict is taken out of the street culture and given a new view of life within the group. In this structure, group members, including ex-addict leaders, constantly confront each behavior in an attempt to help the participants gain insight and find a new and more successful life-style for coping with problems. Most large cities in the United States have programs run on the Synanon or Day Top models.[96] Unfortunately, there has been very little controlled evaluation of this approach.

It is difficult to compare results from TCs and methadone maintenance, as the patients in the former tend to be young and Caucasian, whereas those in the latter tend to be older and are more often minority-group members.[98] However, individuals assigned to methadone maintenance are more likely to appear at the clinic for actual care (29 vs. 18% for TCs in one series) and may be 50% more likely to stay in treatment for 1 year.[98] As is true in other treatment approaches, the best prognosis in TCs is for those who are employed; who have higher levels of school completion, less intense involvement with heroin, and less extensive jail records; and who stay in treatment for 2 months or longer.[98−102] The most usual retention rate in a TC is approximately 50% or less at 12 months, but some studies reveal figures of less than 20%.[98,103]

15.3.5. The Medical Abuser

The middle-class individual who is primarily abusing prescription opiates may be more similar to the alcoholic in general life outlook and history than to the street abuser of opiates. There is little good information on the best rehabilitation mode for this population, and the final program should be tailored to the specific patient, perhaps using the same approach applied to the alcoholic. Some of the patients will have chronic pain problems that must be addressed as part of their rehabilitation.

15.4. A SPECIAL CASE: REHABILITATION STIMULANT ABUSE
(e.g., 304.40, 304.20, 305.70, or 305.60 in DSM-III-R)

Amphetamines and cocaine are in some ways a special case for rehabilitation efforts. This reflects in part the relative intensity and persistence of craving for these drugs and the prolonged secondary abstinence syndrome. Such problems probably relate to the powerful behavioral reinforcement that can be seen with stimulants [whether taken intranasally (IN) or IV or smoked] as well as the persistence of pharmacological changes, including relatively long-term problems with adjustment of brain levels of norepinephrine, dopamine, and possibly serotonin. These latter issues are discussed in Chapter 5 in the sections on pharmacology (5.1.1) and on withdrawal from stimulants (5.2.6).

While acute withdrawal from stimulants can last weeks, it is likely that this phenomenon blends into a protracted abstinence or "extinction phase."[104] This period can persist for many months, during which the patient is likely to demonstrate a normal mood and ability to enjoy surroundings, along with periods of craving. The drug-seeking can be intense and probably reflects both the behavioral and the biological factors described above.

Rehabilitation efforts aimed at stimulant abusers follow the same general principles outlined in preceding sections. The need for early identification, gathering information from resource persons as well as patients, and the importance of careful physical examinations must be emphasized. As is true of all substance-abuse problems, the mainstay of rehabilitation efforts often boils down to using approaches that increase and maintain high levels of motivation for abstinence while working closely with patients to help them rebuild their lives without abusing any substances. While the specific implementation of these general rules differs with each individual, a careful rereading of Section 15.2 can be most helpful, because issues similar to those experienced in alcoholic rehabilitation are experienced with patients entering rehabilitation for cocaine or amphetamine abuse.

As is true for abuse of other substances, patients will often respond well to outpatient rehabilitation efforts. While the indications to hospitalize for detoxification and rehabilitation have not been carefully worked out, some specific suggestions have been made in the literature.[105] Similar to the guidlines used for alcoholism, hospitalization would seem appropriate for patients with severe psychiatric disturbances (e.g., psychoses or depressions) secondary to their drug abuse, those dependent on multiple drugs, and individuals with such severe social impairment that their survival on a day-to-day basis could be jeopardized, as well as those who, in their outpatient participation, seemed unable or unwilling to stop their stimulant abuse. It is also probable that individuals with histories of more intensive drug abuse might require at least short-term hospitalization.

Counseling and brief, relatively superficial forms of psychotherapy are also important in the treatment of stimulant abusers. This treatment most usually takes the form of discussing issues such as relationships with relatives and friends, the need to establish a drug-free peer group, the importance of structuring and using active free time, and so on. A more intense form of interpersonal psychotherapy has also been proposed, focusing on the need to decrease impulsiveness by carefully thinking about events before acting and the need to recognize the context in which craving is most likely to be intense and the cues that stimulate the craving so that these situations can be avoided.[106]

While offering general supports, it is important to recognize the potential role of self-help groups. Cocaine Anonymous, or similar groups such as Narcotics Anonymous or AA, can complement other treatment efforts. Because many stimulant abusers also abuse alcohol and other drugs, the selection of the specific type of organization often reflects the individual's own wishes as well as the specific groups available. A point similar to that made in Section 15.2.4.3 is that through such groups, cocaine abusers are likely to meet people who are willing to help them 24 hours a day, are able to develop a cohort of drug and alcohol-free friends, and to learn that it is possible to enjoy oneself while free of drugs and alcohol. For individuals seeking such additional supports, these groups can also offer a structured series of steps to follow in maintaining abstinence and freedom from drugs, while offering a belief system that for some can be quite comforting.

Consistent with my general philosophy, I prefer to treat drug and alcohol rehabilitation without medications, unless there is convincing evidence that a specific pharmacological approach offers significantly more assets than liabilities. On the other hand, some recent work indicates that at least one type of medication *might* be worth considering in the future, after more specific data have accrued from controlled studies. In response to the frequent complaint of mood swings and feelings of depression voiced by stimulant abusers during the first months of abstinence, several laboratories have investigated the possibility that antidepressant medication might help alleviate some of these symptoms and might thereby increase the chances for remaining drug-free.[107,108] With the use of the tricyclic antidepressants imipramine (Tofranil) or desipramine (Norpramin) in doses of 25–400 mg/day (most subjects take 150–250 mg), there are some data to suggest that some patients may function better. It is not clear whether imipramine itself is important or whether any antidepressant-type drug would be likely to work. Much less impressive and generally negative results have been reported regarding the use of some other types of medications during rehabilitation, including relatively weak stimulants such as methylphenidate (Ritalin), and the use of lithium.

In summary, efforts aimed at rehabilitation of stimulant-drug abusers, including those who abuse cocaine, follow the same general supportive and commonsense approaches suggested for rehabilitation of abusers of other types of drugs. As is true of abuse of substances in the two other categories known to be physically addicting (brain depressants and opiates), rehabilitation efforts are jeopardized by the probability of a secondary, less intense abstinence phase likely to last many months and even up to 1 year. At present, clinicians should focus on general supports, supportive psychotherapy, outreach to families, and the use of self-help groups such as Cocaine Anonymous. It is hoped that by the time the fourth edition of this text is developed, there might be available more definitive information on the relatively safety and efficacy of more specific pharmacological agents for use in stimulant rehabilitation. Until suitable data accrue, however, such medications should probably not be used in usual clinical practice.

15.5. A SPECIAL CASE: HALLUCINOGEN, DEPRESSANT, AND MULTIDRUG ABUSE (e.g., 304.30, 305.20, 304.50, 305.30, 304.10, 305.40, or 304.90 in DSM-III-R)

It is rarely necessary to establish specific rehabilitation efforts for individuals who are "casual" users of marijuana or hallucinogens. However, there can be serious consequences when hallucinogens are used regularly or in high doses and when depressants are regularly ingested. Because there is a high level of correlation between the heavy use of any one of these substances and the use of multiple drugs, I will present a discussion that is aimed primarily at the multidrug user but that can also be applied to those individuals who use only one type of substance.

After establishing the diagnosis, carrying out detoxification, if necessary, and ruling out the possibility of any major preexisting psychiatric disorder, the next step is to determine the answers to the following questions:

1. Is the individual primarily abusing street drugs or taking medications prescribed by a physician?

2. Is there a primary or preferred drug of use?
3. Under what circumstances does the individual use multiple drugs?
4. Is the client a member of a street subculture of drug users or a middle-class, blue-collar or white-collar working person?

In a program dealing primarily with street users, the middle-class individual may be referred to a more appropriate program. This type of flexibility is of great importance in giving the patient an adequate and comfortable milieu. The actual treatment protocol chosen will resemble either the efforts described for alcoholism (Section 15.2) or, for the person more heavily involved in the street culture, those described in the drug-free program for opiates (Section 15.3). Each individual client's needs, of course, must be considered in designing patient rehabilitation plans.

15.6. A SPECIAL CASE: SMOKING (e.g., 305.10 in DSM-III-R)

15.6.1. Some General Comments

Treatment of chronic smokers involves blending many of the efforts outlined in this chapter. The goal, as always, is to alleviate withdrawal symptoms, use counseling and education to enhance and maintain high levels of motivation, and use behavioral therapies when needed. Section 15.6.3 outlines several pharmacological approaches that are also worth considering.

Confrontation and rehabilitation efforts with smokers should focus on abstinence. Some cigarette users will try changing to other forms of tobacco, but because they will probably continue to inhale, it may do little good to advise them to switch to a pipe or a cigar. Others may turn to low-yield or smaller cigarettes or might attempt to smoke only part of a cigarette. Unfortunately, this approach seems rarely to work to the patient's advantage because he or she is likely to inhale more deeply or use more of the low-yield brands than they would of the high-yield, the result being an only moderate (if any) decrease in tar, carbon monoxide, and nicotine, but a possible increase in inhalation of a variety of other toxins.[109]

A possible treatment approach is to use dilution filters—cigarette appliances that progressively mix more air with the smoke in the hope that this will help the user decrease the amount of actual smoke inhaled.[110] Once again, unfortunately, the result is likely to be an increase in the number of puffs per cigarette or more intense inhalation with little convincing overall benefit.

15.6.2. Behavioral Approaches

While many cigarette users seem to be able to stop at least temporarily on their own and some actually achieve and maintain abstinence without help, a significant percentage turn to specialized smoking clinics. There is some debate about the overall cost-effectiveness of these specialized "treatment" approaches,[111] but there is some evidence of benefit. Most of these "rehabilitation" programs focus their efforts on behavioral approaches. All can be expected to result in some fairly rapid level of improvement (if abstinence is used as a measure), but it is unlikely that this level will be maintained for extended periods unless the patient is given "refresher" courses.

One type of behavior modification involves self-control strategies. In this approach, the smoker is asked to keep reminding himself why he wants to stop and to smoke in the least pleasurable way possible. For instance, he may be told never to smoke after meals, always to smoke entirely alone, or to begin smoking his least-preferred brand.[112]

Other behavioral approaches center on aversive conditioning, coupling an unpleasant event with the nicotine intake. The use of mild electric shocks to the hands while smoking does not appear to be as effective as aversions more directly related to the smoking itself. Many programs use a forced consumption of 2–3 times the usual amount of tobacco, having stale and warm smoke blown in the smoker's face, or enforced rapid chain smoking. As a result of these types of approaches, as many as 50% of smokers may maintain abstinence after 6 months if they complete the entire original program.[113] As is true with all forms of behavior modification, the results are probably enhanced when the patient has a warm relationship with the counselor.[112]

15.6.3. Pharmacological Approaches

In the interval between the second and third editions of this text, much information has been generated on a pharmacological adjunct to the treatment of chronic smokers. *Nicorette Gum* contains 2 mg of nicotine bound to an ion-exchange resin in each piece. Smokers consuming approximately 15 or more cigarettes per day who have otherwise had difficulty stopping can be advised to stop smoking immediately and begin chewing Nicorette Gum, taking care to chew each piece slowly for approximately 30 minutes to avoid overly rapid release of the nicotine, with a final consumption of usually 10–20 pieces of gum per 24 hours.[59,114,115] The philosophy of use of this substance is to minimize nicotine withdrawal symptoms with the thought that patients may have to continue taking Nicorette Gum for several months or more. Careful evaluations of this substance have documented a significant decrease in symptoms of nicotine withdrawal over the first 4 weeks for active drug vs. placebo.[116] Two recent reviews have also documented significantly higher levels of abstinence at 6 months and 12 months for Nicorette Gum users than for placebo users, but *only* when the Nicorette Gum is given as part of a balanced treatment program in a speciality clinic.[114,117] For example, a review of 14 random double-blind controlled studies demonstrated that at 12 months 23% of the Nicorette Gum users versus 13% of controls had maintained abstinence from cigarettes.

Of course, all treatments have dangers, and Nicorette Gum cannot be viewed as totally safe.First, physical addiction to the gum itself can develop after protracted use (e.g., several months), and patients should be slowly weaned off.[116] Second, there are a number of contraindications to prescription of this substance, including recent myocardial infarctions, evidence of vasospastic disease, and cardiac arrythmias.[115] The drug should also not be used by patients with inflammations of the mouth or throat, those with esophagitis, or individuals with peptic ulcer disease. Third, use of more Nicorette Gum per day than prescribed can result in a toxic reaction, similar to that described in Section 12.3.4.3. Finally, side effects that can be expected with this treatment include some nausea, possible vomiting, and hiccups.

One other type of drug has been discussed for helping alleviate withdrawal and perhaps helping patients achieve abstinence. Clonidine (Catapres) has been reported to significantly decrease feelings of tension, anxiety, irritability, and restlessness as well as to decrease feelings of craving.[118] While this drug does appear to help, the paucity of information on its use and the lack of data on the optimal length of treatment, as well as the potentially significant side-effect profile of this drug, mitigate against its prescription until more data accumulate.

In summary, considering the huge amounts of morbidity and mortality associated with tobacco use (see Section 12.3), treatment of heavy smokers and users of smokeless tobaccos would appear to be warranted. Much of the general information regarding rehabilitation applies here because the most prominent therapeutic efforts involve treatment of withdrawal along with education, behavioral techniques, and the judicious use of medications. Tobacco users should first be encouraged to stop on their own, and physicians as well as other health-care deliverers should do all they can to help them achieve and maintain abstinence. However, for those individuals for whom these approaches do not appear to be enough, referral to a specialized smoking clinic would appear to be worth consideration. Such clinics do seem to have enhanced levels of effectiveness over efforts given in the physician's office, at least as results apply to Nicorette Gum.

15.7. PREVENTION OF SUBSTANCE PROBLEMS

15.7.1. Some Preliminary Thoughts

This text has focused on the recognition and treatment of a variety of substance-related difficulties. I have introduced the reader to a scheme for placing substances of abuse into categories based on the usual effects at the usual doses. This classification in turn has served as the basis for the discussion of the history, pharmacology, and recognition and treatment of emergency problems related to each of the categories of drugs. My hope has been to offer a book from which interested readers can gain greater general knowledge of substances of abuse and to develop a handbook of immediate use in clinical situations.

This chapter, focusing on rehabilitation, is a general introduction to maneuvers to be invoked once the initial emergency has passed. I hope that increasing your

understanding of rehabilitation efforts will encourage you to either institute rehabilitation yourself or refer the patient to an established rehabilitation program and
self-help group.

I have attempted to ensure that all the information directed to this point is
pragmatic by avoiding topics that lack immediate relevance to patient care. Thus, if
you have worked your way through the text to this point, you have accomplished all
that I have set out for you. It is my hope that by this point you understand some of
my biases in the recognition and treatment of substance-related problems.

From this general perspective, the remaining several pages of this third edition
are an indulgence. Because there are limited amounts of data from which I can draw
conclusions, this section offers some preliminary considerations on ways to head off
substance-related problems before they occur.

15.7.2. Some General Thoughts on Primary Prevention

Because our work is done and the following discussion is heuristic, I have not
forced myself into a disciplined and broad-based discussion of prevention as a
whole. Those interested in more scholarly reviews are offered several references
that are worth detailed and careful consideration.[119,120]

The emphasis here is limited to thoughts about *primary prevention* of substance abuse.[120] Because of space limitations, I also emphasize examples related to
alcohol. While they are equally important, I have chosen not to discuss secondary
prevention strategies such as those that attempt to intervene early in the course of
substance problems[119] or efforts aimed at increasing access to clean needles and
purer drugs in order to decrease the incidence of AIDS, hepatitis, and bacterial
endocarditis.[95] The thoughts offered here center on issues regarding primary prevention efforts aimed at the general population, as well as thought relating to a
group in which I have a special interest, health-care professionals.

At present, primary prevention can be divided into at least four categories.[119]
First, the general availability or supply of alcoholic beverages can be limited
through price controls or taxation, control of the number of sales outlets, and
restrictions on production. A recent review of consumption trends between 1955
and 1980 revealed a probable correlation between per capita consumption of alcoholic beverages and the level of restrictiveness of relevant laws,[121] a conclusion
supported by predictions made through computer modeling.[122] On the other hand,
decreases in consumption are not necessarily paralleled by commensurate changes
in problem patterns, especially when the changes in availability occur through
relatively limited restrictions such as those on the sales of wine or beer in grocery
stores or those that regulate prices during ''happy hours.''[123–125]

A second primary prevention strategy, one closely related to the first, is to
partially restrict the availability of alcohol to specific high-risk groups. A good
example of this approach is the movement to increase the legal drinking age from 18
to 21 in North America.[126] This effort followed the observation that in many locales
an increase in the drinking age was accompanied by a tendency for 18- to 20-year-

olds to avoid drinking and driving, with a subsequent decrease in alcohol-related traffic deaths in that age group.[127] A comparison of student self-reports of drinking practices in states with legal drinking ages of 21 versus those in which drinking is allowed at an age of less than 21 demonstrated some trends that support these conclusions.[126] This included evidence of fewer students who drank while driving in the restrictive states (56 versus 63%), as well as evidence that students in the more restrictive states were less likely to miss class because of drinking (35 versus 44%), less likely to get lower grades (10 versus 14%), and less likely to think that they had a drinking problem (17 versus 22%).

A third approach to primary prevention aims at attempting to shape drinking practices among drinkers. This approach is based on the assumption that increasing levels of education regarding alcohol and drugs among both the general population and young people, along with attempts at teaching clarification of values and decision-making processes, will result in decreased intake of substances and associated problems.[128] There is a general feeling that the overall leveling off of drug and alcohol intake patterns among students reported in the epidemiological subsections of the chapters in this book might relate to many of these efforts.[122] However, the relationship between education and changes in drinking, drug use, or associated problems is difficult to prove.[128] A related tack is that of attempting to control the amount as well as the content of advertisements. Once again, while this stratagem has some commonsense merit, research experiments observing drinking habits among young people after exposure to a number of different types of advertisements have given little evidence of a close and immediate association between advertising practices and alcohol consumption.[129,130]

The fourth general strategy for primary prevention of alcohol- and substance-related problems is to attempt to decrease the risks associated with use of substances.[119] For example, Gussfield has commented on the folly of allowing popular bars to be located along crowded highways in locales where drinkers have limited, if any, access to public transportation.[131] This implies that in addition to the steps outlined above, one might help prevent accidents involving drunk driving by regulating the location of bars or by improving public transportation. Similarly, it might be possible to decrease the risk for vitamin-related medical problems such as Wernicke–Korsakoff's disease by adding relevant vitamins such as thiamine to alcoholic beverages.[132,133]

A brief review of the sections on epidemiology makes it apparent that despite our best efforts, substance use and related problems remain a major source of morbidity, mortality, and lost productivity in all Western societies. The efforts to date might well have contributed to the general leveling off and even slight decreases in the prevalence of use of many of these substances, but it is also obvious that there is still room for great improvement.

I *believe* that one logical way to increase the effectiveness of primary prevention is to increase our understanding of the causes that contribute to use and related problems. In many ways, investment in careful research in these areas is like putting money in the bank—while immediate benefits are not likely to be apparent, in the long run this research can potentially lead to a revolution in our abilities to prevent problems before they develop.

One example of the potential future impact of research on primary prevention of substance-related problems is offered in Section 3.5.4. Research over this last decade has documented the probable importance of genetic factors in alcoholism, and more recent studies are attempting to refine methodologies appropriate for identifying the genetic factors that might increase the alcoholism risk.[134,135] *If* we are able to identify markers associated with a predisposition to this disorder, it makes sense that this could lead to improved prevention efforts. For example, knowledge of which children of alcoholics are at highest risk and observation of environmental and psychological factors that seem to be associated with the actual development of alcoholism *or its absence* in these high-risk children could lead to the development of programs that attempt to change the environment or enhance psychological functioning in relevant areas. It is also possible that behavior-modification programs can help individuals at exceptionally high risk avoid the development of alcohol-related problems or that the research could identify biological processes (e.g., characteristic levels of enzyme activities) that might also be modified to change the risk. In any of these theoretical instances, new and as yet unimagined prevention efforts could accrue from presently ongoing research and markedly change our approaches and levels of effectivness in primary prevention in the substance-abuse areas.

My final general thought regarding primary prevention is the *belief* that no single prevention effort in isolation is likely to produce major changes in patterns of use or abuse of any substance by the general population. I recognize that for alcoholism, for instance, increasing cost or decreasing availability can contribute to a modest decrease in per capita consumption and decreasing availability of alcohol to 18- to 20-year-olds appears to have a reductive impact on arrests for driving while intoxicated, with a subsequent beneficial effect on serious alcohol-related accidents in that age group. Furthermore, attempts at minimizing the supply of illicit drugs such as heroin might help prevent such "epidemics" of new users as were observed in the Eastern metropolitan areas of the United States in the 1960s. These efforts might actually have placed a partial lid on an expansion of substance use and problems. The approaches are certainly better than doing nothing, but I feel that much more will be required before we have any major impact on substance problems.

As a nonexpert in prevention issues, I am impressed with the decreases in heart disease observed during the last 10–15 years in most Western countries. While no one knows why this trend has occurred, it might reflect the confluence of a number of major changes. During these years, the Heart Society has established a campaign to help people recognize the need to identify and treat high blood pressure, most countries have experienced a "fad" of heightened interest in slimness and exercise, and the Tuberculosis Society as well as other health groups have mounted strong antismoking campaigns. While only some of these efforts were specifically aimed at decreasing the prevalence of heart disease, all these as well as other efforts may have combined to have a significant impact on the rate of this disorder.

Similarly, I look forward to an increasing awareness, generated by *many sources*, of the need to refrain from heavy use of substances. Some insurance companies give discounts for nonsmokers and nondrinkers and those who pledge nonuse of other substances. In addition, television programs and the movies are beginning to portray intoxication or drug use as potentially serious behaviors that are not to be tolerated, governments are enacting laws to require us to take responsibility for the subsequent actions of people who become intoxicated in our businesses or homes, physicians and other health-care deliverers are beginning to recognize the massive impact that heavy substance intake can have on physical and mental health, and so on. It is my hope that the combination of these efforts, each with its own underlying motivations, might contribute to a steady decrease in abuse and misuse of substances over the next decade.

15.7.3. Application to the Health-Care Field

I have special concern regarding alcohol and drug use and associated difficulties that occur within the health-care professions. It is likely that the lifetime risk for at least temporary alcohol problems may be as high as 1 in 3 and that the risk for actual alcohol dependence is probably about 10% for men and 3–5% for women in the helping professions.[136,137] Perhaps reflecting the ready availability of most substances (including alcohol) as well as the stresses incurred by health-care deliverers, it has been hypothesized that rates of temporary and more persistent substance problems may even be higher among health-care delivers than among the general population.[138,139] A recent survey revealed that 18% of medical students had at some point met the Research Diagnostic Criteria for alcohol abuse during their first two years of medical school, with evidence that there is an association between the increase in alcohol consumption and related problems and use or misuse of other drugs. No matter what the actual rate of alcohol-related problems or of alcohol dependence among medical students, nurses, physicians, and other health-care deliverers, any level of emotional or cognitive impairment in these groups could seriously affect decision making in life-or-death matters.

For these reasons, it appears appropriate to consider the need for the development of careful prevention strategies for students and practitioners in the health-care system.[139] Briefly, these can include the need for increased levels of education about alcohol, drug use, and associated problems within medical schools and allied professions; the need for increased numbers of counseling and discussion groups for staff in nursing programs and in relevant schools; increased education of professionals about the need to recognize and help colleagues when they seem to be facing problems in these areas; and a requirement for periodic anonymous surveys within medical schools, hospitals, and similar facilities to determine the rate of use and identify associated problems and to give feedback to the staff on the results of such surveys.

REFERENCES

1. McGuire, F. L. Alcohol rehabilitation: Fact or myth? *American Journal of Drug and Alcohol Abuse 8:*131–135, 1981.
2. Schuckit, M. A., & Cahalan, D. Evaluation of alcohoholism treatment programs. In W. J. Filstead, J. J. Rossi, & M. Keller (Eds.), *Alcohol and Alcohol Problems: New Thinking and New Directions.* Cambridge, Masschusetts: Ballinger, 1976, pp. 267–292.
3. Schuckit, M. A., Schwei, M. G., & Gold, E. Prediction of outcome in inpatient alcoholics. *Journal of Studies on Alcohol 47:*151–155, 1986.
4. Slater, E. J., & Linn, M. W. Predictors of rehospitalization in a male alcoholic population. *American Journal of Drug and Alcohol Abuse 9:*211–220, 1983.
5. Moos, R. J., Finney, J. W., & Chan, D. A. The process of recovery from alcoholism. *Journal of Studies on Alcohol 42:*383–420, 1981.
6. Schuckit, M. A. Treatment of alcoholism in office and outpatient settings. In J. H. Mendelson & N. K. Mello (Eds.), *Diagnosis and Treatment of Alcoholism* (2nd ed.). New York: McGraw-Hill, 1984, pp. 295–324.
7. Cole, S. G., Lehman, W. E., Cole, E. A., *et al.* Inpatient vs. outpatient treatment of alcohol and drug abusers. *American Journal of Drug and Alcohol Abuse 8:*329–345, 1981.
8. Stinson, D. J., Smith, W. G., Amidjaya, I., *et al.* Systems of care and treatment outcomes for alcoholic patients. *Archives of General Psychiatry 36:*535–539, 1979.
9. Zweben, A., Pearlman, S., & Selina, L. A comparison of brief adverse and conjoint therapy in the treatment of alcohol abuse. *British Journal of Addiction 83:*899–916, 1988.
10. Ojehagen, A., Skjaerris, A., & Berglund, M. Prediction of posttreatment drinking outcome in a 2-year out-patient alcoholic treatment program: A follow-up study. *Alcoholism: Clinical and Experimental Research 12:*46–49, 1988.
11. Stein, L. I., Newton, J. R., & Bowman, R. S. Duration of hospitalization for alcoholism. *Archives of General Psychiatry 32:*247–252, 1975.
12. Brandsma, J. M., & Pattison, E. M. The outcome of group psychotherapy alcoholics: An empirical review. *American Journal of Drug and Alcohol Abuse 11:*151–162, 1985.
13. Nirenberg, T. D., Sobell, L. C., & Sobell, M. B. Effective and inexpensive procedures for decreasing client attrition in an outpatient alcohol treatment program. *American Journal of Drug and Alcohol Abuse 7:*73–82, 1980.
14. Irwin, M., Baird, S., Smith, T. L., & Schuckit, M. A. Monitoring heavy drinking in recovering alcoholic men. *American Journal of Psychiatry 145:*595–599, 1988.
15. Schuckit, M. A., & Irwin, M. Diagnosis of alcoholism. In Geokas, M. (Ed.), *Medical Clinics of North America 72:*1133–1153, 1988.
16. McCrady, B. S., Noel, N. E., Abrams, D. B., *et al.* Comparative effectiveness of three types of spouse involvement in outpatient behavioral alcoholism treatment. *Journal of Studies on Alcohol 47:*459–467, 1986.
17. Helzer, J. E., Robins, L. N., Taylor, J. R., *et al.* The extent of long-term moderate drinking among alcoholics discharged from medical and psychiatric treatment facilities. *New England Journal of Medicine 312:*1678–1662, 1985.
18. Schuckit, M. A. Inpatient and residential approaches to the treatment of alcoholism. In J. H. Mendelson & N. K. Mello (Eds.), *Diagnosis and Treatment of Alcoholism* (2nd ed.). New York: McGraw-Hill, 1984, pp. 325–354.
19. Edwards, G., Orford, J., Egert, S., *et al.* Alcoholism: A controlled trial of ''treatment'' and ''advice.'' *Journal of Studies on Alcohol 38:*1004–1031, 1977.

20. Goodwin, D. W., & Guze, S. B. (Eds.). *Psychiatric Diagnosis* (4th ed.). New York: Oxford University Press, 1988.

21. Baldessarini, R. J. *Chemotherapy in Psychiatry.* Cambridge: Harvard University Press, 1977.

22. Fawcett, J. A double-blind placebo controlled trial of lithium for alcoholism. *Archives of General Psychiatry 44:*248–256, 1987.

23. Berger, F. Alcoholism rehabilitation. *Hospital and Community 34:*1017–1021, 1983.

24. Bloom, J. D., Bradford, J., & Kofoed, L. An overview of psychiatric treatment approaches to three offender groups. *Hospital and Community Psychiatry 39:*151–158, 1988.

25. Forrest, G. G. *The Diagnosis and Treatment of Alcoholism.* Springfield, Illinois: Charles C. Thomas, 1975.

26. Brown, S., & Yalom, I. D. Interactional group therapy with alcoholics. *Journal of Studies on Alcohol 38:*426–456, 1977.

27. U.S. Department of Health and Human Services. *Chemical Aversion Therapy for the Treatment of Alcoholism.* Washington, D.C. U.S. Government Printing Office. DHHS Publication Number 88-3425, 1988, pp. 1–24.

28. Nathan, P. Learning theory and alcoholism. In G. Vaillant (Ed.), *Psychiatry Update III.* Washington, DC: APA Press, 1984, pp. 328–337.

29. Pendery, M. L., Maltzman, I. M., & West, L. J. Controlled drinking by alcoholics? New findings and a reevaluation of a major affirmative study. *Science 217:*169–175, 1982.

30. Moos, R. H., & Moos, B. S. The process of recovery from alcoholism. III. Comparing functioning in families of alcoholics and matched control families. *Journal of Studies on Alcohol 45:*111–118, 1984.

31. Kitson, T. M. The disulfiram–ethanol reaction. *Journal of Studies on Alcohol 38:*96–113, 1977.

32. Iber, F. L., Lee, K., Lacoursiere, R., & Fuller, R. Liver toxicity encountered in the Veterans Administration trial of disulfiram in alcoholics. *Alcoholism: Clinical and Experimental Research 11:*301–304, 1987.

33. Branchey, L., Davis, W., Lee, K. K., & Fuller, R. K. Psychiatric complications of disulfiram treatment. *American Journal of Psychiatry 144:*1310–1312, 1987.

34. Rainey, J. M. Disulfiram toxicity and carbon disulfide poisoning. *American Journal of Psychiatry 134:*371–378, 1977.

35. Jacobsen, D., Sebastian, S., Blomstrand, R., McMartin, K. E. 4-Methylpyrazole: a controlled study. *Alcoholism: Clinical and Experimental Research 12:*516–520, 1988.

36. Fuller, R. K., Branchey, L., Brightwell, D. R., et al. Disulfiram treatment of alcoholism: A Veterans Administration Cooperative Study. *Journal of the American Medical Association 256:*1449–1455, 1986.

37. Schuckit, M. A. A one-year follow-up of men alcoholics given disulfiram. *Journal of Studies on Alcohol 46:*191–195, 1985.

38. Johnson, J., Stowell, A., Bache-Wiig, J. E., et al. A double-blind placebo controlled study of male alcoholics given a subcutaneous disulfiram implantation. *British Journal of Addiction 82:*607–713, 1987.

39. Spinosa, G., Perlanski, E., Leenen, F. H. H. et al. Angiotensin converting enzyme inhibitors: Animal experiments suggest a new pharmacological treatment for alcohol abuse in humans. *Alcoholism: Clinical and Experimental Research 12:*65–68, 1988.

40. Naranjo, C. A., Sellers, E. M., & Lawrin, M. O. Modulation of ethanol intake by serotonin uptake inhibitors. *Journal of Clinical Psychiatry 47:*16–22, 1986.

41. Lawrin, M. O., Naranjo, C. A., & Sellers, E. M. Identification and testing of new drugs for modulating alcohol consumption. *Psychopharmacology 22:*1020–1025, 1986.

42. Lader, M. Assessing the potential for buspirone dependence or abuse and effects of its withdrawal. *American Journal of Medicine 82:*20–26, 1987.

43. Griffith, J. D., Jasinski, D. R., Casten, G. P., & McKinney, G. R. Investigation of the abuse liability of buspirone in alcohol-dependent patients. *American Journal of Medicine 80:*30–35, 1986.

44. Trice, H. M., & Beyer, J. M. Work-related outcomes of the constructive-confrontation strategy in a job-based alcoholism program. *Journal of Studies on Alcohol 45:*393–404, 1984.

45. Beaumont, P., & Allsop, S. An industrial alcohol policy. *British Journal of Addiction 79:*315–318, 1984.

46. Miletich, J. *Work and Alcohol Abuse.* New York: Greenwood Press, 1987.

47. Schuckit, M. A. Genetic and clinical implications of alcoholism and affective disorder. *American Journal of Psychiatry 143:*140–147, 1986.

48. Vaillant, G. E. Natural history of male alcoholism. V. Is alcoholism the cart to sociopathy or the horse? Paper presented at the American Psychiatric Association Meeting in Toronto, May 1982.

49. Schuckit, M. A. Alcoholism and sociopathy: Diagnostic confusion. *Quarterly Journal of Studies on Alcohol 34:*157–164, 1973.

50. Emrick, C. D. Alcoholics Anonymous affiliation processes and effectiveness as treatment. *Alcoholism: Clinical and Experimental Research 11:*416–423, 1987.

51. Galanter, M., Castaneda, R., & Salamon, I. Institutional self-help therapy for alcoholism: Clinical outcome. *Alcoholism: Clinical and Experimental Research 11:*424–429, 1987.

52. Goldstein, A. Heroin addiction: Sequential treatment employing pharmacologic supports. *Archives of General Psychiatry 33:*353–358, 1976.

53. Sells, S. B., & Simpson, D. D. Role of alcohol use by narcotic addicts as revealed in the DARP research on evaluation of treatment for drug abuse. *Alcoholism: Clinical and Experimental Research 11:*437–439, 1987.

54. McClellan, A. T., Ball, J. C., Rosen, L., et al. Pretreatment source of income and response to methadone maintenance: A follow-up study. *American Journal of Psychiatry 138:*785–789, 1981.

55. Simpson, D. D., & Savage, L. J. Drug abuse treatment readmissions and outcomes. *Archives of General Psychiatry 37:*896–901, 1980.

56. Stephens, R. C., & Weppner, R. S. Legal and illegal use of methadone: One year later. *American Journal of Psychiatry 130:*1391–1394, 1973.

57. Ball, J. C., Corty, E., Bond, H. R., et al. The reduction of intravenous heroin use, non-opiate abuse and crime during methadone maintenance treatment—Further findings. Paper presented at the Annual Meeting of the Committee on Problems of Drug Dependency, Philadelphia, June 14–19, 1987.

58. McLellan, A. T., Luborosky, L., O'Brien, C. P., et al. Is treatment for substance abuse effective? *Journal of the American Medical Association 247:*1423–1428, 1982.

59. Jaffe, J. H., Drug addiction and drug abuse. In A. G. Gilman, L. S. Goodman, T. W. Rall, & F. Murad, (Eds.), *The Pharmacological Basis of Therapeutics* (7th ed.). New York: Macmillan, 1985, pp. 532–581.

60. Rounsaville, B. J., Kosten, T. R., & Kleber, H. D. The antecedents and benefits of achieving abstinence in opioid addicts: A 2.5 year follow-up study. *American Journal of Drug and Alcohol Abuse 13:*213–229, 1987.

61. Brown, B. S., Watters, J. K., & Iglehart, A. S. Methadone maintenance dosage levels and program retention. *American Journal of Drug and Alcohol Abuse 9:*129–139, 1983.

62. McGlothlin, W. H., & Anglin, M. D. Long-term follow-up of clients of high- and low-dose methadone programs. *Archives of General Psychiatry 38:*1055–1063, 1981.

63. Ling, W., Charuvastra, V. C., Kaim, S. C., et al. Methadyl acetate and methadone as maintenance treatments for heroin addicts. *Archives of General Psychiatry 33:*709–720, 1976.

64. Tennant, F. S. LAAM maintenance for opioid addicts who cannot maintain with methadone. Paper presented at the Research Society on Alcoholism Meeting, San Francisco, June 1986.

65. Razani, J., Chilholm, D., Glasser, M., et al. Self-regulated methadone detoxification of heroin addicts: An improved technique in an inpatient setting. *Archives of General Psychiatry 32:*909–911, 1975.

66. Newman, R. G. Methadone treatment. *New England Journal of Medicine 317:*447–450, 1987.

67. Senay, E. C., Dorus, W., Goldberg, F., et al. Withdrawal from methadone maintenance: Rate of withdrawal and expectation. *Archives of General Psychiatry 34:*361–368, 1977.

68. Kreek, M. J. Health consequences associated with methadone. In J. Cooper & F. Altman (Eds.), *Research on the Treatment of Narcotic Addiction. NIDA Research Monograph Series.* Department of Health and Human Services Publication (ADM) 83–1281. Washington, D.C.: U.S. Government Printing Office, 1983, pp. 456–482.

69. Newman, R. G. Methadone maintenance: It ain't what it used to be. *British Journal of Addictions 71:*183–186, 1976.

70. Stimmel, B. *Heroin Dependency: Medical, Economic, and Social Aspects.* New York: Stratton Intercontinental Medical Book Corporation, 1975.

71. Weissman, M. M.,Slobetz, F., Prusoff, B., *et al.* Clinical depression among narcotic addicts maintained on methadone in the community. *American Journal of Psychiatry 133:*1434–1438, 1976.

72. Croughan, J. L., Miller, J. P., Koepke, J., *et al.* Depression in narcotic addicts—A prospective study with a five-year follow-up. *Comprehensive Psychiatry 22:*428–433, 1981.

73. Kosten, T. R., Rounsaville, B. J., & Kleber, H. D. Predictors of 2.5-year outcome in opioid addicts: Pretreatment source of income. *American Journal of Drug and Alcohol Abuse 13:*19–32, 1987.

74. Rounsaville, B. J., Kosten, T. R., Weissman, M. M., & Kleber, H. D. Prognostic significance of psychopathology in treated opiate addicts. *Archives of General Psychiatry 43:*739–745, 1986.

75. Kosten, T. R. A 2.5 year follow-up of cocaine use among treated opiate addicts (the relationship with depression). *Archives of General Psychiatry 44:*281–284, 1987.

76. Green, J., & Jaffe, J. H. Alcohol and opiate dependence: A review. *Journal of Studies on Alcohol 38:*1274–1293, 1977.

77. Simpson, D. D. Treatment for drug abuse. *Archives of General Psychiatry 38:*875–880, 1981.

78. Kosten, T. R., Schaumann, B., Wright, D., *et al.* A preliminary study of desipramine in cocaine abuse. *Journal of Clinical Psychiatry 48:*442–444, 1987.

79. McGlothlin, W., & Anglin, D. Shutting off methadone: Costs and benefits. *Archives of General Psychiatry 38:*885–892, 1981.

80. Schecter, A. The role of narcotic antagonists in the rehabiliation of opiate addicts: A review of naltrexone. *American Journal of Drug and Alcohol Abuse 7:*1–18, 1980.

81. Charney, D. S., Heninger, G. R., & Kleber, H. D. The combined use of clonidine and naltrexone as a rapid, safe, and effective treatment of abrupt withdrawal from methadone. *American Journal of Psychiatry 143:*831–837, 1986.

82. O'Brien, C. P. A new approach to the management of opioid dependence: Naltrexone. *Journal of Clinical Psychiatry 45:*57–58, 1984.

83. Brahan, L. S., Capone, T., Wiechert, V., *et al.* Naltrexone and cyclazocine: A controlled treatment study. *Archives of General Psychiatry 34:*1181–1184, 1977.

84. Volavka, J., Resnick, R. B., Kestenbaum, R. S., *et al.* Short-term effects of naltrexone in 155 heroin ex-addicts. *Biological Psychiatry 11:*679–685, 1976.

85. Greenstein, R. A., O'Brien, C. P., McLellan, A. T., *et al.* Naltrexone: A short-term treatment of opiate dependence. *American Journal of Drug and Alcohol Abuse 8:*291–300, 1981.

86. Atkinson, R. L. Endocrine and metabolic effects of opiate antagonists. *Journal of Clinical Psychiatry 45:*20–24, 1984.

87. Kosten, T. R., & Kleber, H. D. Strategies to improve compliance with narcotic antagonists. *American Journal of Drug and Alcohol Abuse 10:*249–266, 1984.

88. Crowley, T. J., Wagner, J. E., Zerbe, G., & Macdonald, M. Naltrexone-induced dysphoria in former opioid addicts. *American Journal of Psychiatry 142:*1081–1984, 1985.

89. Tennant, F. S., Rawson, R. A., Cohen, A. J., & Mann, A. Clinical experience with naltrexone in suburban opioid addicts. *Journal of Clinical Psychiatry 45:*42–45, 1984.

90. Greenstein, R. A., Arndt, I. C., McLellan, A. T., *et al.* Naltrexone: A clinical perspective. *Journal of Clinical Psychiatry 45:*25–28, 1984.

91. Wandzel, L., & Falicki, Z. Heroin addiction treated by atropine coma. *American Journal of Psychiatry 144:*1243, 1987.

92. Tennant, F. S., Jr. Propoxyphene napsylate for heroin addiction. *Journal of the American Medical Association 226:*1012, 1973.

93. Grosz, H. J. Propranolol in the treatment of heroin dependence. In H. Bostrum (Ed.), *Skandia International Symposia: Drug Dependence, Treatment and Treatment Evaluation.* Stockholm: Bastrum, 1974, pp. 17–33.

94. Lidz, C. W., Lewis, S. H., Crane, L. E., *et al.* Heroin maintenance and heroin control. *International Journal of the Addictions 10:*35–52, 1975.

95. Robertson, J. R., & Skidmore, C. A. Management of drug addicts. *Lancet 1:*1322, 1987.

96. Pompi, K. F., & Resnick, J. Retention of court-referred adolescents and young adults in the therapeutic community. *American Journal of Drug and Alcohol Abuse 13:*309–325, 1987.

97. Gossop, M., Green, I., Phillips, G., & Bradley, B. What happens to opiate addicts immediately after treatment: A prospective follow-up study. *British Medical Journal 294:*1377–1380, 1987.

98. Bale, R. N., Van Stone, W. W., Kuldau, J. M., *et al.* Therapeutic communities vs. methadone maintenance. *Archives of General Psychiatry 37:*179–193, 1980.

99. Simpson, D. D., Savage, L. J., & Lloyd, M. R. Follow-up evaluation of treatment of drug abuse during 1969 to 1972. *Archives of General Psychiatry 36:*772–780, 1979.

100. Bracy, S. A., & Simpson, D. D. Status of opioid addicts 5 years after admission to drug abuse treatment. *American Journal of Drug and Alcohol Abuse 9:*115–127, 1983.

101. Simpson, D. D., Joe, G. W., & Bracy, S. A. Six-year follow-up of opioid addicts after admission to treatment. *Archives of General Psychiatry 39:*1318–1323, 1982.

102. De Leon, G. Alcohol use among drug abusers: Treatment outcomes in a therapeutic community. *Alcoholism: Clinical and Experimental Research 11:*430–436, 1987.

103. De Leon, G., & Schwartz, S. Therapeutic communities: What are the retention rates? *American Journal of Drug and Alcohol Abuse 10:*267–284, 1984.

104. Gawin, F. H., & Kleber, H. D. Abstinence symptomatology and psychiatric diagnosis in cocaine abusers. *Archives of General Psychiatry 43:*107–113, 1986.

105. Kozel, N. J., & Adams, E. H. Cocaine use in America: Epidemiologic and clinical perspectives. *NIDA Research Monograph 61:*130–150, 1985.

106. Rounsaville, B. J., Gawin, F., & Kleber, H. Interpersonal psychotherapy adapted for ambulatory cocain abusers. *American Journal of Drug and Alcohol Aubse 11:*171–191, 1985.

107. Kleber, H., & Gawin, F. Psychopharmacology trials in cocaine abuse treatment. *American Journal of Drug and Alcohol Abuse 12:*235–246, 1986.

108. Kosten, T. R., Schumann, B., Wright, D., *et al.* A preliminary study of desipramine in the treatment of cocaine abuse in methadone maintenance patients. *Journal of Clinical Psychiatry 48:*442–444, 1987.

109. Benowitz, N. L., Jacob, P., Kozlowski, L. T., & Yu, L. Influence of smoking fewer cigarettes on exposure to tar, nicotine, and carbon monoxide. *New England Journal of Medicine 315:*1310–1313, 1986.

110. Henningfield, J. E. Pharmacologic basis and treatment of cigarette smoking. *Journal of Clinical Psychiatry 45:*24–34, 1984.

111. Chapman, S. Stop-smoking clinics: A case for their abandonment. *Lancet 1:*918–920, 1985.

112. Capman, R. F., Smith, J. W., & Layden, T. Elimination of cigarette smoking by punishment. *Behavioral Research and Therapy 9:*255–264, 1971.

113. DeChacek, T. An overview of smoking behavior and its modification. In N. A. Krasnegor (Ed.), *Behavioral Analyses and Treatment of Substance Abuse: Research Monograph 25.* Rockville, Maryland: National Institute on Drug Abuse, 1979.

114. Editorial: Nicotine chewing gum. *Lancet 1:*320–322, 1985.

115. Fielding, J. E. Smoking: Health effects and controls. *New England Journal of Medicine 313:*491–498, 1985.

116. Hughes, J. R., Gust, S. W., Keenan, R. M., *et al.* Efficacy of nicotine gum in general practice: One year follow-up. In L. Harris (Ed.), *Problems of Drug Dependence.* Rockville, Maryland; National Institute on Drug Abuse Research Monograph Series, (in press).

117. Lam, W., Sacks, H. S., Sze, P. C., & Chalmers, T. C. Meta-analysis of randomized controlled trials of nicotine chewing-gum. *Lancet 2:*27–30, 1987.

118. Glassman, A. H., Jackson, W. K., Walsh, T., *et al.* Cigarette craving, smoking withdrawal and clonidine. Paper presented at the American College of Neuropsychopharmacology, San Juan, Puerto Rico, December 1984.

119. Gerstein, D. Alcohol policy: Preventive options. In L. Grinspoon (Ed.), *Psychiatry Update III.* Washington, D.C.: American Psychiatric Association, 1984, pp. 359–371.

120. Secretary of Health and Human Services. *Sixth Special Report to Congress on Alcohol and Health.* Rockville, Maryland: United States Department of Health and Human Services, ADAMHA, 1987, pp. 97–119.

121. Hoadley, J. F., Fuch, B. C., & Holder, H. D. The effect of alcohol beverage restrictions on consumption: A 25-year longitudinal analysis. *American Journal of Drug and Alcohol Abuse 10:*375–401, 1984.

122. Holder, H. D., & Blose, J. O. Reduction of community alcohol problems: Computer simulation experiments in three countries. *Journal of Studies on Alcohol 48:*1124–1135, 1987.

123. Smart, R. G. Changes in alcohol problems as a result of changing alcohol consumption: A natural experiment. *Drug and Alcohol Dependence 19:*91–97, 1987.

124. Smart, R. G. The impact on consumption of selling wine in grocery stores. *Alcohol and Alcoholism 21:*233–236, 1986.

125. Smart, R. G., & Adlaf, E. M. Banning happy hours: The impact on drinking and impaired-driving charges in Ontario, Canada. *Journal of Studies on Alcohol 47:*256–258, 1986.

126. Engs, R. C., & Hanson, D. J. Age-specific alcohol prohibition and college students' drinking problems. *Psychology Report 59:*979–984, 1986.

127. Hingson, R. W., Scotch, N., Mangione, T., *et al.* Impact of legislation raising the legal drinking age in Massachusetts from 18 to 20. *American Journal of Public Health 73:*163–170, 1983.

128. Kivlahan, D. R., Coppel, D. B., Fromme, K., *et al.* Secondary prevention of alcohol-related problems in young adults at risk. In K. D. Craig & S. M. Weiss (Eds.), *Prevention and Early Intervention: Biobehavioral Perspectives.* New York: Springer (in press).

129. Sobell, L. C., Sobell, M. B., Riley, D. M., *et al.* Effect of television programming and advertising on alcohol consumption in normal drinkers. *Journal of Studies on Alcohol 47:*333–340, 1986.

130. Kohn, P. M., & Smart, R. G. The impact of television advertising on alcohol consumption: An experiment. *Journal of Studies on Alcohol 45:*295–301, 1984.

131. United States Department of Health and Human Services. Chapter VI: Prevention and intervention. In *Alcohol and Health, 6th Special Report to the U.S. Congress.* Rockville, Maryland: Department of Health and Human Services Publication No. (ADM) 87-1519, 1987, pp. 97–120.

132. Meilgaard, M. C. Wernicke's encephalopathy. *New England Journal of Medicine 313:*637, 1985.

133. Reuler, J., Gurard, D., & Cooney, T. Wernicke's encephalopathy. *New England Journal of Medicine 312:*1035–1039, 1985.

134. Monteiro, M. G., & Schuckit, M. A. Populations at high alcoholism risk—Recent findings. *Journal of Clinical Psychiatry* (in press).

135. Schuckit, M. A. Biological vulnerability to alcoholism. *Journal of Consulting and Clinical Psychology 55:*301–309, 1987.

136. Clark, D. C., Eckenfels, E. J., Daugherty, S. R., & Fawcett, J. Alcohol-use patterns through medical school. *Journal of the American Medical Association 257:*2921–226, 1987.

137. McCue, J. The effects of stress on physicians and their medical practice. *New England Journal of Medicine 306:*458–463, 1982.

138. Brewster, J. M. Prevalence of alcohol and other drug problems among physicians. *Journal of the American Medical Association 255:*1913–1920, 1986.

139. Seigle, R. D., Schuckit, M. A., & Plumb, D. Availability of personal counseling in medical schools. *Journal of Medical Education 58:*542–546, 1983.

Index